全国高等院校医学整合教材

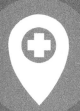

组织学与胚胎学实验教程（双语版）

HISTOLOGY AND EMBRYOLOGY LABORATORY MANUAL (BILINGUAL)

周雯　谢小薰　主编

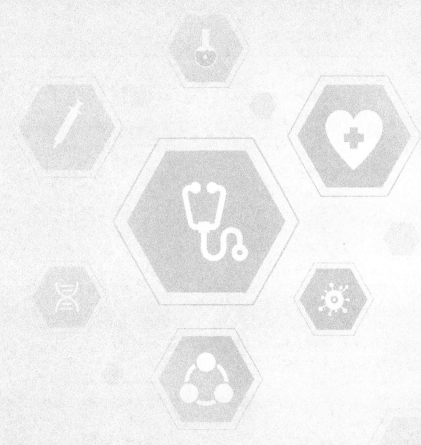

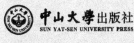 中山大学出版社
SUN YAT-SEN UNIVERSITY PRESS

·广州·

图书在版编目（CIP）数据

组织学与胚胎学实验教程：双语版/周雯，谢小薰主编. —广州：中山大学出版社，2024.11

（全国高等院校医学整合教材）

ISBN 978 - 7 - 306 - 08026 - 4

Ⅰ. ①组… Ⅱ. ①周… ②谢… Ⅲ. ①人体组织学—实验—医学院校—教材 ②人体胚胎学—实验—医学院校—教材 Ⅳ. ①R32 - 33

中国国家版本馆 CIP 数据核字（2024）第 033574 号

出 版 人：王天琪

策划编辑：吕肖剑

责任编辑：谢贞静

封面设计：林绵华

责任校对：郑雪漫

责任技编：靳晓虹

出版发行：中山大学出版社

电　　话：编辑部 020 - 84110283，84113349，84111997，84110779，84110776
　　　　　发行部 020 - 84111998，84111981，84111160

地　　址：广州市新港西路 135 号

邮　　编：510275　　传　真：020 - 84036565

网　　址：http://www.zsup.com.cn　E-mail：zdcbs@mail.sysu.edu.cn

印 刷 者：广东虎彩云印刷有限公司

规　　格：787mm×1092mm　1/16　21 印张　　600 千字

版次印次：2024 年 11 月第 1 版　2024 年 11 月第 1 次印刷

定　　价：88.00 元

编写委员会名单

主　编　周　雯　谢小薰

副主编　陈雄林　黄文峰　张　巍　张庆梅　魏　霞

编　委　（按姓氏拼音排序）

陈雄林（九江学院）　　　　　　陈志强（海南医科大学）

崔志刚（海南医科大学）　　　　葛盈盈（广西医科大学）

洪　灯（海南医科大学）　　　　黄文峰（湖北三峡职业技术学院）

陆海霞（海南医科大学）　　　　马百成（九江学院）

滕　藤（海南医科大学）　　　　王艳华（三峡大学）

魏　霞（三峡大学）　　　　　　谢小薰（广西医科大学）

岳晓阳（广西医科大学）　　　　张庆梅（广西医科大学）

张　巍（天津医科大学）　　　　周　雯（海南医科大学）

前　言

　　欢迎来到组织与胚胎学实验室！本书旨在为读者学习组织学和胚胎学领域的实践课程提供全面的帮助。

　　在组织学部分，读者将学习如何准备组织样本、在显微镜下观察它们，并识别对理解生理过程至关重要的关键组织学特征。而在胚胎学部分，则通过详细的插图、实验步骤和解剖特点描述，使读者深入了解不同物种胚胎发育中的形态发生事件。

　　本书以清晰的指导、丰富的插图、深入的解释、激发思考的问题以及实用的临床案例为特色，构建起组织学和胚胎学知识与临床实践之间的桥梁，帮助读者深入研究不同物种的微观结构和发育过程，从而带来更好的学习体验。

　　实验室安全至关重要。请确保遵守本手册中概述的所有安全指南，包括正确处理实验室设备、处理危险材料和佩戴适当的防护装备。

　　我们希望本书能够增进读者对医学基本领域的理解和欣赏。祝愿读者在探索知识的旅程中收获满满！

周雯　谢小薰

Preface

Welcome to the Histology and Embryology Laboratory! This guide accompanies your practical sessions in the fascinating fields of histology and embryology. Here, you will explore microscopic structures and developmental processes that underpin the complexity of living organisms.

Understanding Histology

Histology, or microscopic anatomy, delves into the examination of tissues and their arrangement within organs. Through the scrutiny of cellular structures, histologists unveil the complex organization and roles of different bodily components. In this guide, you will discover techniques for tissue sample preparation, microscopy observation, and identification of crucial histological characteristics vital for comprehending physiological mechanisms.

Exploring Embryology

Embryology investigates the journey of organisms from fertilization to birth, elucidating the genesis of tissues, organs, and systems throughout embryonic and fetal phases. Through intricate illustrations, experiments, and dissections, you'll acquire a deeper understanding of the morphogenetic processes and molecular pathways governing embryonic development.

Structure of the book

This book is crafted to enhance your learning journey through clear instructions, labeled diagrams, and insightful explanations for every laboratory exercise. Each section is dedicated to distinct topics, enabling a methodical exploration of histological structures and embryonic development.

Key Features

1. Comprehensive protocols for tissue preparation, staining techniques, and microscopy.

2. Guided procedures for observing embryonic development, presented step by step.

3. Illustrative diagrams and images to facilitate structure identification.

4. Clinical correlations to underscore the significance of histology and embryology in medical contexts.

Safety Precautions

Safety is of utmost importance in the laboratory. Please strictly follow all safety protocols provided in this manual, which include handling laboratory equipment with care, disposing of hazardous materials properly, and always wearing suitable protective gear.

As you delve into the fascinating worlds of histology and embryology, embrace the chance to uncover the intricacies of life at both the cellular and developmental scales. We trust that this book will enrich your comprehension and admiration for these essential pillars of biology.

Let the exploration begin!

Wen Zhou, Xiaoxun Xie

Contents

目 录

第 1 章　组织学绪论 ·· 1

Chapter 1　INTRODUCTION TO HISTOLOGY ················ 6

第 2 章　上皮组织 ··· 10

Chapter 2　EPITHELIAL TISSUE ································· 19

第 3 章　固有结缔组织 ·· 25

Chapter 3　CONNECTIVE TISSUE PROPER ················ 31

第 4 章　软骨和骨 ··· 35

Chapter 4　CARTILAGE AND BONE ·························· 41

第 5 章　血液和血细胞发生 ·· 45

Chapter 5　BLOOD AND HEMATOPOIESIS ················ 53

第 6 章　肌组织 ··· 59

Chapter 6　MUSCULAR TISSUE ······························· 64

第 7 章　神经组织 ··· 67

Chapter 7　NERVOUS TISSUE ·································· 74

第 8 章　神经系统 ··· 79

Chapter 8　NERVOUS SYSTEM ································· 86

第 9 章　循环系统 ··· 92

Chapter 9　CIRCULATORY SYSTEM ························· 98

第 10 章　免疫系统 ··· 102

Chapter 10　IMMUNE SYSTEM ································· 107

第 11 章　内分泌系统 ·· 111

Chapter 11　ENDOCRINE SYSTEM ··························· 117

第 12 章　眼和耳 ·· 121

Chapter 12　EYE AND EAR ···································· 127

第 13 章　皮肤 ··· 132

Chapter 13　SKIN ··· 137

第 14 章　消化管 ··· 141

Chapter 14　DIGESTIVE TRACT ··· 150

第 15 章　消化腺 ··· 156

Chapter 15　DIGESTIVE GLANDS ·· 162

第 16 章　呼吸系统 ·· 166

Chapter 16　RESPIRATORY SYSTEM ··· 172

第 17 章　泌尿系统 ·· 177

Chapter 17　URINARY SYSTEM ·· 183

第 18 章　男性生殖系统 ·· 188

Chapter 18　MALE REPRODUCTIVE SYSTEM ·· 195

第 19 章　女性生殖系统 ·· 200

Chapter 19　FEMALE REPRODUCTIVE SYSTEM ······································· 211

第 20 章　胚胎学绪论 ··· 219

Chapter 20　INTRODUCTION TO EMBRYOLOGY ······································ 222

第 21 章　胚胎学总论 ··· 226

Chapter 21　GENERAL EMBRYOLOGY ·· 232

第 22 章　颜面的发生 ··· 235

Chapter 22　FORMATION OF FACE ··· 241

第 23 章　心血管系统的发生 ··· 244

Chapter 23　DEVELOPMENT OF CARDIOVASCULAR SYSTEM ·················· 251

第 24 章　消化系统和呼吸系统的发生 ·· 255

Chapter 24　DEVELOPMENT OF DIGESTIVE AND RESPIRATORY SYSTEM ···· 268

第 25 章　泌尿生殖系统的发生 ·· 275

Chapter 25　DEVELOPMENT OF THE UROGENITAL SYSTEM ··················· 287

第 26 章　神经系统的发生 ·· 295

Chapter 26　DEVELOPMENT OF NERVOUS SYSTEM ································· 305

第 27 章　眼和耳的发生 ·· 311

Chapter 27　DEVELOPMENT OF EYES AND EARS ···································· 317

参考文献（References）·· 323

致谢 ··· 325

Acknowledgments ··· 326

第1章 | 组织学绪论

组织学是研究机体微细结构及其相关功能的科学。四种基本组织是上皮组织、结缔组织、肌组织和神经组织。每种类型的组织都由细胞和细胞外基质组成。不同组织按照一定的规律有机结合形成器官。

学习目标

（1）能用光学显微镜观察标本。
（2）了解石蜡切片和 HE 染色的基本原理。
（3）能够将理论知识与实验室观察分析联系起来。
（4）了解组织学实验的一些基本要求。

课前问题

你会为组织学实验课做哪些准备？
光学显微镜的结构和使用

1. 光学显微镜结构

一台光学显微镜主要由两部分组成：机械部分、光学部分（图 1-1）。

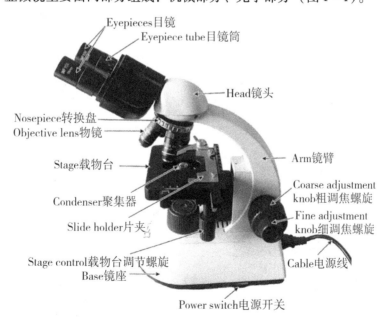

图 1-1 光学显微镜

Fig. 1-1 Light microscope

➢ **机械部分**

镜头、目镜筒、屈光度调节螺旋；镜臂、物镜转换盘、粗调焦螺旋、细调焦螺旋；镜座、亮度调节、电源开关；载物台、片夹、载物台调节螺旋。

➢ **光学部分**

目镜，物镜，聚光器，光圈，照明。

2. 如何使用光学显微镜

➢ **使用方法**

（1）打开显微镜电源开关。打开光圈。

（2）始终从低倍镜开始（4×物镜），把载物台降到最低。

（3）将载玻片放在载物台上，并用片夹固定。确保样品位于物镜下方。

（4）透过目镜观察，使用粗调焦螺旋缓慢升高载物台，直到观察到清晰的图像。观察视野中的结构，了解切片的全貌。

（5）使用载物台调节螺旋移动片夹，把要观察的切片部位放在视野中央。无须进一步调整，将物镜倍数切换到10×。然后使用粗调焦螺旋进行对焦。

（6）将要观察的部位移到视野中央，换成高倍镜（40×物镜）。使用细调焦螺旋进行对焦。**切勿在高倍镜下使用粗调焦螺旋**。观察视野中的微观结构，观察细胞的形态和染色特点。

（7）观察完一张玻片后，切换到低倍镜（4×物镜），放上另一张玻片。

（8）实验结束后，将载物台降到最低。将物镜放置成"八"字。取下玻片，用防尘罩盖上显微镜。

➢ **注意事项**

（1）切勿在高倍镜下使用粗调焦螺旋，否则可能会压碎玻璃并刮伤镜头。

（2）若在高倍镜下用细调焦螺旋前后旋转1圈也无法清楚对焦，则换成低倍镜并使用粗调焦螺旋重新聚焦。

（3）若发现显微镜头有污渍，应用专用擦镜纸轻轻擦拭。切勿用自己的纸巾或手擦拭镜头。

（4）搬运显微镜时始终使用双手，一只手抓住镜臂，另一只手托住镜座底部。

组织制备和 HE 染色

1. 石蜡包埋的组织制备

➢ **固定**

组织在4 ℃的固定液中固定24 h。

➢ **脱水**

在40 ℃将组织在梯度乙醇（70%、90%、90%、100%、100%）中分别浸泡1 h。

➢ **澄清**

将组织转移到二甲苯中并在40 ℃下浸泡1 h。用新鲜的二甲苯重复此步骤。

➢ **浸蜡**

将组织转移到石蜡中并在63 ℃下浸泡45 min。用新鲜石蜡重复此步骤3次。将组织放入充满熔融蜡的模具中。冷却后，用切片机进行切片。

2. 苏木精－伊红染色（HE 染色）

➤ **脱蜡**

切片在二甲苯中脱蜡 5 min。用新鲜二甲苯重复此步骤 2 ～ 3 次。

➤ **水化**

切片在梯度乙醇（100%、100%、95%、75%）中水化，各 3 min。

➤ **染色**

①苏木精染色 30 s。在显微镜下观察染色情况（细胞核应该是蓝色的，带有淡蓝色的组织基质）；②在流动的自来水中冲洗 1 min；③在酸性酒精中分化 8 ～ 12 s；④用自来水冲洗 3 h，显微镜下观察；⑤用 1% 伊红溶液染色 10 s；⑥用自来水冲洗以去除多余的污渍；⑦用 70% 乙醇清洗，显微镜下观察，直到组织基质和细胞成分被差异染色。

➤ **脱水**

通过梯度乙醇（95%、95%、100%、100%）快速脱水切片。

➤ **澄清**

在两个二甲苯瓶中各澄清 1 min。

➤ **封固**

在组织片上滴 1 滴中性树胶，放上盖玻片封盖。

组织学实验的基本要求

1. 从大体结构到微观结构

观察组织时，首先用肉眼了解组织切片的外观，然后用低倍镜观察切片的概貌，最后用高倍镜观察特征性结构和细胞。

2. 有序观察

按一定顺序进行观察：对于实质性器官，从表到里进行观察；对于中空性器官，由内向外逐层观察。

3. 联系和比较

首先，将器官的微观结构与大体结构联系起来，这样可以全面了解正常结构。其次，将微观结构与其功能联系起来，结构是功能的物质基础。最后，对相似的结构（如骨骼肌和心肌）进行比较，找出异同。

4. 将平面形状与实体形状联系起来

细胞、组织和器官是三维立体形状，而我们从光学显微照片中得到的显微照片是平面图像。因此，由于切面方向、视图不同，平面形状可能会有所不同（图 1-2 和图 1-3）。

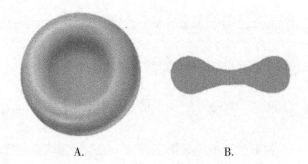

A. 表面观（Surface view）；B. 侧面观（Lateral view）。

图 1-2 红细胞
Fig. 1-2 Different view of the erythrocyte

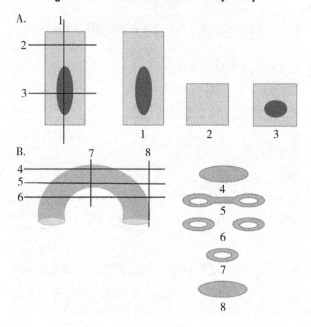

A. 柱状细胞（Columnar cell）；B. 中空性器官（hollow organ）。

图 1-3 不同切面的形态
Fig. 1-3 The shapes in different cut surfaces

5. 绘图和标注

绘画和标注可以帮助理解结构的基本特征。相比随意观察，绘图需要对切片进行更准确、更仔细的观察。

课后作业

画一个细胞的光镜结构模式图。

病例教学

法国解剖学家 Marie François Xavier Bichat（1771 年 11 月 14 日—1802 年 7 月 22 日）被誉为"现代组织学之父"。"观察疾病和解剖尸体的次数越多，他就越会相信有必要考虑局部疾病，不是从复杂器官的角度，而是从单个组织的角度。" Marie François Xavier Bichat 说。Marie François Xavier Bichat 引入了"组织"（tissue）一词，并提出疾病是由各种组织的病变引起的。

（1）请查找更多关于 Xavier Bichat 的故事和贡献。

（2）人体由哪四种基本组织构成？

（谢小薰，岳晓阳）

Chapter 1   INTRODUCTION TO HISTOLOGY

Histology is the study of the microanatomy of cells, tissues, and organs as seen through a microscope. It examines the correlation between structure and function. There are four types of fundamental tissues: epithelial tissue, connective tissue, muscular tissue, and nervous tissue.

Each type of tissue consists of cells and extracellular matrix. And an organ is a collection of tissues that structurally form a functional unit specialized to perform a particular function.

Learning Objectives

(1) Be able to use light microscopy to observe the specimen.

(2) Be able to understand the basic mechanisms of paraffin section and H & E staining.

(3) Be able to understand some basic requirements for histology lab.

Pre-class Questions

What would you do to get yourself prepared for histology lab?

Structure and Operation of Light Microscope

1. Microscope Structure

A light microscope mainly consists of 2 parts: mechanical parts, optical parts (Fig. 1 –1).

➤ Mechanical parts

head, eyepiece tube（目镜筒）, diopter adjustment; arm（镜臂）, nosepiece, coarse adjustment knob（粗调焦螺旋）, fine adjustment knob（细调焦螺旋）; base（镜座）, brightness adjustment, power switch; stage（载物台）, slide holder（片夹）, stage control.

➤ Optical parts

eyepiece（目镜）, objective lens（物镜）, condenser（聚光器）, diaphragm（光圈）, illumination.

2. How to Use a Light Microscope

➤ Step-by-step tutorial

(1) Switch on the power of microscope. Open the diaphragm.

(2) Always start at lowest power objective lens（4 ×）. Put the stage down as low as possible.

(3) Place the slide on the stage, and lock it with the slide holder. Make sure the slide is un-

derneath the objective lens.

(4) Look through the eyepieces, and use the coarse adjustment knob to raise the stage slowly until you can obtain a clear focus under the low power objective lens. Observe the structures in the field of view, and you can get a general overview of the organ.

(5) Use the stage control to move the slide holder until the part of the specimen you are interested in is centered in the field of view. Without any further adjustments, turn the nosepiece and switch to the objective lens (10 ×). Then you should refocus the image using the coarse adjustment knob.

(6) Once you have the specimen focused and centered on medium power, you can change to a high objective lens (40 ×). You can only use the fine adjustment knob to adjust carefully until the image comes into focus and you have a clear image. **Never use the coarse adjustment knob when the slide was under a high objective lens.**

(7) When you have finished viewing the slide, click the low power objective lens (4 ×) into viewing position. Then take off this slide and put on another slide.

(8) When finishing observation of the slide, put the stage back down as low as possible. Then turn the nosepiece to the lowest power of the lens. After that, remove the slide from the slide holder carefully, and protect your microscope with a cover.

➢ **Tips and Precautions**

(1) Never use the coarse adjustment knob when you are using the high objective lens (e. g. 40 × or 100 ×), or you may crush the glass and scratch the lens.

(2) If you cannot see the specimen clearly under a high objective lens. You might need to turn back to the low objective lens, and then refocus the specimen with the coarse adjustment knob.

(3) If the microscopic lens is found to be stained, you should wipe it gently with special lens tissue. Do not wipe the lens with your own hands or napkin.

(4) Always use both hands when carrying a microscope, with one hand on the arm and the other under the base.

Tissue Preparation and Haematoxylin & Eosin staining

1. Tissue Preparation with Paraffin-embedding

➢ **Fixation**

Place tissue in fixation solution for 24 h at 4 ℃.

➢ **Dehydration**

Incubate tissue in gradient concentrations of ethanol (乙醇) (70%, 90%, 90%, 100%, 100%) for 1 h at 40 ℃ each.

➢ **Clearing**

Transfer tissue to xylene (二甲苯) and incubate for 1 h at 40 ℃. Repeat this step with fresh xylene.

➢ **Paraffin Infiltration & Embedment**

Transfer tissue to paraffin and incubate for 45 min at 63 ℃. Repeat this step three times with fresh paraffin. Place the tissue into a mold filled with molten paraffin. After cooling down, the tissue can be cut with a microtome.

2. Haematoxylin and Eosin Staining

➤ **Deparaffinization**

Place slides into xylene for 5 min. Repeat this step with fresh xylene for 2 or 3 times.

➤ **Rehydration**

Rehydrate sections in gradient concentrations of ethanol （100%, 100%, 95%, 75%) for 3 min each.

➤ **Staining**

（1） Stain in haematoxylin for 30 s. Watch how stain develops and check the slide under microscope （nuclei should be blue with a pale blue tissue matrix）.

（2） Wash in running tap water for 1 min.

（3） Differentiating in acid alcohol for 8 – 12 s.

（4） Wash in tap water again for 3 h and check under the microscope.

（5） Stain with the 1% eosin solution for 10 s.

（6） Rinse in tap water to remove the excess stain.

（7） Wash in 70% ethanol and check microscopically until the tissue matrix and cellular components are differentially stained.

➤ **Dehydration**

Rapidly dehydrate the sections through graded ethanol （95%, 95%, 100%, 100%).

➤ **Clearing**

Put the slide separately in two bottles of xylene for 1 min.

➤ **Mounting**

Put a coverslip onto the slide with neutral resin.

Basic Requirements for Histology Lab

1. Microstructure vs Gross Structure

First, you should inspect a slide using just your naked eyes to determine the shape of the tissue section. Then, get an overview of the section with a lower objective lens. And finally identify the characteristic microstructures and cells with a high objective lens.

2. The order of slide observation

When observing a slide, we should follow a certain order. That is, for a slide of solid organs, observing it from its outer surface to its inner structure. And for a slide of hollow organs, it is better to observe it layer by layer from its inside to its outside.

3. Connection and comparison

First, connect the microstructure with the gross structure of an organ so that you can get a thorough view of normal structure. Second, relate the microstructure to its functions because the structure is the material basis of function. Third, summarize the similarities and differences through comparison of those similar structures such as the structures in both skeletal and cardia muscle.

4. Relation between the plain appearance and solid shape

The cells, tissues and organs have 3-dimensional shape, while the micrographs we get from the light micrograph are 2-dimensional. Thus, due to difference of sectioning and view direction, the microscopic image we get may vary (Fig. 1 – 2, Fig. 1 – 3).

5. Drawing and Labelling

Drawing a diagram with labeling detail structures can help you understand the basic features of characteristic structures. It requires accurate observation rather than casual examination to draw a diagram.

Post-class Task

Draw a diagram of a cell under light microscope.

Case-based Learning

A French anatomist, Marie François Xavier Bichat (Nov. 14, 1771 to Jul. 22, 1802), is well-known as "Father of the Modern Histology". "The more one will observe diseases and opens cadavers, the more he will be convinced of the necessity of considering local diseases not from the aspect of complex organs but from that of the individual tissues." Stated Marie François Xavier Bichat. Marie François Bichat introduced the term "tissue" and suggested that diseases result from the lesions of various tissues.

(1) Could you find more stories and legacies of Xavier Bichat?

(2) What are four types of fundamental tissues in human body?

(谢小薰，岳晓阳)

第 2 章 | 上皮组织

上皮组织是四种基本组织之一，基本特征有：①细胞密集，细胞外基质少；②无血管；③有极性；④富含神经末梢。

学习目标

（1）能够识别各种被覆上皮，并将每种类型的形态特征与功能相联系。
（2）能够区分外分泌腺的黏液性腺细胞和浆液性腺细胞。

课前问题

（1）上皮组织的基本特征是什么？
（2）被覆上皮的分类标准是什么？

实验观察与思考

1. 单层扁平上皮

1）单层扁平上皮（平铺片）

➢ **材料**
青蛙肠系膜平铺片（银染）。

➢ **肉眼观察**
标本被染成棕褐色。

➢ **低倍镜**
细胞轮廓不规则或呈多边形，细胞核呈椭圆形，位于细胞中央。相邻细胞间的细胞外基质被染成黑色。

➢ **高倍镜**
细胞边缘呈棕色的锯齿状（图 2-1）。

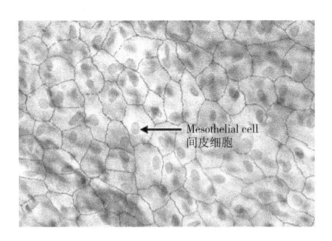

图 2 - 1 肠系膜（镀银染色，400 ×）

Fig. 2 - 1 Mesentery（silver stain, 400 ×）

2）单层扁平上皮（切片）

➤ **材料**

人阑尾切片（HE 染色）。

➤ **肉眼观察**

阑尾的横切面。

➤ **低倍镜**

阑尾壁的最外层染色浅，单层扁平上皮位于此处。

➤ **高倍镜**

单层扁平上皮非常薄。上皮细胞胞质呈粉红色，细胞核呈椭圆形或扁平，有时凸出表面（图 2 -2）。

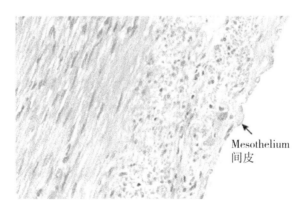

图 2 -2 阑尾（HE 染色，400 ×）

Fig. 2 - 2 Appendix（H & E stain, 400 ×）

2. 单层立方上皮

➤ **材料**

狗甲状腺（HE 染色）。

➤ **肉眼观察**

标本染成红色。

➤ **低倍镜**

甲状腺表面有疏松结缔组织被膜。实质由大量甲状腺滤泡组成。滤泡的大小和形状各不相同，但都有一个腔。滤泡壁由单层立方上皮组成。

➤ **高倍镜**

单层立方上皮由一层细胞构成，细胞呈立方形，胞质淡粉色，核圆形，细胞边界不清（图 2 – 3）。

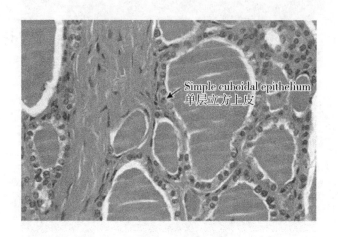

图 2 – 3　甲状腺（HE 染色，400 ×）

Fig. 2 – 3　Thyroid（H & E stain，400 ×）

思考题

（1）组织极性是什么意思？

（2）你能识别甲状腺中单层立方上皮的游离面和基底面吗？

---

3. 单层柱状上皮

➤ **材料**

狗胆囊（HE 染色）。

➤ **肉眼观察**

标本一侧被染成蓝色，另一侧被染成粉红色。蓝色部分是胆囊的黏膜，将其放在视野中央。

➤ **低倍镜**

单层柱状上皮位于胆囊黏膜表面。

➤ **高倍镜**

单层柱状上皮的细胞排列成单层，细胞呈柱状，细胞核椭圆形，位于细胞底部，细胞核的长轴与细胞的长轴平行（图 2 – 4）。

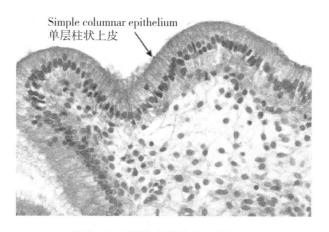

图 2-4　胆囊（HE 染色，400×）

Fig. 2-4　Gallbladder（H & E stain，400×）

4. 假复层纤毛柱状上皮

➤ **材料**

人气管（HE 染色）。

➤ **肉眼观察**

组织切片呈"C"字形。凹面被染成紫色。将凹面置于视野中央。

➤ **低倍镜**

假复层纤毛柱状上皮位于气管的内表面。该上皮的顶端和基底面平坦。

➤ **高倍镜**

上皮细胞的游离面可以看到纤毛（图 2-5）。所有上皮细胞都位于基底膜上，但细胞核处于不同的水平。柱状细胞的细胞核靠近细胞的游离面。梭形细胞的细胞核位于中间。锥形细胞的细胞核位于底部。还有较多的杯状细胞。基底膜位于上皮下方，通常比较明显。

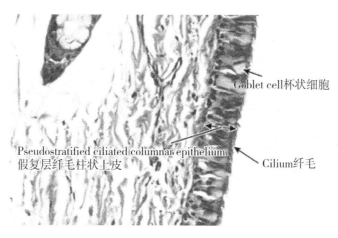

图 2-5　气管（HE 染色，400×）

Fig. 2-5　Trachea（H & E stain，400×）

思考题

（1）假复层纤毛柱状上皮的功能是什么？

（2）光镜下如何区分单层柱状上皮和假复层纤毛柱状上皮？

5. 复层扁平上皮

1）角化的复层扁平上皮

➤ **材料**

人手指皮（HE染色）。

➤ **肉眼观察**

标本一侧染色较深，一侧染色较浅。

➤ **低倍镜**

深色部分为角化的复层扁平上皮，构成皮肤表皮，浅色部分为结缔组织，构成皮肤真皮和皮下组织。复层扁平上皮的基底面凹凸不平（图2-6）。

➤ **高倍镜**

角化的复层扁平上皮细胞层数多。基底层细胞呈柱状，胞质呈强嗜碱性。中间层的细胞呈多边形。靠近表层的细胞逐渐变平。角质层很厚，由多层死细胞构成，细胞呈扁平状，细胞质粉红色，内有角蛋白，无细胞核。

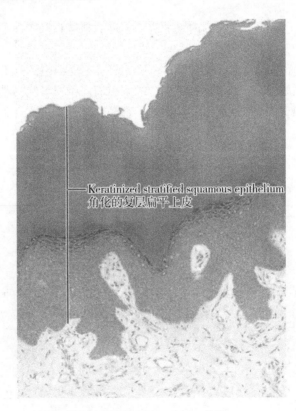

图2-6　皮肤（HE染色，100×）

Fig.2-6　Skin（H & E stain, 100×）

2）未角化的复层扁平上皮

➢ **材料**

狗食管（HE 染色）。

➢ **肉眼观察**

食管管腔不规则。将管腔内表面置于通光孔中央。

➢ **低倍镜**

未角化的复层扁平上皮覆盖食道管腔表面。上皮的基底面不平整（图 2 - 7）。

➢ **高倍镜**

表层细胞扁平形，细胞核呈扁椭圆形。

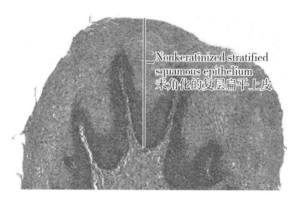

图 2 - 7　食管（HE 染色，100 ×）

Fig. 2 - 7　Esophagus（H & E stain，100 ×）

思考题

（1）复层扁平上皮的功能是什么？

（2）如何区分角化和未角化的复层扁平上皮？

（3）角化和未角化的复层扁平上皮分别分布在哪里？为什么角化的复层扁平上皮能对身体外表面提供更好的保护？

---

6. 复层立方上皮

➢ **材料**

人手指皮（HE 染色）。

➢ **肉眼观察**

标本一侧染色深，一侧染色浅。将浅色部分放在通光孔中央。

➢ **低倍镜**

浅色部分是真皮和皮下组织，汗腺分布在此。汗腺的分泌部染色较浅。导管染色较深，导管壁由复层立方上皮构成。

➢ **高倍镜**

复层立方上皮由两层细胞组成。顶层由立方细胞组成（图 2 - 8）。

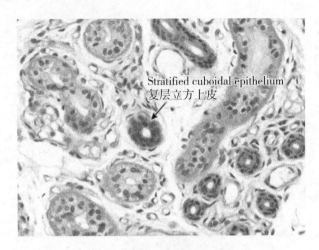

图2-8 汗腺（HE 染色，400×）

Fig. 2-8 Sweat gland（H & E stain，400×）

7. 复层柱状上皮

> **材料**

人下颌下腺（HE 染色）。

> **肉眼观察**

被染成深蓝色的是腺体实质，被染成浅粉色的是被膜和间质。

> **低倍镜**

腺体实质被结缔组织分隔成多个小叶。下颌下腺的主导管位于标本一侧的间质中。

> **高倍镜**

下颌下腺主导管的管腔面被覆了复层柱状上皮（图2-9）。上皮的表层细胞呈柱状，上皮内有散在的杯状细胞和纤毛细胞。

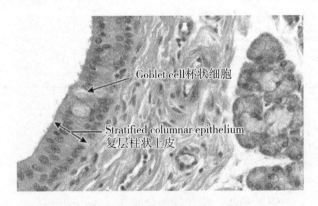

图2-9 下颌下腺（HE 染色，400×）

Fig. 2-9 Submandibular gland（H & E stain，400×）

8. 变移上皮

> **材料**

兔子膀胱（HE 染色）。

> ➤ **肉眼观察**

样本的一侧被染成蓝色，将其放在通光孔中央。

> ➤ **低倍镜**

变移上皮具有多层细胞。上皮基部表面平整。

> ➤ **高倍镜**

（1）排空状态。变移上皮具有多层细胞（图 2 - 10）。顶层细胞称为盖细胞，体积大，呈圆穹状，覆盖下方 2 ～ 3 个细胞。一些盖细胞有 2 个细胞核。中间层的细胞呈多边形。基底层细胞呈低柱状。

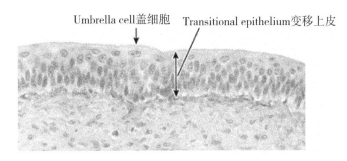

图 2 - 10 膀胱（排空状态，HE 染色，400 ×）

Fig. 2 - 10 Urinary bladder, in relaxed state (H & E stain, 400 ×)

（2）充盈状态。充盈状态的上皮比排空状态的薄（图 2 - 11）。盖细胞被拉长并变平。

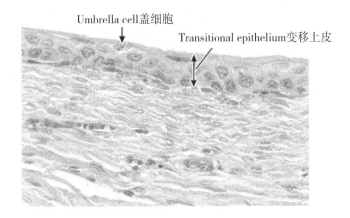

图 2 - 11 膀胱（充盈状态，HE 染色，400 ×）

Fig. 2 - 11 Urinary bladder in extended state (H & E stain, 400 ×)

9. 腺上皮

> ➤ **材料**

人下颌下腺（HE 染色）。

> ➤ **肉眼观察**

标本被染成蓝色。

➢ **低倍镜**

腺体里有许多腺泡。大多数腺泡是深色的浆液性腺泡。有些是浅色的黏液性腺泡和混合性腺泡。

➢ **高倍镜**

（1）浆液性腺泡。其仅包含浆液细胞。细胞核位于基底部，呈圆形。

（2）黏液性腺泡。其仅包含黏液细胞。细胞染色浅，细胞核扁平或不规则。

（3）混合性腺泡。其包含浆液细胞和黏液细胞。一些黏液细胞被浆液细胞包绕，形成新月形的"浆半月"（图 2 -12）。

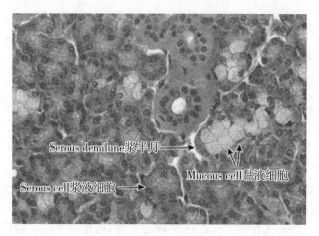

图 2 –12　下颌下腺（HE 染色，400 ×）

Fig. 2 –12　Submandibular gland（H & E stain, 400 ×）

课后作业

画单层柱状上皮光镜结构模式图。

病例教学

患者，男，21 岁，因腹部不适和体重减轻 3 个月就诊。CT 发现回肠末端一个 4.5 cm × 9 cm 的肿块，进行了腹腔镜肿块切除术。病理检查结果显示囊性病变，内衬假复层纤毛柱状上皮，少部分区域有复层扁平上皮和单层柱状上皮。患者被诊断为肠重复囊肿。

（1）假复层纤毛柱状上皮正常分布在哪些部位？

（2）复层扁平上皮正常分布在哪些部位？

（3）单层柱状上皮正常分布在哪些部位？

（4）回肠内表面被覆了什么上皮？

（周雯，洪灯）

Chapter 2　EPITHELIAL TISSUE

The epithelial tissue is one of four basic tissues. It has some basic features:

(1) It has tightly packed cells and a small amount of extracellular matrix.

(2) It is avascular.

(3) It has tissue polarity（极性）.

(4) It is rich in nerve endings.

Learning Objectives

(1) Be able to identify various covering epithelium, and relate the functions to the morphological features of each type.

(2) Be able to differentiate mucous cell and serous cell of exocrine gland.

Pre-class Questions

(1) What are the basic features of epithelial tissue?

(2) What are the classification criteria of covering epithelial?

Observation and Reflection

1. Simple Squamous Epithelium（单层扁平上皮）

1) Simple squamous epithelium, whole mount

➢ Material

Frog's mesentery, whole mount (silver stain).

➢ Gross observation

The specimen is stained brown.

➢ Low power

The outlines of mesothelial cells are irregular or polygonal. Adjacent cells are separated by black lines, which is the intercellular substance (not the cell membrane). The nucleus is oval in shape and located in the center.

➢ High power

The cell edges are brown and serrated or wavy lines (Fig. 2-1).

2) Simple squamous epithelium, section

> Material

Human appendix, section (H & E stain).

> Gross observation

This is a transverse section of appendix.

> Low power

The outmost layer of appendix wall is palely stained. Find the simple squamous epithelium at the outermost surface of appendix.

> High power

The simple squamous epithelium is very thin. The cytoplasm of epithelial cell is pink, and the nucleus is oval or flattened and sometimes bulges out (Fig. 2 – 2).

2. Simple Cuboidal Epithelium （单层立方上皮）

> Material

Canine thyroid (H & E stain).

> Gross observation

The specimen is stained red.

> Low power

Thyroid is a parenchymal organ wrapped by loose connective tissue capsule. This organ is comprised mostly of thyroid follicles （甲状腺滤泡）. Although the follicles vary in size and shape, each of them is made up of a central cavity filled with colloid （胶质） and a wall of simple cuboidal epithelium.

> High power

The follicular wall is made up of simple cuboidal epithelium (Fig. 2 – 3). This epithelium consists of one single layer of cells. The epithelial cells are cuboidal, with pale-pink cytoplasm and round nucleus. The cell boundaries are not clear.

Reflection

(1) What does tissue polarity mean?

(2) Can you identify the apical and basal surface of simple cuboidal epithelium in thyroid?

---

3. Simple Columnar Epithelium （单层柱状上层）

> Material

Canine gallbladder (H & E stain).

> Gross observation

The specimen is stained blue at one side and pink at the opposite side. The blue part is the mucosa of the gallbladder. Place the surface of blue part in the central view.

> Low power

Simple columnar epithelium is at the surface of the gallbladder mucosa.

➢ High power

Simple columnar epithelium has one single layer of columnar cells. The cell nuclei are elongated and near the bottom of the columnar cell (Fig. 2 – 4).

4. Pseudostratified Ciliated Columnar Epithelium (假复层纤毛柱状上皮)

➢ Material

Human trachea (H & E stain).

➢ Gross observation

The specimen is C-shaped. The concave surface is purple. Put the concave surface in the central view.

➢ Low power

The pseudostratified ciliated columnar epithelium is at the innermost surface of trachea. The apical and basal surface of this epithelium are flat.

➢ High power

A number of cilia can be seen at the apical surface of this epithelium (Fig. 2 – 5). All epithelial cells rest on the basement membrane, but the nuclei are at different levels. The nuclei of columnar cells are near the free surface, while those of fusiform cells are in the middle. And The nuclei of pyramidal cells are at the bottom. Goblet cells are also present inside this epithelium. The basement membrane is usually obvious and underneath the epithelium.

Reflection

(1) What are the functions of pseudostratified ciliated columnar epithelium?

(2) How can you distinguish between simple columnar epithelium and pseudostratified ciliated columnar epithelium under light microscope?

---

5. Stratified Squamous Epithelium (复层扁平上皮)

1) Keratinized stratified squamous epithelium

➢ Material

Human finger skin (H & E stain).

➢ Gross observation

The specimen has a blue part and a light-stained part. Place the blue part in the central view.

➢ Low power

The dark-stained part is keratinized stratified squamous epithelium which makes up the **epidermis** (表皮) of skin, while the light-stained part is connective tissue which forms the **dermis** (真皮) of skin. The basal surface of keratinized stratified squamous epithelium is uneven (Fig. 2 – 6).

➢ High power

The keratinized stratified squamous epithelium has several layers. The basal cells are columnar with strongly basophilic cytoplasm. The cells of the middle layers are polygonal. The cells of upper layers become flattened gradually. The cells of superficial layers are compact, flattened, and dead，with keratin（角蛋白）inside the pink cytoplasm and without nuclei.

2）Nonkeratinized stratified squamous epithelium

➢ **Material**

Canine esophagus（H & E stain）.

➢ **Gross observation**

The lumen of esophagus is irregular. Place the luminal surface of esophagus in the central view.

➢ **Low power**

The nonkeratinized stratified squamous epithelium is covering the luminal surface of esophagus. The basal surface of keratinized stratified squamous epithelium is uneven（Fig. 2 – 7）.

➢ **High power**

The superficial cells are flattened with basophilic nuclei.

Reflection

（1）What are the functions of stratified squamous epithelium?

（2）How can you distinguish between keratinized stratified squamous epithelium and nonkeratinized stratified squamous epithelium?

（3）Where is keratinized and nonkeratinized stratified squamous epithelium found respectively? Why does keratinized stratified squamous epithelium provide better protection for the external surface of the body than nonkeratinized one?

---

6. Stratified Cuboidal Epithelium（复层立方上皮）

➢ **Material**

Human finger skin（H & E stain）.

➢ **Gross observation**

The specimen has one blue part and another light-stained part. Place the light-stained part in the central view.

➢ **Low power**

The light-stained part of the skin is dermis and hypodermis. Find out the coiled sweat gland in the view. The secretory portions of sweat gland are stained pale. The ducts are stained darker and have a wall of stratified cuboidal epithelium.

➢ **High power**

The ductal wall is made up of two cell layers. The apical layer is made up of cuboidal cells （Fig. 2 – 8）.

7. Stratified Columnar Epithelium（复层柱状上皮）

➢ **Material**

Human submandibular gland（H & E stain）.

➢ **Gross observation**

The parenchyma of the gland is stained dark blue. The capsule and stroma are stained pink.

➢ **Low power**

The parenchyma is divided into lobules by connective tissue septum. Find the main duct of submandibular gland in the stroma at a lateral side of the specimen.

➢ **High power**

The epithelium lining the main duct of the submandibular gland is stratified columnar epithelium (Fig. 2 – 9). The apical cells of the epithelium are columnar. Some goblet cells and ciliated cells are scattered in the epithelium.

8. Transitional Epithelium (变移上皮)

➢ **Material**

Rabbit urinary bladder (H & E stain).

➢ **Gross observation**

One side of the specimen is stained blue. Place the blue side in the central view.

➢ **Low power**

Transitional epithelium has multiple cell layers. The basal surface of the epithelium is even.

➢ **High power**

(1) Relaxed state. The transitional epithelium has multiple layers of cells (Fig. 2 – 10). The apical cells are called **umbrella cells**, which are large, dome-shaped, covering 2 – 3 underlying cells. Some umbrella cells have two nuclei. The cells in the middle layer are polyhedral, while the cells in the basal layer are low columnar.

(2) Extended state. The transitional epithelium in extended state is thinner than that in relaxed state (Fig. 2 – 11). The umbrella cells are elongated and flattened.

9. Glandular Epithelium (腺上皮)

➢ **Material**

Human submandibular gland (H & E stain).

➢ **Gross observation**

The specimen is stained blue.

➢ **Low power**

Numerous acini are present in the view. Most of the acini are dark-stained serous acini. Some are pale-stained mucous acini or seromucous acini.

➢ **High power**

(1) Serous acini. Serous acini contain only serous cells. Serous cell is darkly stained with a round nucleus at the base.

(2) Mucous acini. Mucous acini contain only mucous cells. Mucous cell is palely stained with a flattened or irregular nucleus at the base.

(3) Seromucous acini. Seromucous acini contain both serous and mucous cells. Some mucous cells are capped by serous cells forming crescent-shaped serous demilunes (Fig. 2 – 12).

Post-class Task

Draw a diagram of simple columnar epithelium under light microscope.

Case-based Learning

A 21-year-old male presented with a 3-month history of abdominal discomfort and weight loss. He was later found to have a 4.5 cm×9 cm mass in the distal ileum（回肠）on CT imaging. He was submitted to a diagnostic laparoscopy with mass resection. Microscopic evaluation of the resected mass revealed a cystic lesion lined by pseudostratified ciliated columnar epithelium, with patchy areas of stratified squamous epithelium and simple columnar epithelium. The patient was diagnosed with enteric duplication cyst（肠重复囊肿）.

（1）Where is pseudostratified ciliated columnar epithelium normally found in human body?

（2）Where is stratified squamous epithelium normally found?

（3）Where is simple columnar epithelium normally found?

（4）What type of epithelium is lining the ileum?

（周雯，洪灯）

第 3 章 固有结缔组织

结缔组织是四种基本组织之一。结缔组织分为 4 种类型：固有结缔组织、血液、骨、软骨。固有结缔组织又分为 4 种类型：疏松结缔组织、致密结缔组织、网状组织、脂肪组织。结缔组织的基本特征与上皮组织几乎相反：

（1）细胞排列松散，细胞外基质多。

（2）血管丰富。

（3）无组织极性。

（4）有丰富的神经末梢，这点与上皮组织相同。

学习目标

（1）能够识别和描述疏松结缔组织中常驻细胞和纤维的微观结构特点。

（2）能够识别和描述致密结缔组织、脂肪组织和网状组织的微观结构特点。

（3）能够将疏松结缔组织中各成分的结构和功能联系起来。

课前问题

（1）疏松结缔组织由什么成分构成？

（2）疏松结缔组织分布在哪里？

实验观察与思考

1. 疏松结缔组织

1）疏松结缔组织（平铺片）

➤ **材料**

大鼠肠系膜平铺片（台盼蓝注射，偶氮红和醛品红染色）。

➤ **肉眼观察**

肉眼可见纤维交错成网状。

➤ **低倍镜**

标本的一些部分较薄，一些部分较厚。选择较薄的部分进行观察。纤维交织成网，细胞散布在其中。

➤ **高倍镜**

胶原纤维粗大，呈浅粉色，很少见分支。弹性纤维细，呈紫色，末端卷曲。网状纤维在此切片不着色。

成纤维细胞数量最多，细胞核椭圆形，细胞质染色浅。巨噬细胞体积较大，形状不规则，胞质内有明显的嗜碱性颗粒。肥大细胞数量较少，呈椭圆形或圆形，胞质内有致密的嗜碱性颗粒（图 3 - 1）。

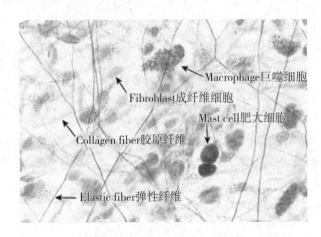

图 3 - 1　疏松结缔组织（平铺片，HE 染色，400 ×）

Fig. 3 - 1　Loose connective tissue（whole mount, H & E stain, 400 ×）

2）疏松结缔组织（切片）

➤ **材料**

人疏松结缔组织切片（HE 染色）。

➤ **肉眼观察**

标本被染成粉红色。

➤ **低倍镜**

胶原纤维被染成粉红色，成波浪状，排列松散。细胞散布在纤维之间。血管丰富。

➤ **高倍镜**

成纤维细胞呈梭形，数量最多。浆细胞呈卵圆形，细胞质嗜碱性，细胞核圆形并位于细胞一侧，细胞核的异染色质聚集在核膜下方形成轮辐状。巨噬细胞体积较大，呈卵圆形或圆形，胞质嗜酸性，核小，核呈卵圆形或肾形。

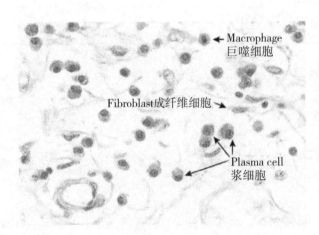

图 3 - 2　疏松结缔组织（切片，HE 染色，400 ×）

Fig. 3 - 2　Loose connective tissue, section（H & E stain, 400 ×）

思考题

（1）哪些细胞永久定居在疏松结缔组织？

（2）哪些细胞可以从血液中迁移到疏松结缔组织？

（3）上皮组织和结缔组织的形态特点有何区别？

（4）成纤维细胞有哪些功能？

（5）巨噬细胞有哪些功能？

（6）肥大细胞有哪些功能？

（7）浆细胞有哪些功能？

（8）白细胞在什么情况下会大量聚集在疏松结缔组织？

2. 致密结缔组织

1）规则的致密结缔组织

➤ **材料**

牛肌腱（HE 染色）。

➤ **肉眼观察**

切片被染成粉红色。

➤ **低倍镜**

胶原纤维平行，排列紧密。胶原纤维间的细胞是腱细胞。

➤ **高倍镜**

腱细胞排列成行。细胞长，细胞核位于中央，核仁明显（图 3 - 2）。

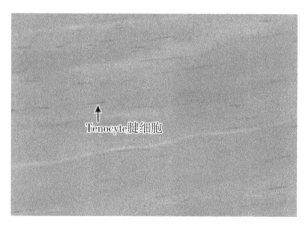

图 3 - 3　肌腱（HE 染色，200×）

Fig. 3 - 3　Tendon（H & E stain, 200×）

（2）不规则的致密结缔组织

➤ **材料**

人皮肤（HE 染色）。

> **肉眼观察**

标本呈半月形。凸面为掌面。

> **低倍镜**

不规则的致密结缔组织位于上皮组织下方，富含纤维和血管。胶原纤维束粗大（图3-4）。

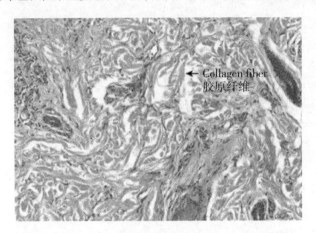

图3-4　不规则的致密结缔组织（HE染色，100×）

Fig. 3-4　Dense irregular connective tissue（H & E stain, 100×）

> **高倍镜**

可见胶原纤维束的纵断面和横切面。成纤维细胞附着在胶原纤维上或散布在胶原纤维之间。弹性纤维也被染成粉色，在切片中，与胶原纤维不易区分。

思考题

（1）规则和不规则的致密结缔组织分别分布在哪里？

（2）规则的致密结缔组织和不规则的致密结缔组织的微观结构和功能有什么区别？

---

3. 网状组织

> **材料**

狗淋巴结（镀银染色）。

> **肉眼观察**

切片被染成黑色，呈扁豆形。

> **低倍镜**

淋巴结中的黑色纤维是网状纤维，其构成淋巴结的支架。

> **高倍镜**

网状纤维纤细，交织成网。网状细胞有多个突起，相邻的细胞突起相互连接成网（图3-5）。

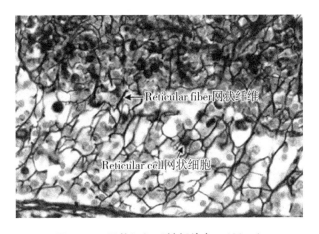

图 3 - 5　网状组织（镀银染色，400 × ）

Fig. 3 - 5　Reticular tissue（silver stain，400 × ）

思考题

（1）网状组织分布在哪里？

（2）网状细胞的功能是什么？

（3）你能在 HE 染色切片中找到网状纤维吗？

4. 脂肪组织

➤ **材料**

人白色脂肪组织（HE 染色）。

➤ **肉眼观察**

标本染色浅淡。

➤ **低倍镜**

白色脂肪组织被疏松结缔组织分隔成多个小叶。脂肪细胞大而圆，呈白色。脂肪组织中可见血管和神经束。

➤ **高倍镜**

白色脂肪细胞胞质空泡状，胞质中的脂滴在制片过程中被溶解了，细胞核位于细胞边缘（图 3 - 6）。

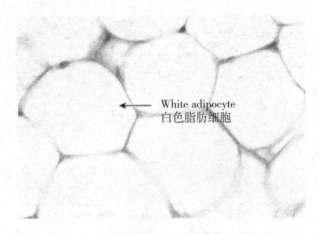

图 3-6　白色脂肪组织（HE 染色，400×）
Fig. 3-6　White adipose tissue（H & E stain，400×）

思考题
脂肪组织分布在哪里？

课后作业
画疏松结缔组织平铺片的结构模式图。

病例教学
患者，男，70 岁，左臀部疼痛进行性加重 1 个月。患者被诊断为金属全髋关节置换术后高度磨损。患者之后接受了左髋关节置换修复术。手术中取下左髋关节的滑膜，进行组织学分析。结果表明滑膜表面有大量的纤维蛋白，巨噬细胞大量聚集，胞质内含有大量的磨损颗粒，滑膜组织中有大量金属磨损碎屑，血管周围可见散在的淋巴细胞聚集。

（1）滑膜由哪些组织构成？
（2）巨噬细胞的功能是什么？
（3）滑膜中的淋巴细胞来自哪里？

（周雯，陈志强）

Chapter 3 CONNECTIVE TISSUE PROPER

Connective tissue is one of four types of fundamental tissues. Connective tissue is classified into four types: connective tissue proper, blood, bone, cartilage. Connective tissue proper is subdivided into four types: loose connective tissue, dense connective tissue, reticular tissue, adipose tissue.

Connective tissue proper has some basic characteristics which are almost opposite to those of epithelial tissue:

(1) It has loosely arranged cells and a large amount of extracellular matrix.

(2) It is rich in blood vessels.

(3) It has no tissue polarity.

(4) It is as rich in nerve endings as epithelial tissue.

Learning Objectives

(1) Be able to identify and describe the microstructural features of the resident cells and fibers in loose connective tissue.

(2) Be able to identify and describe the microstructural features of dense connective tissue, adipose tissue, and reticular tissue.

(3) Be able to relate the functions to the morphological features of each component in loose connective tissue.

Pre-class Questions

(1) What components does loose connective tissue consist of?

(2) Where is loose connective tissue found in human body?

Observation and Reflection

1. Loose Connective Tissue (疏松结缔组织)

1) Loose connective tissue, whole mount

➤ Material

Rat mesentery, whole mount (Trypan blue injection, Azo Red & Aldehyde Fuchsin stain).

➤ Gross observation

Fibers are interwoven together.

➤ Low power

Some parts of the specimen are thin, while some parts are a little thick. Choose the thinner part for observation. Fibers are interwoven with cells scattered between them.

> ➤ High power

Collagen fibers（胶原纤维）are coarse, palely pink, and branching rarely. **Elastic fibers**（弹性纤维）are fine, purple, with coiled endings. **Reticular fibers**（网状纤维）cannot be seen in this slide.

The **fibroblast**（成纤维细胞）is the most numerous cell type in loose connective tissue. It has an oval nucleus and weakly stained cytoplasm. The **macrophage**（巨噬细胞）is larger than fibroblast, and irregular in shape with distinctive basophilic granules inside the cytoplasm. **Mast cells**（肥大细胞）are less than macrophages. Mast cell is oval or round in shape, with dense basophilic granules in the cytoplasm（Fig. 3 – 1）.

2）Loose connective tissue, section

> ➤ Material

Human loose connective tissue, section（H & E stain）.

> ➤ Gross observation

Specimen is stained pink.

> ➤ Low power

Collagen fibers are stained pink and loosely arranged into wavy bundles. Cells and blood vessels are scattered between fibers.

> ➤ High power

Fibroblast is fusiform in shape. It is the most common cell in loose connective tissue. Plasma cell has basophilic cytoplasm, a round and eccentric nucleus, and coarse clumps of heterochromatin appearing like a clock face. Macrophage is large ovoid or spherical, with acidophilic cytoplasm and a small ovoid or kidney-shaped nucleus（Fig. 3 – 2）.

Reflection

（1）Which cells are permanent in the loose connective tissue?

（2）Which cells can migrate from blood into the loose connective tissue?

（3）What are the morphological differences between epithelial tissue and connective tissue?

（4）What functions do fibroblasts have?

（5）What functions do macrophages have?

（6）What functions do mast cells have?

（7）What functions do plasma cells have?

（8）In what condition can leukocytes be found to aggregate in loose connective tissue?

2. Dense Connective Tissue（致密结缔组织）

1）Dense regular connective tissue（规则致密结缔组织）

> ➤ Material

Bovine tendon（H & E stain）.

> Gross observation

The specimen is stained pink.

> Low power

Collagen fibers are parallelly oriented and tightly packed together. The cells between collagen fibers are tenocytes （腱细胞）（Fig. 3 – 3）.

> High power

Tenocytes are elongated, with a long, spindle-shaped nucleus. These cells line up in parallel rows.

2）Dense irregular connective tissue （不规则致密结缔组织）

> Material

Human skin （H & E stain）.

> Gross observation

The specimen is half-moon shaped. The convex side is the palm surface.

> Low power

Dense irregular connective tissue is underneath the epithelium and rich in fibers and blood vessels. Thick collagen fibers are interwoven together （Fig. 3 – 4）.

> High power

Longitudinal section and cross section of collagen fibers are seen. Fibroblasts are attaching on or scattered between collagen fibers.

Reflection

（1）Where can dense regular connective tissue and dense irregular connective tissue be found?

（2）What are the microstructural and functional differences between dense regular connective tissue and dense irregular connective tissue?

---

3. Reticular Tissue （网状组织）

> Material

Canine lymph node （silver stain）.

> Gross observation

The specimen is black and bean-shaped.

> Low power

Black fibers in the lymph node are reticular fibers which form the framework of lymph node.

> High power

Reticular fibers are delicate and intertwined to form a meshwork. Reticular cells are stellate with several processes. These cells are connected to each other through the processes （Fig. 3 – 5）.

Reflection

(1) Where is reticular tissue found?

(2) What is the function of reticular cell?

(3) Can you identify reticular fibers in loose connective tissue using H & E staining?

4. Adipose Tissue（脂肪组织）

➢ **Material**

Human white adipose tissue（H & E stain）.

➢ **Gross observation**

The specimen is palely stained.

➢ **Low power**

White adipose tissue is divided into several lobules by loose connective tissue septa. Adipocytes are round and white. In adipose tissue, blood vessels and nerve bundles can be seen.

➢ **High power**

White adipocyte appears empty because lipids are removed by tissue preparation. The cell nucleus is compressed to the cell edge（Fig. 3 – 6）.

Reflection

Where is adipose tissue found?

Post-class Task

Draw a diagram of loose connective tissue（whole mount）at high magnification.

Case-based Learning

A 70-year-old man complained of increasing left hip pain for around 1 month. After diagnosed with high wear of a metalonmetal total hip arthroplasty（全髋关节置换），he was given left hip arthroplasty revision surgery. Synovium（滑膜）of the left hip was harvested during the revision surgery and analyzed histologically. Light microscopy showed replacement of the synovial surface by fibrin, prominent infiltrates of macrophages containing wear particles, variable amounts of metallic wear debris, and scattered perivascular lymphocyte aggregates.

(1) What tissue is synovium normally made up of?

(2) What are the functions of macrophages?

(3) Where are lymphocytes in synovium coming from?

（周雯，陈志强）

第4章 | 软骨和骨

软骨和骨是两种特殊的结缔组织。

（1）软骨由软骨组织和软骨膜组成。

（2）骨由骨组织、骨膜和骨髓组成。

学习目标

（1）能够描述软骨和长骨骨干的主要结构。

（2）能够识别透明软骨和骨组织。

（3）了解软骨成骨的过程。

课前问题

（1）软骨的主要类型有哪几种?

（2）骨组织内的细胞组成有哪些?

实验观察与思考

1. 透明软骨

➤ **材料**

大鼠气管横切面（HE染色）。

➤ **肉眼观察**

软骨部分被染为紫色，呈"C"字形。

➤ **低倍镜**

软骨周边被覆薄层致密结缔组织是软骨膜，染成粉红色。软骨基质呈蓝色的均质状，从外侧到中心颜色逐渐加深。软骨组织外周的软骨细胞小而幼稚，且单一分布。越靠近软骨中央，软骨细胞变大而成熟，且2～6个成群分布，称为同源细胞群。

➤ **高倍镜**

软骨组织周边的软骨细胞较小，呈扁圆形；中央成熟的软骨细胞呈圆形或椭圆形，核圆，核仁清晰，胞质少，弱嗜碱性，软骨细胞所在的腔隙称为软骨陷窝，陷窝周围的软骨基质染色较深，称为软骨囊。软骨细胞由于制片原因常皱缩变形，可显现出空白的软骨陷窝。（图4-1）

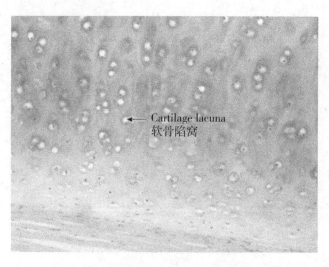

图 4 – 1　透明软骨（HE 染色，200 ×）
Fig. 4 – 1　Hyaline cartilage（H & E stain，200 ×）

思考题

（1）透明软骨不同位置的软骨基质颜色有什么变化，思考一下可能的原因？

（2）软骨基质中含有血管和纤维吗？为何镜下看不到纤维？

（3）软骨细胞在透明软骨的不同位置有什么形态的变化？

（4）透明软骨如何获得营养？

---

2. 弹性软骨

➤ **材料**

人耳郭（醛复红染色）。

➤ **肉眼观察**

呈蓝紫色的带状组织。

➤ **低倍镜**

标本周围浅染的是皮肤，中央被染成蓝紫色的带状组织为弹性软骨。

➤ **高倍镜**

软骨基质中可见大量染成蓝紫色的弹性纤维，交织成网，其他结构与透明软骨相似（图 4 – 2）。

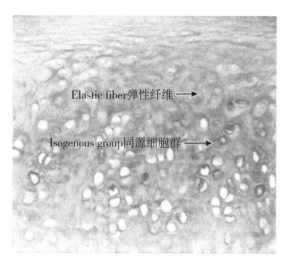

图4-2 弹性软骨（醛复红染色，200×）

Fig. 4-2 Elastic cartilage（elastic stain，200×）

思考题

（1）透明软骨、弹性软骨和纤维软骨的主要异同点是什么？

（2）透明软骨如何获取营养？

---

3. 密质骨

➤ **材料**

人长骨骨磨片（硫堇染色）。

➤ **肉眼观察**

切面中弧形光滑的一面为外表面，对侧不规则的一面为内表面。

➤ **低倍镜**

（1）外环骨板位于骨干外表面，较厚，是数层或十几层较整齐平行排列的骨板；内环骨板位于骨髓腔内表面，较薄，为几层不规则的骨板，可见骨小梁。

（2）骨单位（哈弗斯系统）位于内、外环骨板之间，呈圆形、卵圆形或不规则形，大小不一，由数层至数十层哈弗斯骨板围绕中央管形成。

（3）间骨板位于骨单位之间或骨单位与内、外环骨板之间的不规则骨板。

（4）福尔克曼管（穿通管）是纵行或斜形横穿内、外环骨板的管道，或骨单位中央管之间连接的管道（图4-3）。

➤ **高倍镜**

骨板之间或骨板内可见蜘蛛状的小黑点，为骨陷窝（骨细胞胞体所在的腔隙）；从陷窝向四周发出细小的放射状突起为骨小管（骨细胞突起所在的腔隙），相邻骨小管彼此相通，近中央管的骨小管与中央管连通；每个骨单位表面有折光性较强的黏合线，骨小管在此终止。

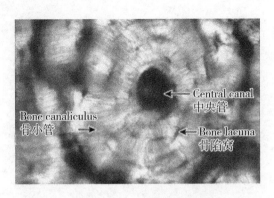

图 4-3　骨单位（硫堇染色，400×）

Fig. 4-3　Osteon（Thionin acetate stain, 400×）

思考题
(1) 骨组织与固有结缔组织的组织学区别是什么，它为什么坚硬？
(2) 骨组织内有血管吗？骨细胞怎么获取营养？

4. 长骨发生（软骨内成骨）

➤ **材料**

新生儿指骨纵切面（HE 染色）。

➤ **肉眼观察**

指骨两端膨大，染色呈浅蓝色的是软骨组织骨骺，中间染成深红色的是骨干表面的骨组织（骨领），和内部的骨髓腔，聚焦其交界染成灰蓝处（软骨内成骨的部位），从软骨组织向骨组织的方向进行观察。

➤ **低倍镜**

从骨骺侧到骨干侧可以观察到以下区域（图 4-4）：

(1) 软骨贮备区：透明软骨组织，软骨细胞小，基质弱嗜碱性。

(2) 软骨增生区：软骨细胞分裂增大，形成同源细胞群，一个同源细胞群的软骨细胞排列成纵行的细胞柱。

(3) 软骨成熟区：软骨细胞变大变圆，周边基质相对变薄。

(4) 软骨钙化区：软骨细胞肥大，逐渐退化死亡；有的细胞已消失，留下空洞状的软骨陷窝。软骨基质钙化，呈强嗜碱性。

(5) 软骨成骨区：蓝色残存钙化软骨基质，表面被覆薄层红色的新生骨组织，形成过渡性骨小梁，其表面常可见成骨细胞。

➤ **高倍镜**

(1) 成骨细胞：细胞呈立方形或矮柱状，单层排列于过渡性骨小梁表面，胞质嗜碱性。

(2) 破骨细胞：常散在分布于软骨钙化区的软骨陷窝或骨小梁凹陷处，胞体较大，形状多不规则，胞质嗜酸性，常见多个核（图 4-5）。

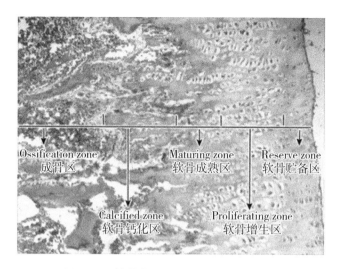

图 4 - 4　软骨内骨化（HE 染色，100 ×）

Fig. 4 - 4　Endochondral ossification（H & E stain，100 ×）

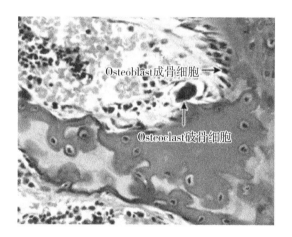

图 4 - 5　成骨细胞和破骨细胞（HE 染色，400 ×）

Fig. 4 - 5　Osteoblast and osteoclast（H & E stain，400 ×）

思考题

软骨内成骨和膜内成骨的主要步骤是什么？

课后作业

画骨单位模式图。

病例教学

一名男子因交通事故住院，被诊断为胫骨脆性骨折和软组织损伤。

（1）损伤部位包括哪些组织类型？

（2）骨组织如何修复？

（魏霞，黄文峰）

Chapter 4　CARTILAGE AND BONE

The cartilage and bone are two kinds of special connective tissue.

(1) The cartilage is composed of the cartilage tissue and perichondrium.

(2) The bone is composed of the osseous tissue, periosteum and bone marrow.

Learning Objectives

(1) Be able to describe the main structures of the cartilage and long bone.

(2) Be able to identify hyaline cartilage and bone tissue.

(3) Understand the process of endochondral ossification.

Pre-class Questions

(1) What's the classification of cartilage?

(2) What cells can be identified within the bone tissue?

Observation and Reflection

1.　Hyaline cartilage （透明软骨）

➢　Material

Rat trachea, cross section （H & E stain）.

➢　Gross observation

The purple and "C" shaped portion is hyaline cartilage.

➢　Low power

The **perichondrium** （软骨膜） is a thin layer of dense connective tissue, which covers the surface of the cartilage and is stained in pink color. The matrix of cartilage is basophilic and stained in blue, with its staining density increasing from the periphery to the center. **Chondrocytes** （软骨细胞） are small and immature, distributed dispersedly at the periphery, while those in the center are large and mature, appearing in groups （2 – 6 chondrocytes）, which are called **isogenous group** （同源细胞群）.

➢　High power

The chondrocyte near the perichondrium is small and oblate in shape, while the mature one near the center is large and ovoid or round. Its nucleus is also round with a clear nucleolus. Its cytoplasm is sparse and a little basophilic. The **cartilage matrix** （软骨基质） is homogenous and the fibers in it are invisible, since the fiber is collagen fibril and its refractive index is similar to the matrix. The space where the chondrocyte locates is called cartilage lacuna. The matrix close to the cartilage lacuna shows strong basophilia because of more chondroitin sulfate deposition, which is called **cartilage capsule**（软骨囊）. Because of the cell shrinkage of the chondrocytes during the routine preparation, uncovered lacuna（white）can be found（Fig. 4 – 1）.

Reflection

（1）What are the color changes of cartilage matrix in the different part of hyaline cartilage? And think about the reasons.

（2）Does the cartilage matrix of hyaline cartilage contain fibers and blood vessels? Why the fibers can't be seen within it under light microscope?

（3）What are the morphological changes of chondrocytes in the different part of hyaline cartilage?

（4）How does the hyaline cartilage get nutrition?

---

2. Elastic cartilage（弹性软骨）

➤ **Material**

Human auricle（aldehyde-fuchsin or orcein stain）.

➤ **Gross observation**

The specimen is stained in purple-blue color.

➤ **Low power**

The auricle is covered by skin, which is stained lightly, and elastic cartilage locates in the center of the auricle, which is stained in purple-blue. Basic structures are similar to hyaline cartilage.

➤ **High power**

The dense network of purple-blue stained elastic fibers fills in the matrix of the elastic cartilage. The cells are quite similar to those of hyaline cartilage（Fig. 4 – 2）.

Reflection

（1）What are the main differences among hyaline cartilage, elastic cartilage and fibrocartilage?

（2）How does the hyaline cartilage get nutrition?

---

3. Compact Bone（密质骨）

➤ **Material**

Human long bone, ground section（thionin acetate stain）.

➤ **Gross observation**

The smooth and bracket-shaped surface is the external surface of the long bone. The opposite is its internal irregular surface.

➢ Low power

(1) The **outer circumferential lamellae** （外环骨板）are composed of several layers of parallelly arranged smooth and regular lamellae. They are thick and located on the external surface of the long bone. **Inner circumferential lamellae** （内环骨板）are near to the marrow cavity and have its irregular outline.

(2) The **osteon** （**Haversian system**）（骨单位）, which are round, ovoid or irregular in shape, with different sizes, are located between the outer and inner circumferential lamellae. It consists of a central canal surrounded by 4 – 20 layers of concentric lamellae.

(3) The **perforating canals** （**Volkmann's canals**）（穿通管）are transverse channels that cross the circumferential lamellae or connect the central cannels of adjacent osteons.

(4) The **interstitial lamellae** （间骨板）are irregular lamellae among osteons or between osteons and circumferential lamellae （Fig. 4 – 3）.

➢ High power

Bone lacunae （骨陷窝）are the ovoid housing space of osteocytes, which can be seen within or between bone lamellae. Many delicate channels radiated from the bone lacunae are **canaliculi** （骨小管）, where the cytoplasmic processes of osteocytes project. Bone canaliculi in the adjacent lacunae are connecting with each other. A narrow pale band called **cement line** （黏合线）is present at the periphery of osteon, where canaliculi terminate.

Reflection

(1) What are the differences between the bone tissue and the connective tissue proper? Why is the bone tissue so hard?

(2) Are there many blood vessels in the bone tissue? How do osteocytes get the nutrition?

---

4. Osteogenesis of long bone （endochondral ossification）（长骨骨发生）

➢ Material

Human fetal phalange, longitudinal section （H & E stain）.

➢ Gross observation

Both ends of the phalange are expanded and stained in lightly blue, indicating the cartilage area （epiphysis）. The middle shaft is stained in deep red, indicating the outer bone tissue （**bone collar**, 骨领）and its inner bone marrow cavity. Their boundary is stained in gray-blue, indicating the location of **endochondral ossification** （软骨内成骨）.

➢ Low power

From epiphyseal side to diaphyseal side, the following four zones can be observed （Fig. 4 – 4）:

(1) **Zone of reserve cartilage** （储备区）: It consists of hyaline cartilage, with small chondrocytes and weak basophilic matrix.

(2) **Zone of proliferating cartilage** （增生区）: Chondrocytes grow and proliferate, forming

isogenous groups, whose chondrocytes are densely arranged in longitudinal rows.

(3) **Zone of maturing cartilage** （成熟区）: Chondrocytes furtherly enlarge and are round, while matrix is thinner.

(4) **Zone of calcified cartilage** （钙化区）: Hypertrophic chondrocytes gradually degenerate. Some cells die and only the cartilage lacunae left. Cartilage matrix becomes calcified and shows strong basophilia.

(5) **Zone of ossification** （成骨区）: The relic calcified cartilage matrix is covered by the new bone tissue, forming the transitional bone trabeculae. Osteoblasts are usually found in one layer on the surface of the bone trabecular. Primitive marrow cavities are among the bone trabeculae, filled with hematopoietic tissue.

➢ High power

(1) **Osteoblasts** （成骨细胞）: Osteoblasts are arranged in one layer on the surface of the transitional bone trabeculae, showing cuboidal or irregular in shape, with basophilic cytoplasm.

(2) **Osteoclasts** （破骨细胞）: Osteoclasts are dispersedly distributed within the cartilage lacunae of the zone of calcified cartilage, or on the concave surface of the transitional bone trabeculae. They are very large and irregular in shape. Their cytoplasm is acidophilic, and multi-nuclei are often found （Fig. 4 – 5）.

Reflection

What are the main steps of endochondral ossification and intramembranous ossification?

Post-class Task

Draw a diagram of an osteon.

Case-based Learning

A man was hospitalized because of a traffic accident. He was diagnosed with tibia fracture and soft tissue injury.

(1) Which tissue types are included in the injury portion?

(2) How does the bone tissue repair?

（魏霞，黄文峰）

第5章 | 血液和血细胞发生

血液是一种特殊的结缔组织,由血细胞和血浆组成。对于成人,造血发生在骨髓和胸腺。

学习目标

(1) 能够使用油镜进行观察。
(2) 能够识别每种类型的血细胞,并将细胞的结构特征与功能相联系。
(3) 能够描述骨髓的微细结构。
(4) 能够识别骨髓中红系、髓系和血小板系列的造血细胞。

课前问题

(1) 血液中有哪些成分?
(2) 血液中每种细胞类型的微细结构特征是什么?
(3) 白细胞的分类标准是什么?
(4) 骨髓中有哪些造血前体细胞?

实验观察与思考

1. 血涂片

➤ **材料**

人血涂片 (瑞氏染色)。

➤ **肉眼观察**

血膜薄,呈舌状。

➤ **低倍镜**

大量的粉红色小点是红细胞。红细胞中有几个紫色小点,是白细胞。

➤ **高倍镜**

选择白细胞集中的区域,换成 40× 物镜,用细调焦螺旋获得清晰的图像。然后将一滴油滴到盖玻片上,油滴的厚度要能接触到油镜的镜头,换成油镜 (100×),使用细调焦螺旋对焦获得清晰的图像。

(1) 红细胞 (图 5-1):直径 7 ~ 8 μm,圆盘形,无细胞核,呈橙色至粉红色,中央染色较浅。红细胞是血液中数量最多的细胞类型。

(2) 中性粒细胞 (图 5-1):直径 10 ~ 12 μm,细胞核分 2 ~ 5 叶,细胞质呈粉红色,含有许多细小的红色颗粒。少数细胞有杆状核。中性粒细胞是数量最多的白细胞,6 岁后占白细胞总数的 50% ~ 70%。

(3) 嗜酸性粒细胞 (图 5-2):直径 10 ~ 15 μm,细胞核通常为 2 叶,胞质内充满大而鲜红色或橙色的颗粒。嗜酸性粒细胞占白细胞总数的 1%～3%。

（4）嗜碱性粒细胞（图 5-3）：数量很少，占白细胞总数的 0%～1%。细胞质内充满粗大、大小不一的深紫色颗粒。细胞核一般被颗粒遮蔽。

（5）淋巴细胞（图 5-4）：淋巴细胞数量较多，6 岁后占白细胞总量的 25%～30%。外周血中的淋巴细胞多为直径 6～8 μm 的小淋巴细胞。小淋巴细胞，核呈圆形或一侧有小凹陷，深蓝色，染色质致密成团；胞质呈深蓝色边缘，有少量嗜天青颗粒。反应性淋巴细胞为中型或大型，直径 10～30 μm，通常不到外周血淋巴细胞总数的 10%。反应性淋巴细胞的细胞核染色较浅，有时可见核仁，细胞质呈清晰的蔚蓝色或呈淡天蓝色，在与其他细胞接触的边缘胞质染色较暗。

（6）单核细胞（图 5-5）：体积大，直径 14～20 μm。单核细胞有 1 个不规则形、肾形或马蹄铁形的核，细胞核染色比淋巴细胞浅。胞质丰富，呈灰蓝色，有许多细小的嗜天青颗粒和一些液泡。

（7）血小板（图 5-6）：小，直径 2～4 μm，常聚集成群。呈圆形、椭圆形或不规则形状，无核，中央含有紫蓝色颗粒。

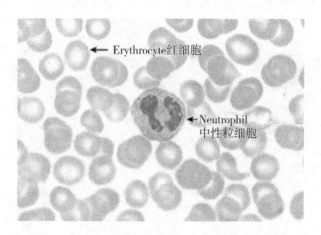

图 5-1　红细胞和白细胞（血涂片，瑞氏染色，1000×）

Fig. 5-1　Erythrocyte and neutrophil（blood smear, Wright's stain, 1000×）

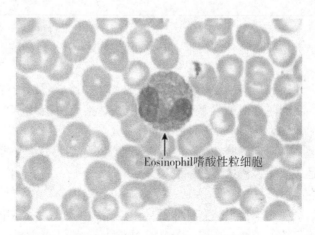

图 5-2　嗜酸性粒细胞（血涂片，瑞氏染色，1000×）

Fig. 5-2　Eosinophil（blood smear, Wright's stain, 1000×）

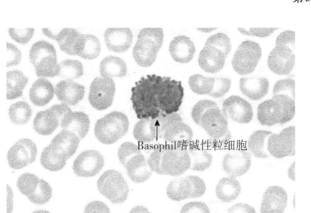

图 5 - 3　嗜碱性粒细胞（血涂片，瑞氏染色，1000×）

Fig. 5 - 3　Basophil（blood smear，Wright's stain，1000×）

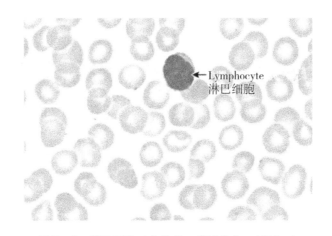

图 5 - 4　淋巴细胞（血涂片，瑞氏染色，1000×）

Fig. 5 - 4　Lymphocyte（blood smear，Wright's stain，1000×）

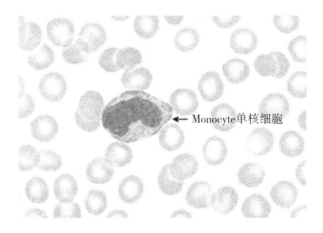

图 5 - 5　单核细胞（血涂片，瑞氏染色，1000×）

Fig. 5 - 5　Monocyte（blood smear，Wright's stain，1000×）

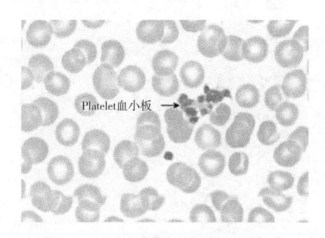

图5-6 血小板（血涂片，瑞氏染色，1000×）
Fig. 5-6 Platelets（blood smear，Wright's stain，1000×）

思考题

（1）红细胞的形态特征是什么？成熟红细胞的细胞质内有什么？成熟红细胞的功能是什么？它的寿命有多长？

（2）白细胞中数量最多的细胞类型是什么？

（3）白细胞根据什么分为有粒白细胞和无粒白细胞？哪些细胞是有粒白细胞？哪些细胞是无粒白细胞？

（4）每种白细胞的形态特征和功能有何不同？

（5）血涂片在临床上有何作用？

2. 血涂片制作和染色

➤ **血涂片制作**

（1）取 2～3 μL（直径 1～2 mm）血液滴在载玻片上，靠近磨砂边缘处。

（2）将另一张玻片作为推片，把推片以约成45°角放在血滴前面，然后将推片向后拉入血滴中，让血液沿推片的边缘散开（图5-7）。

（3）推片平稳向前推动，产生舌状血膜。

（4）血涂片自然晾干。

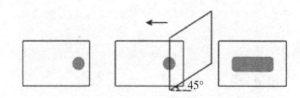

图5-7 血涂片制作
Fig. 5-7 Blood smear preparation

➢ **May-Grunwald-Giemsa 染色**

May-Grunwald-Giemsa 染色是两种染色的组合：May-Grunwald 染色由亚甲基蓝和伊红组成，Giemsa 染色由亚甲基蓝、伊红和天青 B 组成。

（1）血涂片在 May-Grunwald 溶液中染色 5 min。

（2）竖立血涂片以去除多余的染液，无须清洗。

（3）在 Giemsa 工作液中染色 15 min，然后在 Sorensen 缓冲液中漂洗 10 ～ 20 s。

（4）用流水冲洗血涂片至少 2 min，直至涂片最薄处呈粉红色。

（5）让载玻片在室温下倾斜风干。

（6）根据需要盖上盖玻片，在显微镜下观察。

3. 红骨髓

➢ **材料**

人骨髓（HE 染色）。

➢ **肉眼观察**

切片染成深蓝色，其中有许多白色小点。

➢ **低倍镜**

造血细胞的细胞核染成蓝色，脂肪细胞的胞质呈白色。

➢ **高倍镜**

造血细胞聚集成群形成血细胞岛。这些血细胞岛靠近血窦。血窦是一种毛细血管，管壁薄，直径为 15 ～ 100 μm。在血窦附近可以看到巨核细胞（图 5 - 8）。巨核细胞是骨髓中最大的细胞（40 ～ 100 μm），胞质嗜酸性，细胞核有多个分叶。

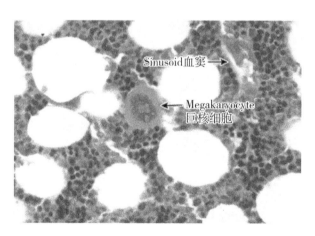

图 5 - 8　红骨髓（HE 染色，400 ×）
Fig. 5 - 8　Red bone marrow (H & E stain, 400 ×)

思考题
红骨髓和黄骨髓分布在哪里？

4. 骨髓涂片

➤ **材料**

人骨髓（瑞氏染色）。

➤ **肉眼观察**

标本被染成浅粉色。

➤ **低倍镜**

红色小点是红细胞，蓝色小点是造血细胞。

➤ **高倍镜**

视野中的多数细胞是成熟的红细胞。选择造血细胞集中的区域，使用 40×物镜获得清晰的图像，然后换成油镜进行观察。

成红细胞、成髓细胞和淋巴母细胞形态相同，均较大，核圆形或卵圆形，核仁可见，胞浆呈蓝色。

（1）红系细胞具有以下特征（图 5-9）：

A. 原红细胞，呈圆形，直径 15～30 μm，胞质边缘呈强嗜碱性。核大圆形，染色质细而分散，有多个核仁。

B. 早幼红细胞，又称嗜碱性成红细胞，直径 10～18 μm，无核仁，胞质内无颗粒，胞质嗜碱性比原红细胞更强。

C. 中幼红细胞，直径 10～12 μm，核染色深，胞质因血红蛋白积累增多并且多核糖体减少而呈灰绿色。

D. 晚幼红细胞，直径 8～10 μm，核小而深，胞质淡粉色。脱核发生在这个阶段的最后，有时镜下可见正在脱核的晚幼红细胞。

E. 网织红细胞，直径 7～8 μm，有核糖体，胞浆粉红色，无细胞核。

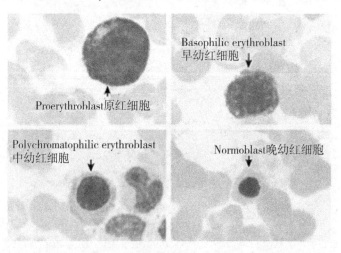

图 5-9　红系细胞（骨髓涂片，瑞氏染色，1000×）

Fig. 5-9　Erythroid cells（bone marrow smear, Wright's stain, 1000×）

（2）髓系细胞具有以下特征（图 5-10）：

A. 早幼粒细胞，是髓系中最大的细胞，直径 15～25 μm。胞质嗜碱性，核大而圆，核仁明显，胞质中有较大的深紫色嗜天青颗粒。

B. 中幼粒细胞，比早幼粒细胞小，直径 15 ～ 18 μm。细胞核位于一侧，胞质呈轻度嗜碱性，紫色嗜天青颗粒减少，特殊颗粒增多。中性粒细胞、嗜碱性粒细胞和嗜酸性粒细胞具有不同的特异性颗粒。

C. 晚幼粒细胞，细胞核一侧凹陷或呈肾形，凹陷程度小于细胞核的半径。其他看起来都像成熟的粒细胞。

D. 杆状核粒细胞，有马蹄形的核，凹陷程度大于细胞核的半径，胞质内有特殊颗粒。

E. 骨髓中成熟的中性粒细胞、嗜酸性粒细胞和嗜碱性粒细胞与外周血相同。

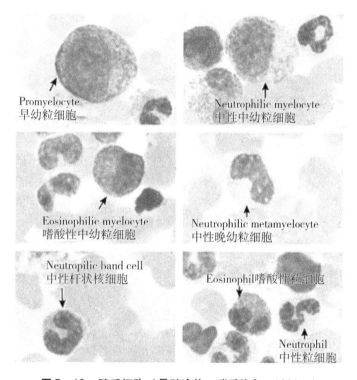

图 5 - 10　髓系细胞（骨髓涂片，瑞氏染色，1000 ×）
Fig. 5 - 10　Myeloid cells（bone marrow smear，Wright's stain，1000 ×）

（3）单核细胞系具有以下特征：

A. 幼单核细胞，在正常骨髓中很少见到，因为它在短时间内分裂成单核细胞。细胞质蓝灰色，有细小的嗜天青颗粒，通常有液泡，细胞核呈分叶状或有褶皱（图 5 - 11）。与成熟的单核细胞相比，染色质比较疏松，有时可见核仁。

B. 成熟的单核细胞不易在骨髓中找到，因为它们很快进入外周血循环，不储存在骨髓中。

（4）血小板系细胞比较容易识别。

A. 幼巨核细胞，又称为嗜碱性巨核细胞。核多叶或马蹄形，体积大（25 ～ 50 μm），胞质深嗜碱性。

B. 巨核细胞，是骨髓中最大的细胞（40 ～ 100 μm），核呈多叶，胞浆嗜酸性（图 5 - 8）。通常位于血窦边缘。它具有拉长的细胞质突起，称为前血小板。血小板从细胞周围脱落。

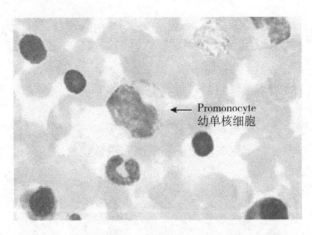

图 5 - 11　幼单核细胞（骨髓涂片，瑞氏染色，1000 × ）

Fig. 5 - 11　Promonocyte（bone marrow smear, Wright's stain, 1000 × ）

思考题

（1）红细胞、粒细胞、单核细胞、血小板的生成过程中分别发生哪些形态学变化？

（2）骨髓涂片在临床上有何应用？

课后作业

画血细胞光镜结构模式图。

病例教学

男性，77 岁，牙龈出血 12 ～ 13 h。患者无外伤或血液病史，也未服用可能改变出血指数的药物。患者有原发性高血压，服用氨氯地平 10 年，血压一直控制好。第 14 和 15 颗牙齿周围有血块，敲击无疼痛。血常规结果显示中性粒细胞减少，贫血，血小板减少。血涂片检查显示存在原始细胞，原粒细胞中偶见红色 Auer 小体。患者被诊断为急性粒细胞白血病。

（1）为什么急性粒细胞白血病会导致该患者出血？

（2）外周血中每种细胞的形态特征和功能是什么？

（3）为什么急性粒细胞白血病会导致中性粒细胞减少、贫血和血小板减少？

（4）正常外周血中有原始细胞吗？

（5）急性粒细胞白血病患者外周血中会发现什么类型的原始细胞？

（周雯）

Chapter 5　BLOOD AND HEMATOPOIESIS

Blood is a special type of connective tissue that consists of cells and plasm. For adults, hematopoiesis takes place in bone marrow and thymus.

Learning Objectives

(1) Be able to use the oil-immersion objective lens.

(2) Be able to identify each type of the blood cells based on the microstructural features and relate the structural features to the functions of each cell type.

(3) Be able to describe the microstructural features of bone marrow.

(4) Be able to identify the cells in the erythroid, myeloid, and platelet series in bone marrow.

Pre-class Questions

(1) What components does the blood have?

(2) What are the microstructural features of each cell type in the blood?

(3) What are the classification criteria of white blood cells (WBCs)?

(4) What hematopoietic precursor cells are inside the bone marrow?

Observation and Reflection

1. Blood Smear（血涂片）

➤ Material

Human blood smear (Wright's stain).

➤ Gross observation

The stained blood film is thin and tongue-shaped.

➤ Low power

A large number of pink dots are erythrocytes（红细胞）. Among the erythrocytes are a few purple dots which are leukocytes（白细胞）.

➤ High power

Choose a region where the leukocytes are concentrated. Make sure to focus on the sample and get a clear image using 40 × objective. Then drip a drop of oil onto the coverslip before turning to oil-immersion objective (100 ×). The oil drop should be thick enough to immerse the 100 × objective lens. View the sample and focus using only the fine adjustment knob.

(1) Erythrocytes (Fig. 5-1): 7-8 μm in diameter, round and biconcave shaped, no nucleus, appearing orange to pink with a lighter center. Erythrocytes are the most numerous cell type of blood.

(2) Neutrophils（中性粒细胞）(Fig. 5-1): 10-12 μm in diameter. The nucleus consists of 2-5 lobes. The cytoplasm is pinkish and contains many fine red granules. A few cells may have band nucleus. Neutrophils are the most numerous leukocytes, making up 50%-70% of the total leukocytes as for people older than 6 years.

(3) Eosinophils（嗜酸性粒细胞）(Fig. 5-2): 10-15 μm in diameter. The nucleus is usually bilobate, and the cytoplasm is full of large, bright red or orange granules. Eosinophils make up 1%-3% of the total leukocytes.

(4) Basophils（嗜碱性粒细胞）(Fig. 5-3): Rare and hard to be found. The cytoplasm is filled with coarse dark-purple granules, size and distribution of which are varying. The nucleus is often obscured by granules. Basophils make up 0%-1% of the total leukocytes.

(5) Lymphocytes（淋巴细胞）(Fig. 5-4): Lymphocytes are the second numerous leukocytes, making up 25%-30% of the total leukocytes as for people older than 6. Most of the lymphocytes in peripheral blood are small lymphocytes which are 6-8 μm in diameter. A small lymphocyte has a dark blue nucleus which is round or indented, dense and clumped. There is a rim of deep blue cytoplasm with a few azurophilic granules. Reactive lymphocytes are medium-sized or large, 10-30 μm in diameter, which usually represent less than 10% of the total number of lymphocytes. The reactive lymphocyte has less dense nucleus and more cytoplasm that is clear and deep or pale sky-blue with darker edges at contact points with other cells. Sometimes the nucleolus is prominent in reactive lymphocytes.

(6) Monocytes（单核细胞）(Fig. 5-5): Large, 14-20 μm in diameter. A monocyte has an ovoid, kidney or horseshoe shaped nucleus which is more lightly stained than that of lymphocytes. The cytoplasm is abundant and stained bluish-gray with many fine azurophilic granules（嗜天青颗粒）and some vacuoles. Monocytes make up 3%-8% of the total leukocytes.

(7) Platelets（血小板）(Fig. 5-6): Small, 2-4 μm in diameter, no nucleus, often in clumps. They are round, oval or irregular in shape and contain purple granules in the center.

Reflection

(1) What are the morphological features of erythrocyte? What are inside the cytoplasm of a mature erythrocyte? What are the functions of a mature erythrocyte? How long is its lifespan?

(2) What is the most numerous cell type among WBCs?

(3) On what basis is WBCs divided into granulocytes and agranulocytes? What cells are granulocytes? What cells are agranulocytes?

(4) What are the differences in morphological feature and function for each type of leukocytes?

(5) What is the blood smear used for?

2.   Blood Smear Preparation and Staining

➢   Blood smear preparation

(1) Place $2 - 3$ μL blood ($1 - 2$ mm in diameter) on top of a slide near the frosted edge.

(2) Put another spreader slide at an angle of around 45° in front of the drop, and then bring the spreader backwards into the drop of blood, allowing the blood to spread along the edge (Fig. $5 - 7$).

(3) Push the spreader forward steadily to produce a tongue-shaped film.

(4) Allow the smear to air dry.

➢   May-Grunwald-Giemsa stain

May-Grunwald-Giemsa stain is a combination of two stains: May-Grunwald stain composed of methylene blue and eosin, and Giemsa stain composed of methylene blue, eosin and azure B.

(1) Stain the smear slide in May-Grunwald solution for 5 min.

(2) Remove stain by holding slide vertically without washing.

(3) Stain the smear slide in Giemsa working solution for 15 min before rinsing in Sorensen's buffer for $10 - 20$ s.

(4) Rinse the smear slide with running water for at least 2 m until the thinnest parts of the film are pinkish red.

(5) Let the slide air dry in tilted position at room temperature.

(6) Mount a coverslip if desired, and examine under microscope.

3.   Red Bone Marrow

➢   Material

Human bone marrow (H & E stain).

➢   Gross observation

The specimen is stained dark blue with many white dots.

➢   Low power

The nuclei of hematopoietic cells are stained blue. The white dots are adipocytes.

➢   High power

Clusters of hematopoietic cells are widely distributed as hematopoietic islands. These islands are next to sinusoids (血窦). Sinusoid is thin-walled capillary with a diameter of $15 - 100$ μm. Megakaryocytes (巨核细胞) can be seen near the sinusoids (Fig. $5 - 8$). This cell is multilobed and the largest cell of the bone marrow ($40 - 100$ μm) with eosinophilic cytoplasm.

Reflection

Where is red bone marrow and yellow bone marrow found respectively in an adult?

4.   Bone Marrow Smear

➢   Material

Human bone marrow smear (Wright's stain).

> **Gross observation**

The specimen is stained slightly pink.

> **Low power**

The red dots in the field are mature erythrocytes. The dark dots are erythroid and myeloid precursors.

> **High power**

Most of the cells are mature erythrocytes. Choose a region where the nucleated precursors are concentrated. Make sure to focus on the sample and get a clear image using $40 \times$ objective. Then drip a drop of oil onto the coverslip before turning to oil-immersion objective （$100 \times$）.

Erythroblasts （成红细胞）, myeloblasts （成髓细胞） and lymphoblasts （淋巴母细胞） look the same. They are all large with round or ovoid nuclei and visible nucleoli, and they all have abundant blue cytoplasm.

（1） Erythroid lineage cells from CFU-E （colony-forming unit-erythrocyte） have the following characteristics （Fig. 5 – 9）：

A. Proerythroblast （原红细胞） is round, 15 – 18 μm in diameter, with a rim of intensely basophilic cytoplasm and a pale perinuclear halo. It has large round nuclei with fine dispersed chromatin and many small nucleoli.

B. Basophilic erythroblast （嗜碱性幼红细胞或早幼红细胞） is 10 – 17 μm in diameter with no nucleolus, no granules and intensely basophilic cytoplasm. The nucleus usually has dark-staining chromatin and light-staining area. A perinuclear halo is usually present.

C. Polychromatophilic erythroblast （中幼红细胞） is 10 – 12 μm in diameter with a dark nucleus and grayish-green cytoplasm due to the increasing accumulation of hemoglobin and decreased polysomes.

D. Normoblast （orthochromatophilic erythroblast） （晚幼红细胞） is 8 – 10 μm in diameter with a smaller and darker nucleus and pale pink cytoplasm. Nuclear expulsion occurs at the end of this stage.

E. Reticulocyte （网织红细胞） is 7 – 8 μm in diameter with many ribosomes, pink cytoplasm and no nucleus.

（2） Myeloid cells from CFU-GM （colony-forming unit-granulocyte-monocyte） have the following features （Fig. 5 – 10）：

A. Promyelocyte （早幼粒细胞） is the largest cell in myeloid series, 15 – 25 μm in diameter. It has basophilic cytoplasm, a large round nucleus and prominent nucleoli as well as large and dark purple azurophilic granules.

B. Myelocyte （中幼粒细胞） is smaller than promyelocyte, 15 – 18 μm in diameter. It contains lightly basophilic cytoplasm, decreasing purple azurophilic granules and increasing specific granules as well as a nucleus on one side. Neutrophilic, basophilic and eosinophilic myelocytes have distinct specific granules.

C. Metamyelocyte （晚幼粒细胞） looks like mature granulocyte except that it has an indented or kidney-shaped nucleus. The indentation of nucleus is less than half of the potential nuclear diameter.

D. Band cell （杆状核细胞） has a horseshoe-shaped nucleus with specific granules. The indentation of nucleus is more than half of nuclear diameter.

E. Mature neutrophil, eosinophil and basophil in the marrow are identical to those in the peripheral blood.

（3） Monocytic cells from CFU-GM have the following features:

A. Promonocyte （幼单核细胞） is rarely seen in normal bone marrow because it divides into monocytes in a short period. It has blue-gray cytoplasm and fine azurophilic granules. Cytoplasmic vacuoles are usually present. The nucleus is lobulated or creased （Fig. 5 – 11）. The chromatin is less condensed than that of a mature monocyte, and nucleoli may be present.

B. Mature monocytes are not easy to be found in the marrow because they go into peripheral circulation quickly and are not retained in the bone marrow as a storage pool.

（4） The thrombocytic lineage can be easily identified.

A. Promegakaryocyte （幼巨核细胞） is also called basophilic megakaryocyte. It is multilobed or horseshoe-shaped, and large （25 – 50 μm） with deep basophilic cytoplasm.

B. Megakaryocyte （巨核细胞） is multilobed and the largest cell of the bone marrow （40 – 100 μm） with strongly eosinophilic cytoplasm （Fig. 5 – 8）. It is usually adjacent to sinuses. It has elongated cytoplasmic extensions （proplatelets）. Strands of platelets are detaching from the periphery of the cell.

Reflection

（1） What morphologic changes occur during erythropoiesis, granulocytopoiesis, monocytopoiesis, thrombocytopoiesis respectively?

（2） What is bone marrow smear used for?

Post-class Task

Draw a diagram of each cell type in blood smear under light microscope.

Case-based Learning

A 77-year-old male complained of bleeding gums （牙龈） for 12 to 13 h. He had no history of trauma or blood dyscrasias and took no medication likely to alter his bleeding indices. The patient had primary hypertension （高血压） and took amlodipine for 10 years. His blood pressure had been well-controlled. He presented with a blood clot around teeth 14 and 15. Both teeth tested vital and neither was particularly tender to percussion （敲击）. FBE （full blood examination） results revealed a moderate neutropenia （中性粒细胞减少症）, a moderate anemia （贫血） but a marked thrombocytopenia （血小板减少症）. Blood film examination revealed the presence of many blast cells and occasional red Auer rods in some myeloblasts. The patient was diagnosed with AML （acute myeloblastic leukemia, 急性粒细胞白血病）.

（1） Why could acute myeloblastic leukemia result in bleeding in this patient?

（2）What are the morphologic features and functions of each cell type in peripheral blood?

（3）Why could acute myeloblastic leukemia result in neutropenia, anemia and thrombocytepenia?

（4）Are there blast cells in normal peripheral blood?

（5）What type of blast cells would be found in peripheral blood as for the patients with AML?

（周雯）

第6章 | 肌组织

肌组织是四种基本组织之一。它的基本特征包括：

（1）肌组织主要由肌细胞组成。

（2）肌细胞细长，因此通常被称为肌纤维。

肌组织分为三种类型：骨骼肌、心肌和平滑肌。

学习目标

（1）能够识别和区分骨骼肌、心肌和平滑肌。

（2）将三种肌组织的特性与功能相联系。

课前问题

（1）三种肌组织的微细结构有何不同？

（2）骨骼肌的收缩机制是什么？

实验观察与思考

1. 骨骼肌

➤ **材料**

兔骨骼肌（HE 染色）。

➤ **肉眼观察**

标本被染成粉红色。

➤ **低倍镜**

纵切面：骨骼肌纤维呈长圆柱形。肌外膜包裹整个肌肉，由结缔组织构成。肌外膜内可见血管。肌束膜和肌内膜也由结缔组织构成，分别围绕每个肌束和每根肌纤维。

横切面：肌纤维呈多边形。肌外膜、肌束膜和肌内膜连接在一起。

➤ **高倍镜**

纵切面（图 6-1）：骨骼肌纤维呈粉红色、长圆柱形，有多个核。细胞核扁平，位于肌膜下方。把显微镜的光圈关闭，可看见骨骼肌纤维有明显的明暗相间的横纹。

横切面（图 6-2）：肌纤维呈多边形或圆形，肌膜下方有许多细胞核。在肌浆内部，多个红点是肌原纤维的横断面。

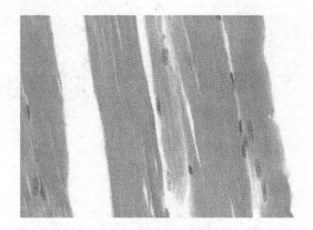

图 6 - 1　骨骼肌（纵切面，HE 染色，400 ×）
Fig. 6 - 1　Skeletal muscle（longitudinal section，H & E stain，400 ×）

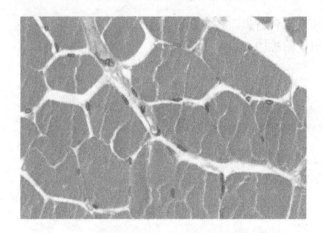

图 6 - 2　骨骼肌（横切面，HE 染色，400 ×）
Fig. 6 - 2　Skeletal muscle（cross section，H & E stain，400 ×）

思考题
（1）骨骼肌的横纹是由什么结构形成的？
（2）你能在骨骼肌横切面上观察到横纹吗？
（3）肌原纤维的结构和功能是什么？
（4）什么类型的运动神经纤维支配骨骼肌？

2. 心肌

➤ **材料**

人心脏（HE 染色）。

➤ **肉眼观察**

切片染成粉红色。

➢ **低倍镜**

心脏主要由心肌组织构成。找到心肌的纵切面、横切面和斜切面。心肌纵切面呈柱状，横切面呈椭圆形。

➢ **高倍镜**

纵切面（图6-3）：心肌呈粉红色，呈柱状，有分支。心肌细胞有1～2个椭圆形核，位于细胞中央，核周肌浆染色浅。与骨骼肌相比，心肌的横纹不明显。心肌纤维之间通过闰盘相互连接。

横切面（图6-4）：心肌呈圆形、椭圆形或不规则形。有些细胞核被切到，细胞核位于细胞的中央。

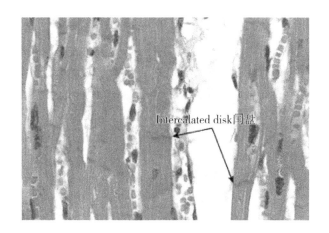

图6-3 心肌（纵切面，HE染色，400×）
Fig. 6-3 Cardiac muscle (longitudinal section, H & E stain, 400×)

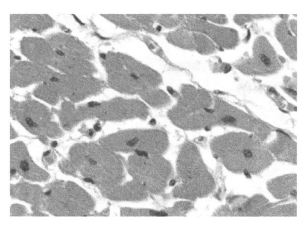

图6-4 心肌（横切面，HE染色，400×）
Fig. 6-4 Cardiac muscle (cross section, H & E stain, 400×)

思考题

（1）闰盘的超微结构是什么？

（2）为什么心肌的横纹不如骨骼肌的明显？

（3）什么类型的运动神经纤维支配心肌？

3. 平滑肌

➢ **材料**

狗空肠（HE染色）。

➢ **肉眼观察**

标本是空肠的横切面。

➢ **低倍镜**

平滑肌靠近空肠壁最外层，有内环外纵两层。平滑肌染成粉红色，密集排列在一起。内环层可见平滑肌纵断面，外纵层可见平滑肌横断面。

➢ **高倍镜**

纵切面（图6-5A）：肌纤维呈粉红色，梭形，中央有1个椭圆形、棒状或扭曲的核，核仁明显。平滑肌没有横纹。

横切面（图6-5B）：平滑肌纤维呈粉红色，圆形或大小不规则。部分细胞中心可见圆形核（图6-3）。

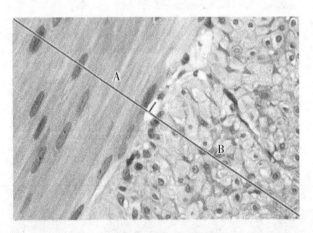

A. 纵切面（Longitudinal section）；B. 横切面（Cross section）。

图6-5 平滑肌（HE染色，400×）

Fig. 6-5 Smooth muscle（H & E stain，400×）

思考题

（1）为什么平滑肌没有横纹？

（2）什么类型的运动神经纤维支配平滑肌？

课后作业

画骨骼肌的纵切面和横切面的光镜结构模式图。

病例教学

患者，男，16岁，足球运动员，体重69.1 kg，身高175.3 cm。在持续8周的季前足球训练后，出现小腿腘绳肌剧烈疼痛和痉挛。无近期疾病史。尿常规检查显示无血红蛋白尿，尿液清澈，呈黄色。血液生化分析显示肌酸激酶 – 肌红蛋白（CK-MB）水平升高至17.2 ng·mL^{-1}（正常为0.6～6.3 ng·mL^{-1}）。患者诊断为轻度劳力性横纹肌溶解症。

（1）腘绳肌属于哪种肌组织？

（2）肌红蛋白的功能是什么？

（3）什么因素可能导致横纹肌溶解？

（周雯，崔志刚）

Chapter 6 MUSCULAR TISSUE

Muscular tissue is one of four basic tissues. It has some basic features:

(1) Muscular tissue is mainly composed of muscle cells.

(2) Muscle cells are elongated so that they are often termed as muscle fibers (myofibers).

Muscular tissue is classified into three types: skeletal muscle, cardiac muscle, and smooth muscle.

Learning Objectives

(1) Be able to identify and differentiate skeletal muscle, cardiac muscle, and smooth muscle.

(2) Relate the functions to the properties of three muscle types.

Pre-class Questions

(1) What are the differences in microstructural features among three types of muscular tissues?

(2) What is the contraction mechanism of skeletal muscle?

Observation and Reflection

1. Skeletal Muscle（骨骼肌）

➤ Material

Rabbit skeletal muscle (H & E stain).

➤ Gross observation

The specimen is stained pink.

➤ Low power

Longitudinal section: Skeletal muscle fibers are long and cylindrical. **Epimysium**（肌外膜）is made of connective tissue which wraps the entire muscle. Blood vessels can be seen inside the epimysium. **Perimysium**（肌束膜）and **endomysium**（肌内膜）are also made of connective tissue which surrounds each muscle fascicle and muscle fiber respectively.

Transverse section: Muscle fibers are polygonal. The epimysium, perimysium and endomysium are connected together.

➤ High power

Longitudinal section (Fig. 6-1): Skeletal muscle fiber is pink, long, cylindrical, and multinucleated. The nuclei are flattened and located underneath the **sarcolemma**（肌膜）. The cross bands are very clear when the iris diaphragm is closed.

Transverse section (Fig. 6 – 2): Muscle fibers are polygonal or round with many nuclei under-neath the sarcolemma. Inside the **sarcoplasm** (肌浆), multiple red dots are cross-sectioned **myo-fibrils** (肌原纤维).

Reflection

(1) What is cross band made of?

(2) Can you find cross band in the transverse section of skeletal muscle?

(3) What is the structure and function of myofibrils?

(4) What type of motor nerve fibers are controlling the function of skeletal muscle?

---

2. Cardiac Muscle (心肌)

➤ Material

Human heart (H & E stain).

➤ Gross observation

The specimen is stained pink.

➤ Low power

Heart wall is mainly comprised of cardiac muscle. Find the longitudinal, transverse, and ob-lique section of cardiac muscle. Cardiac muscles are columnar in longitudinal section and oval in transvers section.

➤ High power

Longitudinal section (Fig. 6 – 3): Cardiac muscle is pink, columnar and branched with 1 ~ 2 oval nuclei in the center of the cell. The perinuclear sarcoplasm is pale-stained. Cardiac muscle has less distinctive cross band than skeletal muscle. Cardiac muscles are anastomosing together through **intercalated disks** (闰盘).

Transverse section (Fig. 6 – 4): Cardiac muscle is round, oval, or irregular. If the nucleus is sectioned, it is in the center of the cell.

Reflection

(1) What ultra-structures are the intercalated disks?

(2) Why is cross band of cardiac muscle not as distinctive as that of skeletal muscle?

(3) What type of motor nerve fibers are controlling the function of cardiac muscle?

---

3. Smooth Muscle (平滑肌)

➤ Material

Canine jejunum (H & E stain).

➤ Gross observation

The specimen is cross section of jejunum.

➤ **Low power**

There are two layers of smooth muscle, inner circular and outer longitudinal, near the outmost layer of jejunum wall. Smooth muscles are stained pink and densely arranged together. Longitudinal sections of smooth muscles can be seen in the inner circular layer, while cross sections of smooth muscles can be seen in the outer longitudinal layer.

➤ **High power**

Longitudinal section (Fig. 6 – 5A): The muscle fiber is pink, spindle-shaped, with 1 oval, rod-shaped or twisted nucleus in the center and prominent nucleoli inside the nucleus. There are no cross band in smooth muscles.

Transverse section (Fig. 6 – 5B): The smooth muscle fibers are stained pink, round or irregular in size. Round nuclei can be seen in the center of some cells.

Reflection

(1) Why is there no cross band in smooth muscle?

(2) What type of motor nerve fibers are controlling the function of smooth muscle?

Post-class Task

Draw a diagram of skeletal muscle in both longitudinal and transverse section under light microscope.

Case-based Learning

A 16-year-old male football player (body mass is 69.1 kg, height is 175.3 cm) complained of severe muscle pain and cramping in his lower legs and hamstrings after preseason football training for previous 8 weeks. He had no history of recent illness. The urinalysis report was negative for hemoglobinuria and the urine was clear and had a straw-colored appearance. Blood analysis revealed elevated creatine kinase-myoglobin (CK-MB) levels at 17.2 ng · mL^{-1} (normal range 0.6 – 6.3 ng · mL^{-1}). The patient was diagnosed with mild exertional rhabdomyolysis (横纹肌溶解症).

(1) Which muscle type is the hamstring comprised of?

(2) What is the function of myoglobin?

(3) What might cause rhabdomyolysis?

（周雯，崔志刚）

第7章 | 神经组织

神经组织是四种基本组织之一,由两种主要细胞类型组成——神经元和神经胶质细胞。

(1)神经元是高度特化(高度分化)的细胞,通过称为突触的特化连接接收信息并将其传递给其他神经元或效应细胞。

(2)神经胶质细胞不传导神经冲动,主要功能是维持体内平衡、形成髓鞘、支持或保护神经元。

学习目标

(1)能够描述神经组织的组成。

(2)能够识别和描述神经元、有髓神经纤维、触觉小体、环层小体、运动终板。

(3)能够理解神经元的结构和功能联系。

课前问题

(1)神经组织由什么构成?

(2)神经系统包括哪些器官?

实验观察与思考

1. 多极神经元

➤ **材料**

人脊髓横断面(HE 染色)。

➤ **肉眼观察**

脊髓的横切面呈扁圆形,中间的小孔是中央管。周围着色较浅,为脊髓白质;中央着色深,呈蝴蝶形(或"H"形)为脊髓灰质。

➤ **低倍镜**

区分脊髓灰质和白质。灰质两个较粗短的突起为前角(又称为腹角),相对的两个细长突起为后角(又称为背角)。前角可看到许多染成紫蓝色,大小不一的多极神经元,其周围有许多较小而圆形的细胞核为神经胶质细胞核。胸髓还有侧角。

➤ **高倍镜**

灰质:运动神经元胞体较大,呈多角形,细胞体向四周发出很多突起,突起因被切断而不完整,细胞核大而圆,常染色质多,着色浅。核仁一个,呈圆形,大而明显。核周质中有许多嗜碱性染色的斑块状结构为尼氏体。轴突和轴丘没有尼氏体(图 7–1)。

白质:有大量神经胶质细胞核和轴突的横断面。

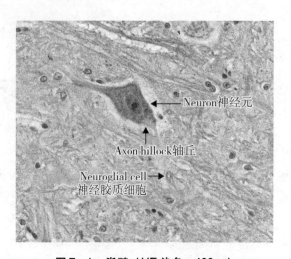

图7-1　脊髓（HE 染色，400×）

Fig. 7-1　Spinal cord（H & E stain，400×）

思考题

（1）哪些解剖结构包绕着脊髓？

（2）光镜下，你能找到脊髓里存在的对称结构吗？

（3）中央管里有什么？

（4）脊髓背侧和腹侧的结构有何区别？

（5）灰质和白质的结构有何不同？

（6）电镜下，尼氏体是什么结构？

（7）光镜下怎么区分轴突和树突？

2. 神经原纤维

➢ **材料**

人脊髓横断面（镀银染色）。

➢ **肉眼观察**

切片染成棕黄色。

➢ **低倍镜**

灰质略深染，白质较浅。

➢ **高倍镜**

神经元胞体和突起里含细小的棕色丝状结构，即神经原纤维（图7-2）。

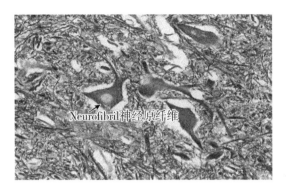

图7-2 脊髓（镀银染色，400×）

Fig. 7-2 Spinal cord（silver stain，400×）

思考题

（1）神经原纤维的电镜结构是什么？

（2）神经原纤维具有什么功能？

---

3. 假单极神经元

➢ **材料**

人脊神经节（HE 染色）。

➢ **肉眼观察**

切片呈卵圆形。

➢ **低倍镜**

神经节外周有结缔组织，节内有大量神经纤维、节细胞和神经胶质细胞。

➢ **高倍镜**

节细胞大小不等，每个节细胞外有一层卫星细胞。

神经节细胞：胞体圆，核呈偏心性分布，核仁明显，突起较难观察到。

卫星细胞：细胞扁平，胞质少（图7-3）。

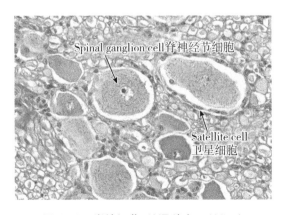

图7-3 脊神经节（HE 染色，400×）

Fig. 7-3 Spinal ganglion（H & E stain，400×）

思考题

（1）除了卫星细胞，脊神经节里还有什么类型的神经胶质细胞？

（2）神经胶质细胞的功能是什么？

4. 有髓神经纤维

➤ **材料**

人坐骨神经纵切面和横切面（HE 染色）。

➤ **肉眼观察**

长条形的为一段坐骨神经的纵切面，椭圆形的为横切面。

➤ **低倍镜**

纵切面：可见大量平行排列的神经纤维。

横断面：致密结缔组织包绕在神经表面形成神经外膜，结缔组织把坐骨神经分隔成大小不等的神经束，包绕在神经束表面的结缔组织称神经束膜。神经外膜由于制片时剥离了，在切片上看不见。

➤ **高倍镜**

纵切面：神经纤维呈长条状，每条神经纤维的中央有一条染色较深的线条为轴突，轴突两侧着色较浅呈空网状是髓鞘，髓鞘外侧着色较深的线条是神经膜。髓鞘和神经膜都呈节段性包在轴突外表，段与段之间为郎飞结（图7-4）。

横切面：神经纤维被切断呈圆形，中央有一着色深的圆点，此即轴突，周围着色浅的部位为髓鞘，外表染色较深的环为神经膜。神经膜外染色浅的疏松结缔组织是神经内膜。

思考题

（1）髓鞘的功能是什么？

（2）坐骨神经里有无髓神经纤维吗？

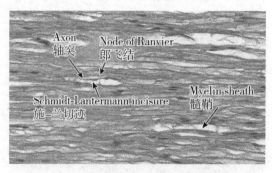

图7-4 坐骨神经（HE 染色，400×）

Fig. 7-4 Sciatic nerve (H & E stain, 400×)

5．触觉小体

➢ **材料**

人手指皮肤（HE 染色）。

➢ **肉眼观察**

标本一侧被染成蓝色，另一侧染色浅淡。

➢ **低倍镜**

染色较深的部分是皮肤的表皮，由角化的复层扁平上皮构成。染色较浅的部分是皮肤的真皮，由结缔组织构成。真皮的结缔组织突入上皮形成真皮乳头，触觉小体位于真皮乳头内，触觉小体的长轴与皮肤表面垂直（图 7 - 5）。

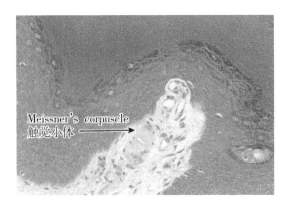

图 7 - 5　皮肤（HE 染色，400 ×）
Fig. 7 - 5　Skin（H & E stain，400 ×）

➢ **高倍镜**

触觉小体表面有结缔组织被囊，内有扁平排列的施万细胞和盘绕于施万细胞的神经纤维。

6．环层小体

➢ **材料**

人手指皮肤（HE 染色）。

➢ **肉眼观察**

标本一侧被染成蓝色，另一侧染色浅淡。

➢ **低倍镜**

环层小体位于结缔组织深面，呈圆形或卵圆形，由较多层同心圆样排列的结缔组织包绕形成，形似洋葱切面。

➢ **高倍镜**

在环层小体中央，有髓神经纤维的轴索沿着其长轴延伸（图 7 - 6）。

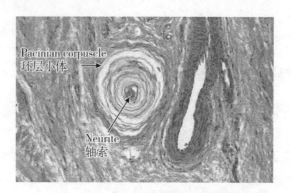

图 7 - 6　皮肤（HE 染色，400 ×）

Fig. 7 - 6　Skin（H & E stain, 400 ×）

思考题

请问还有哪些机械感受器，它们的功能是什么？

7. 运动终板

➤ 材料

人骨骼肌铺片（氯化金染色）。

➤ 肉眼观察

切片被染成黑色。

➤ 低倍镜

骨骼肌纤维被染成黑色，有明显的横纹。神经纤维较细，被染成黑色，末端发出分支。

➤ 高倍镜

神经纤维分支的末端膨大与相连接的骨骼肌形成运动终板（电镜下为突触）（图 7 - 7）。

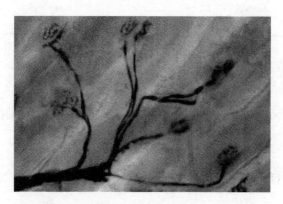

图 7 - 7　运动终板（氯化金染色，400 ×）

Fig. 7 - 7　Motor endplate（gold chloride stain, 400 ×）

思考题

请描述运动终板的超微结构。

课后作业

画一个运动神经元光镜结构模式图。

病例教学

患者，男，35 岁，左腿进行性无力 5 年，加重 2 个月。神经学检查显示，胸髓 T7 平面以下左侧针刺感觉麻痹、触觉丧失。病人无外伤、肿瘤及脊髓蛛网膜炎病史。最终，病人被确诊为脊髓空洞症。

（1）为什么脊髓空洞症会导致以上症状和体征？

（2）该患者的哪一侧的脊髓受损？

（3）该患者的脊髓里的哪些微细结构可能受损？

（4）哪些机械感受器参与针刺感觉和触觉？

（周雯，陆海霞）

Chapter 7 NERVOUS TISSUE

Nervous tissue is one of four basic tissues and it consists of two major cell types—**neurons**（神经元）and **glia**（神经胶质细胞）.

（1）Neurons are highly specialized cells for receiving and transmitting information to other neurons or effector cells via specialized connections called synapses.

（2）Glia do not conduct nerve impulses, and mainly maintain homeostasis, form myelin, support or protect neurons.

Learning Objectives

（1）Be able to describe the components of nervous tissue.

（2）Be able to identify and describe microstructure of a neuron, the myelinated nerve fiber, Meissner corpuscle, Pacinian corpuscle and motor endplate.

（3）Relate nerve function to the properties of neurons and their cell processes.

Pre-class Questions

（1）What structures is nervous tissue comprised of?

（2）What organs is nervous system composed of?

Observation and Reflection

1. Multipolar Neuron（多极神经元）

➢ Material

Human spinal cord, cross section（H & E stain）.

➢ Gross observation

The center of the section is a small pore called **central canal**（中央管）. The **gray matter**（灰质）is relatively darker and appears like H-shape or butterfly. The **white matter**（白质）is brighter and at the periphery.

➢ Low power

Find out the white matter and gray matter. The **anterior**（**ventral**）**horns**（前角，又称腹角）are broad and contain many large neurons. The **posterior**（**dorsal**）**horns**（后角，又称背角）are narrow and have small neurons. The **lateral horns**（侧角）can be found in thoracic segments of spinal cord.

➢ High power

Grey matter: Motor neurons are large and multipolar neurons in the anterior horn. A motor neuron has a large, round and pale stained nucleus and a clear nucleolus（Fig. 7-1）. Inside the

perikaryon （核周质） are numerous basophilic granules called **Nissl bodies** （尼氏体）. The **ax-on** （轴突） and **axon hillock** （轴丘） lack Nissl bodies.

White matter：Find out the nuclei of glial cells and the cross sections of axons.

Reflection

（1） What anatomical structures are surrounding spinal cord?

（2） What symmetrical （对称的） structures can you find in the spinal cord under microscope?

（3） What is inside the central canal?

（4） How is the structure of the dorsal part of the spinal cord different from those of the ventral part?

（5） How is the structure of the gray matter different from that of the white matter?

（6） What ultra-structures at the electron microscopic level are the Nissl bodies?

（7） How can you distinguish an axon from a dendrite under light microscope?

2.　Neurofibril （神经原纤维）

➢　Material

Human spinal cord, cross section （silver stain）.

➢　Gross observation

The specimen is stained brown.

➢　Low power

The gray matter is darker, and the white matter is paler. Identify the neurons and the associated processes.

➢　High power

Neurofilaments are brown threadlike microstructures within cell bodies of neurons and their processes （Fig. 7 – 2）.

Reflection

（1） What ultra-structures at the electron microscopic level are the neurofibrils?

（2） What functions do neurofibrils have?

3.　Pseudounipolar Neuron （假单极神经元）

➢　Material

Human spinal ganglion （H & E stain）.

➢　Gross observation

The specimen is oval.

➢　Low power

Each **spinal ganglion cell** （脊神经节细胞） is encapsulated by one layer of **satellite cells**

（卫星细胞）.

> ➤ **High power**

Spinal ganglion cell: It has a round cell body and an eccentric （偏心性） nuclei with prominent nucleoli. The process of a ganglion cell is hardly seen.

Satellite cell: It is small and flattened with little cytoplasm （Fig. 7 – 3）.

Reflection

（1） Are there other types of neuroglia inside spinal ganglion beside satellite cells?

（2） What are the functions of neuroglia in nervous system?

---

4. Myelinated Nerve Fiber （有髓神经纤维）

> ➤ **Material**

Human sciatic nerve, longitudinal & cross section （H & E stain）.

> ➤ **Gross observation**

The longitudinal-sectioned specimen is longer, and another oval one is transverse-sectioned.

> ➤ **Low power**

Longitudinal section: Many parallel cords containing a central, purple axon are myelinated nerve fibers.

Cross section: The dense connective tissue enclosing the entire nerve trunk is the **epineurium** （神经外膜）. The dense connective tissue surrounding each nerve fascicle is the **perineurium** （神经束膜）. Within the nerve bundles, connective tissue separating each never fiber is the **endoneurium** （神经内膜）. The epineurium is not present on these sections.

> ➤ **High power**

Longitudinal section: **Myelin sheath** （髓鞘） of the myelination nerve fiber is spongy and pale-stained with a purple axon inside. On the surface of myelin sheath are thin lines which are the neurolemma. At the gap between neighboring myelin sheath is an indent called **Nodes of Ranvier** （郎飞结） （Fig. 7 – 4）.

Cross section: The purple dot in the center of a nerve fiber is the axon. The open space outside the axon represents the myelin sheath. The outermost purple circle around the myelin sheath is the neurolemma. The endoneurium is loose connective tissue surrounding each nerve fibers. There capillaries can be seen.

Reflection

（1） What are the functions of myelin sheath?

（2） Are there unmyelinated nerve fibers inside a nerve trunk?

---

5. Meissner's corpuscle (触觉小体)

➤ Material

Human finger skin (H & E stain).

➤ Gross observation

The specimen has a blue part and a light-stained part.

➤ Low power

The dark-stained part is keratinized stratified squamous epithelium which makes up the **epidermis** (表皮) of skin, while the light-stained part is connective tissue which forms the **dermis** (真皮) of skin. The superficial layer of connective tissue projects into the epithelium to form dermal papillae. Inside the dermal papillae, ellipse Meissner's corpuscles can be seen with their long axis oriented perpendicularly to the skin surface (Fig. 7 – 5).

➤ High power

Meissner corpuscle has a connective tissue capsule. Inside the capsule, flattened Schwann cells are organized in stacks. The central axon is hard to see.

6. Pacinian corpuscle (环层小体)

➤ Material

Human finger skin (H & E stain).

➤ Gross observation

The specimen has a blue part and a light-stained part.

➤ Low power

Pacinian corpuscle is round or ovoid and deep in the connective tissue. It appears like a sliced onion and has several concentric lamellae.

➤ High power

In the center of Pacinian corpuscle, a large myelinated nerve fiber called **neurite** (轴索) is running along its long axis (Fig. 7 – 6).

Reflection

Can you list other mechanoreceptors? What are their functions?

---

7. Motor endplate (运动终板)

➤ Material

Human skeletal muscle, spread (gold chloride stain).

➤ Gross observation

The sample is stained black.

➤ Low power

The skeletal muscle fibers are stained black with distinct crossband. Black nerve fibers give branches at the ends and reach the muscle fibers.

➤ High power

The ends of nerve fiber branches are expanded and attached to the surface of muscle fibers forming the motor endplates (synapses in EM) (Fig. 7 – 7).

Reflection

What are the ultrastructural features of a motor end plate?

Post-class Task

Draw a diagram of a typical motor neuron under light microscope.

Case-based Learning

A 35-year-old male had experienced gradually progressive weakness in his left leg since 5 years ago. The weakness worsened in the last 2 months and he needed a cane when walking. He also had hypoesthesia（感觉麻痹）of pinprick（针刺）and light touch sensation below the T7 dermatome on his left side. He had no history of trauma, spinal tumor, or any evidence of spinal arachnoiditis（脊髓蛛网膜炎）. Finally, the patient was diagnosed with syringomyelia（cavitation within the spinal cord，脊髓空洞症）.

（1）Why could cavitation in the spinal cord result in these symptoms in this patient?

（2）Which side of the spinal cord might be affected in this patient?

（3）What microstructures in the spinal cord might be injured in this patient?

（4）What types of mechanoreceptors are participating in sensing pinprick and light touch?

（周雯，陆海霞）

第8章 | 神经系统

神经系统主要由神经组织组成。它可分为中枢神经系统（central nervous system，CNS）和外周神经系统（peripheral nervous system，PNS）。

学习目标

（1）掌握大脑皮质、小脑皮质和脊髓灰质的光镜结构。

（2）了解脊神经节和交感神经节的光镜结构。

课前问题

（1）中枢神经系统和周围神经系统的组成是什么？

（2）神经元的特征性结构是什么？

实验观察与思考

1．大脑

➤ **材料**

猫大脑冠状切面（HE 染色）。

➤ **肉眼观察**

大脑表面皮质凹陷形成脑沟，沟与沟之间隆起处为脑回。切片周边深染处为大脑皮质（灰质），浅染处为大脑髓质（白质）。

➤ **低倍镜**

皮质的表面被覆一薄层结缔组织膜，为软脑膜，含有丰富的小血管。软脑膜下方为脑皮质，主要是神经元胞体、胶质细胞和无髓神经纤维。从外向内，神经元可分层排列，一般为六层，各层分界不清。可先辨别细胞多密集排列的外颗粒层和内颗粒层，然后再向内外辨别（图 8 –1）。

分子层：位于最表层，神经元小而少，染色浅。

外颗粒层：细胞密集排列，主要是颗粒细胞和少量小锥体细胞。

外锥体细胞层：比外颗粒层厚，细胞密度不如外颗粒层，主要是中小型锥体细胞组成，中型多数。

内颗粒层：细胞大小及排列与外颗粒层相似，多为星形细胞。中央前回不明显，中央后回较明显。

内锥体细胞层：主要是大、中型锥体细胞，细胞分布密度较低。

多形细胞层：这层靠近髓质，但是和髓质的分界不明显，以梭形细胞为主，但细胞大小不一。

> **高倍镜**

定位到大脑皮质的内、外锥体细胞层，转到高倍镜观察锥体细胞的形态和结构。细胞体呈锥形，核圆，位于中央，可见浅染的泡状核，核仁清晰，胞浆内可见尼氏体，胞体尖端发出主树突（只见根部），伸向皮质表面，轴突自胞体底部发出，但因切面关系不易见到（图8－2）。

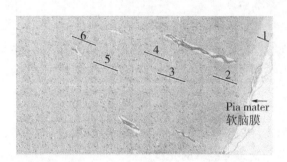

1—分子层（Molecular layer）；2—外颗粒层（External granular layer）；

3—外锥体层（External pyramidal layer）；4—内颗粒层（Internal granular layer）；

5—内锥体细胞层（Internal pyramidal layer）；6—多形细胞层（Polymorphic layer）。

图 8 –1　大脑皮质（HE 染色，40 ×）

Fig. 8 – 1　Cerebral cortex（H & E stain，40 ×）

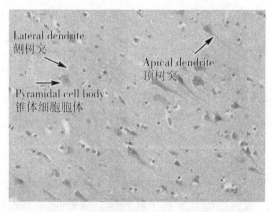

图 8 –2　大脑皮质锥体细胞（HE 染色，200 ×）

Fig. 8 –2　Pyramidal cell in cerebral cortex（H & E stain，200 ×）

2. 大脑皮质锥体细胞

> **材料**

猫大脑（镀银染色）。

> **肉眼观察**

标本被染成棕色。

> **低倍镜**

大脑皮质相当于灰质，主要是神经胞体存在的部位。大脑髓质不含有神经元胞体。定位至大脑皮质外椎体层或内锥体层，转到高倍镜观察典型锥体细胞的结构。

➢ **高倍镜**

锥体细胞的胞体呈锥形或三角形，大小不一，顶树突较粗，从胞体顶端发出，伸向皮质表面，沿途发出一些分枝（图 8 – 3）。胞体基部也发出一些树突。在树突的表面存在树突棘。轴突自胞体底部发出，因切面关系不易见到。

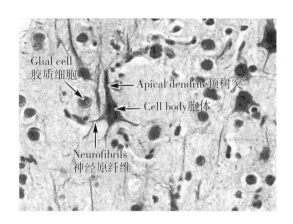

图 8 – 3　大脑皮质锥体细胞（银染，400 ×）
Fig. 8 – 3　Pyramidal cell in cerebral cortex（silver stain，400 ×）

思考题

（1）大脑皮质中颗粒细胞（外颗粒层）和锥体细胞（内锥体细胞层）胞质内尼氏体有何不同？

（2）通过比较大脑皮质的 HE 染色和银染片，理解锥体细胞的典型结构。

（3）在大脑皮质切片中，常常可以见到血管的切面。什么是血脑屏障？

---

3. **小脑**

➢ **材料**

猫小脑冠状切面（HE 染色）。

➢ **肉眼观察**

小脑表面有许多横沟，把小脑分割成许多叶片，每一叶片有表面的皮质和内部的髓质。

➢ **低倍镜**

小脑皮质（灰质）由外向内可分为 3 层，而髓质（白质）主要由神经纤维和神经胶质细胞组成，不含有神经元胞体（图 8 – 4）。在小脑皮质，表面被染成粉红色区域的是分子层，被染成紫蓝色区域的是颗粒层，重点观察皮质的结构。

➢ **高倍镜**

分子层：为皮质最浅层，较厚，主要有星形细胞和蓝状细胞，因神经元少且分散稀疏而染色淡。

蒲肯野细胞层：介于分子层及颗粒层之间，由一层排列规则的蒲肯野细胞胞体组成。细胞体积较大，呈梨形，可见顶端发出的粗大的主树突和 2～3 条次级树突伸向皮质表面，并在分子层反复分支，这在银染的切片中较明显。

颗粒层：位于小脑皮质最深层，细胞小，数目多，密集的细胞核堆积呈颗粒状（图8-5）。

思考题

蒲肯野细胞的树突和树突棘上，可能和什么类型细胞形成突触？

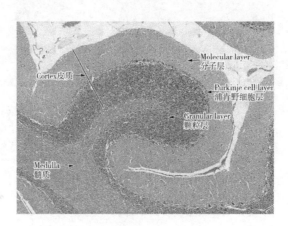

图8-4 小脑（HE染色，40×）

Fig. 8-4 Cerebellum（H & E stain, 40×）

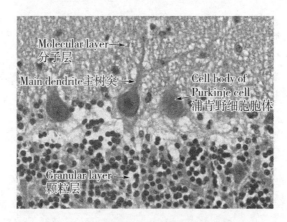

图8-5 小脑皮质（HE染色，400×）

Fig. 8-5 Cerebellar cortex（H & E stain, 400×）

4. 脊髓

➢ **材料**

猫脊髓横切面（HE染色）。

➢ **肉眼观察**

切片中央的小孔为中央管，中央的灰质呈"H"形或蝴蝶状，染色较深，可分为前侧较宽大的前角（又称腹角）和后侧细长的后角（又称背角）。外周的白质染色较浅，在脊髓胸段还可见侧角。

➢ **低倍镜**

脊髓灰质可见大、中、小各型神经细胞。脊髓前角观察有多极运动神经元，白质由许多神经纤维（以有髓神经纤维占多数）和胶质细胞构成（图8-6）。

➤ **高倍镜**

因切面关系，脊髓灰质前角的多极运动神经元胞体大小不一，注意辨别具有典型细胞核、尼氏体的神经元胞体。背角神经元胞体较小，主要是束细胞和中间神经元。中央管腔面被覆的一层上皮样细胞为室管膜细胞。白质的神经纤维以有髓神经纤维为主，且神经纤维厚度不一。

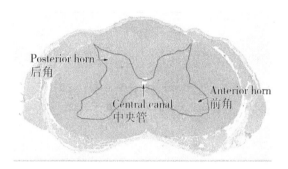

图8-6　脊髓（HE染色，11×）

Fig. 8-6　Spinal cord（H & E stain，11×）

思考题

（1）脊髓周围有什么解剖结构？

（2）脊髓背侧和腹侧的结构有何区别？

（3）脊髓内不同类型神经元中尼氏体的形态会不同吗？

（4）脊髓前角的多极神经元发出的轴突可能终止于哪里？

---

5. 脊神经节

➤ **材料**

狗脊髓背根节（HE染色）。

➤ **肉眼观察**

标本呈椭圆形，脊神经节主要含有假单极神经元。

➤ **低倍镜**

神经节内节细胞成群排列，在细胞群之间分布有平行排列的有髓神经纤维束。

➤ **高倍镜**

节细胞胞体较大，呈圆形或椭圆形，因切面关系大小不一。细胞核圆形，较大，居中，染色浅，核仁清晰。胞质内有呈细砂状的尼氏体。胞体突起在切片中不易见到。节细胞外围环绕一层扁平的卫星细胞，其胞核染色较深（图8-7）。

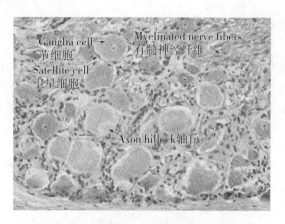

图 8 - 7　脊神经节（HE 染色，400 ×）
Fig. 8 - 7　Spinal ganglia（H & E stain，400 ×）

6. 交感神经节

➢ **材料**

人交感神经节（HE 染色）。

➢ **肉眼观察**

标本形状与脊神经节类似，交感神经节内主要含有多极神经元。

➢ **低倍镜**

结构也与脊神经节类似，但是多极神经元分散分布，不集中成群。在节细胞之间分布有无髓神经纤维。

➢ **高倍镜**

与脊神经节节细胞相比，交感神经节含有多极神经元，神经元胞体较小，切面大小不一，轮廓不规则，可见到突起。细胞核亦呈泡状，常偏位。围绕的卫星细胞比脊神经节略少（图 8 - 8）。

思考题

（1）脊神经节和交感神经节结构的不同是什么？

（2）脊神经节中假单极神经元仅发出一个突起，随后立即呈"T"形分支，这个"T"形分支分别终止于哪里？

（3）交感神经节接受的冲动来自哪里？其轴突终端又指向哪里？

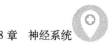

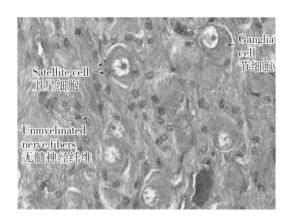

图 8 –8　交感神经节（HE 染色，400 ×）
Fig. 8 –8　Sympathetic ganglia（H & E stain，400 ×）

课后作业

（1）在光镜下辨别大脑皮质的各层结构，并找到一个典型的锥体细胞。

（2）在光镜下辨别小脑皮质的各层结构，并找到一个典型的蒲肯野细胞。

病例教学

男孩，3 岁，1 岁前未规律接种疫苗。2 个月前突然出现高热，3 天后发现左下肢不能活动，以后体温虽然降至正常，但左下肢的运动仍未恢复，且肢体逐渐变细。经检查发现：左下肢完全瘫痪，肌张力减退，膝和跟腱腱反射消失，肌肉明显萎缩，无病理反射。深、浅感觉未发现异常。最后诊断为急性脊髓前角灰质炎（也称小儿麻痹症），脊髓受损伤节段在腰骶膨大（L1—S4）处。请结合图 8 –9，回答以下问题。

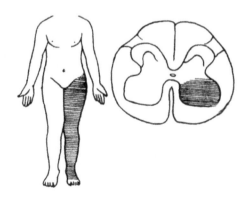

图 8 –9　脊髓损伤部位和受影响区域
Fig. 8 –9　The spinal cord lesion and affected lower limb

（1）脊髓前角有什么神经元，它发出的轴突主要支配什么？

（2）腰骶膨大节段脊髓左侧前角受损为何影响左下肢功能？其结构基础是什么？

（3）该患者有哪些神经学异常？原因是什么？

（张巍）

Chapter 8　NERVOUS SYSTEM

Nervous system mainly consists of the nervous tissue. It can be divided into the **central nervous system** (CNS) and the **peripheral nervous system** (PNS).

Learning Objectives

(1) Be able to grasp the structure of cerebral cortex, cerebellar cortex and gray matter of the spinal cord.

(2) Be able to understand the structural features of spinal ganglia and sympathetic ganglia.

Pre-class Questions

(1) What're the components of the central nervous system and the peripheral nervous system?

(2) What're the characteristic features of the neurons?

Observation and Reflection

1. Cerebrum (大脑)

➤ Material

Cat cerebrum, coronal section (H & E stain).

➤ Gross observation

This is a part of cerebrum. On the surface cerebral cortical pits form sulci, and gyri lie between the sulci. The **cerebral cortex** (大脑皮质) is stained darker than **cerebral medulla** (大脑髓质).

➤ Low power

A delicate connective tissue covers the surface of cerebrum, which is **pia mater** (软脑膜) containing many small vessels. Beneath the pia mater cerebral cortex is found. Cerebral cortex contains glial cell, nerve fibers and neuronal cell body. And from outside to inside, the cerebral cortex can be divided into six indistinct layers (Fig. 8 – 1).

Molecular layer (分子层) is located in the outermost layer and palely stained. Relatively few neurons are found.

External granular layer (外颗粒层) is rich in granular cells, which are densely packed. A few small pyramidal cells are also found.

External pyramidal layer (外锥体细胞层) is thicker than the external granular layer. It is composed of the medium-sized pyramidal cells.

Internal granular layer (内颗粒层) contains numerous stellate cells, whose size and arrangement are similar as those in the external granular layer. This layer is more clearly in the postcentral gyrus than that in the precentral gyrus.

Internal pyramidal layer（内锥体细胞层）is mainly composed of medium and large pyramidal cells.

Polymorphic layer（多形细胞层）is near the cerebral medulla, but their limit is not obvious. Fusiform cells, granule cells and stellate cells are located in this layer. All these cells vary in size.

➤ High power

Choose one field at the external or internal pyramidal layer to observe the morphology and structure of **pyramidal cells**（锥体细胞）under high power. Identify their cell body, one apical and several basal dendrites, a single thin axon, palely-stained nucleus with distinct nucleolus and Nissl bodies within the cytoplasm（Fig. 8 – 2）.

2. Pyramidal cell in cerebral cortex（大脑皮质锥体细胞）

➤ Material

Cat cerebrum（silver stain）.

➤ Gross observation

The specimen is stained in brown.

➤ Low power

Cerebral cortex is the grey matter of cerebrum, which mainly contains the cell bodies of neurons. But cerebral medulla doesn't contain the cell bodies of neurons. The external pyramidal layer and the internal pyramidal layer is chosen to observe the morphology and structure of pyramidal cells.

➤ High power

The bodies of pyramidal cells are triangular in shape and various in size. The typical large vesicular nucleolus with its prominent nucleolus is outlined. The most prominent cell process is the **apical dendrite**（顶树突）, which is directed toward the surface of the cortex. Several collateral dendrites are given off from the apical dendrite along its course to the surface of the cortex. Some dendrites start from the root of cell bodies. Dendritic spines exist on all the dendrites' surface（Fig. 8 – 3）. One single slender axon arises from the base of the cell body and passes into the medulla.

Reflection

（1）Compare the differences of Nissl bodies between external granular layer and internal pyramidal layer in pyramidal cells.

（2）Identify the detailed structure of the pyramidal cells, by comparing those with HE and silver staining sections.

（3）In the slide of cerebral cortex, we can find some sections of vessels. What is blood-brain barrier?

---

3. Cerebellum（小脑）

> Material

Cat cerebellum, coronal section (H & E stain).

> Gross observation

There are numerous transverse grooves on the surface of the cerebellum, which divide cerebellum into manyfolia. Each folium contains outer **cerebellar cortex**（小脑皮层）and inner **cerebellar medulla**（小脑髓质）.

> Low power

The grey matter (the cerebellar cortex) can be distinguished into three layers from outside to inside, while the white matter (the cerebellar medulla) mainly consists of myelinated nerve fibers or axons, which is stained in red color. Within the cerebellar cortex, the pink region on the cortical surface is molecular layer. The layer stained in purple blue is the granular layer (Fig. 8 – 4).

> High power

Molecular layer（分子层）is the superficial layer of the grey matter of the cerebellum, which is thicker than other layers. It is relatively light stained and consists mainly of stellate cells and basket cells. Cells within this layer are few and disperse.

Purkinje cell layer（蒲肯野细胞层）is a thin layer with Purkinje cells, which contains large, pear-shaped cell bodies and are regularly arranged in one layer. Ramified dendrites arising from the cell body extend into the molecular layer.

Granular layer（颗粒层）contains numerous small cells with intensely stained nuclei (Fig. 8 –5).

In-class Reflection

At the dendrites and dendritic spines of the Purkinje cells, what kind of cells do they link to form synapses?

---

4. Spinal cord（脊髓）

> Material

Cat spinal cord, cross section (H & E stain).

> Gross observation

The center of the section is a small pore called **central canal**（中央管）. The **grey matter**（灰质）is stained deeply and appears like H or butterfly in shape. It can be divided into two broad **anterior (ventral) horns**（前角，又称腹角）and two narrow **posterior (dorsal) horns**（后角，又称背角）. The **white matter**（白质）at the periphery is palely stained. The **lateral horns**（侧角）can be found in thoracic segments of spinal cord.

> Low power

Large, medium, or small sizes of nerve cells can be found in gray matter of spinal cord. Note that groups of multipolar neurons lie in ventral horns. White matter consists of glial cells and many nerve fibers in different sizes, most of which are myelinated (Fig. 8 –6).

➤ High power

The section of multipolar neuron in the ventral horn of spinal cord is variable in size. Its pale nucleus with distinct nucleolus, and abundant lump Nissl bodies within the cytoplasm are easy to be found in a large section of neuron. While within the dorsal horn, the nerve cells are relatively small in size, mainly including tract cells and interneurons. The lining cells of the central canal is the ependymal cell, a kind of glia cells in CNS, which appears as a single layer of epithelial cells. White matter consists of glial cells and nerve fibers, most of which are myelinated, although few are unmyelinated. The nerve fibers are variable in thickness.

Reflection

(1) What anatomical structures are surrounding spinal cord?

(2) How are the structures of the dorsal part of the spinal cord different from those of the ventral part?

(3) Are the Nissl bodies' morphologic features different in the different types of neurons?

(4) Where do the axons of the multipolar neurons within the ventral horn of spinal cord terminate?

---

5. Spinal ganglia (脊神经节)

➤ Material

Dog dorsal ganglia (H & E stain).

➤ Gross observation

The specimen has an oval shape. The spinal ganglia mainly contain the pseudounipolar neurons.

➤ Low power

A dense fibrous capsule covers the surface of the spinal ganglia. Cell bodies of pseudounipolar neurons are clumped in the ganglia. Numerous myelinated nerve fibers are located in a parallel pattern among the cell bodies.

➤ High power

The cell bodies of **pseudounipolar neurons** (假单极神经元) can be spherical, ovoid, or angular. The cells are very large and variable in size, which are located in groups separated by bundles of nerve fibers (mainly myelinated). The neuronal body has round central nucleus with a distinct nucleolus, appearing to be a vacuole under microscope. Their processes are difficult to be found in the specimen, since each pseudounipolar neuron has only one process. Their processes start from cell body and then branch into T-shape. Within the cytoplasm, fine Nissl bodies can be found. Each neuronal cell body is surrounded by a layer of flat **satellite cells** (卫星细胞), while its nucleus is stained darker (Fig. 8 – 7).

6. Sympathetic Ganglion（交感神经节）

➤ **Material**

Human sympathetic ganglion（H & E stain）.

➤ **Gross observation**

The specimen is similar as spinal ganglion in shape. But the sympathetic ganglion mainly contains multipolar neurons.

➤ **Low power**

The structure is similar as that of spinal ganglion, however, multipolar neurons are evenly distributed instead of being located in groups. Unmyelinated nerve fibers are present around the neurons.

➤ **High power**

In contrast to spinal ganglion cells, sympathetic ganglion neurons are multipolar neurons. The cells are smaller and more uniform in size. Their outlines and processes appear irregular. Their nuclei are often eccentric and appear to be a vacuole with prominent nucleolus. The surrounding satellite cells are usually less numerous than those in spinal ganglion（Fig. 8 – 8）.

Reflection

（1）What're the structural differences between spinal ganglion and sympathetic ganglion?

（2）In spinal ganglion, where does the T-shaped branch of the pseudounipolar neuron end up?

（3）Where does the neuron of sympathetic ganglia receive impulse from? Where is the end of its axon?

Post-class Task

（1）Identify the layers of the cerebral cortex under light microscope, and find a typical pyramidal cell.

（2）Identify the layers of the cerebella cortex under light microscope, and find a typical Purkinje cell.

Case-based Learning

A 3-year-old boy had not regularly been vaccinated before one year old. He had experienced a sudden high fever two months ago. Three days later, it had been found the left lower limb could not move. After that, although the temperature had dropped to normal, the movement of the left lower limb still hadn't recovered. And his left lower limb had gradually become thinner and thinner. After physical examination, complete paralysis of left lower limb was found, associating with decreased muscular tension. Knee and Achilles tendon reflex disappeared. Muscles of left lower limb showed distinct atrophy. No pathologic reflex was found. Superficial and deep sensations showed no abnormality. Finally, the patient was diagnosed with acute anterior poliomyelitis（急性脊髓前角灰质

炎，也称小儿麻痹症）．The injured segments of spinal cord were at lumbosacral enlargement（腰骶膨大，L1 – S4）．Combining with Fig. 8 – 9，answer the followed questions.

（1）What kind of neurons are located in the anterior horn of spinal cord? Where do the axons of these neurons dominate?

（2）Why did the injured anterior horn of spinal cord at lumbosacral enlargement level affect the function of the patient's left lower limb? What's the structural basis for this abnormality?

（3）What neurological abnormalities does the patient have? And what's the leading cause of this?

（张巍）

第 9 章 | 循环系统

循环系统由心血管系统和淋巴管系统组成。心脏、动脉、静脉和毛细血管等器官组成了心血管系统，同为中空性器官。

学习目标

（1）能够描述血管壁一般结构。
（2）能够识别和区分动脉、静脉的结构区别。
（3）能够理解心脏结构和心脏循环系统。

课前问题

（1）动脉和静脉如何分类？
（2）血管壁的组成有哪些？

实验观察与思考

1. 大动脉

➤ **材料**
人主动脉横断面（HE 染色和弹性染色）。

➤ **肉眼观察**
大动脉的管壁呈规则的圆环形，染色后可以看到明显分层。

➤ **低倍镜**
大动脉又称为弹性动脉，在弹性染色下，可以看到明显的紫蓝色弹性纤维（图 9-1）。大动脉的内膜由游离面的内皮和基底面的内弹性膜夹着少量结缔组织构成。中膜可以看到明显的弹性染色聚集。外膜由结缔组织构成。外弹性膜为中膜和外膜的分界线（图 9-2）。

➤ **高倍镜**
内膜：内膜的内皮为单层扁平上皮，其细胞核向血管的管腔突出。内弹性膜与中膜界限不清晰，平滑肌细胞与纵轴平行。
中膜：中膜富含卷曲状的弹性纤维，并含有一定数量的平滑肌细胞。
外膜：主要为疏松结缔组织构成，富含脂肪和神经。

思考题
（1）如何区分大动脉的内膜、中膜和外膜？
（2）为什么大动脉又称为弹性动脉？

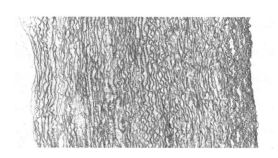

图 9 - 1　大动脉（弹性染色，150×）
Fig. 9 - 1　Aorta（Elastic stain, 150×）

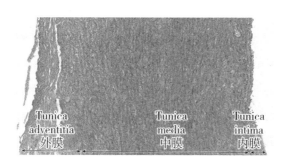

图 9 - 2　大动脉（HE 染色，150×）
Fig. 9 - 2　Aorta（H & E stain, 150×）

2. 中动脉

➤ **材料**

人中动脉横断面（HE 染色和弹性染色）。

➤ **肉眼观察**

规则环形，弹性染色后分层明显。

➤ **低倍镜**

弹性染色下，内弹性膜和外弹性膜清晰可见，能明确区分出三层结构。

➤ **高倍镜**

中动脉的中膜由大量的螺旋分布的平滑肌细胞组成，因此又称肌性动脉。平滑肌的核多为长杆状，染色较浅。

思考题

（1）大动脉和中动脉的结构区别是什么？

（2）他们的结构区别和功能有何相关性？

組织学与胚胎学实验教程（双语版）

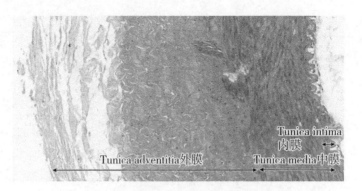

图 9 – 3　中动脉（HE 染色，200 ×）
Fig. 9 – 3　Medium-sized artery（H & E stain, 200 ×）

图 9 – 4　中动脉（弹性染色，200 ×）
Fig. 9 – 4　Medium-sized artery（Elastic stain, 200 ×）

3. 小动脉和小静脉

➤ 材料

人精索（HE 染色）。

➤ 肉眼观察

直径较小的圆环形管壁，细胞层数较少。

➤ 低倍镜

小动脉管壁厚，管径小，小动脉管壁薄，管径大。

➤ 高倍镜

小动脉：内皮细胞明显，可见内弹性膜、弹性纤维、胶原纤维和 10 层以内的平滑肌细胞，外弹性膜消失或不明显（图 9 – 5）。

小静脉：内皮细胞明显，平滑肌细胞层数较少，外膜极薄（图 9 – 5）。

思考题
（1）小动脉和小静脉一般分布于何处？
（2）小动脉和小静脉的功能？

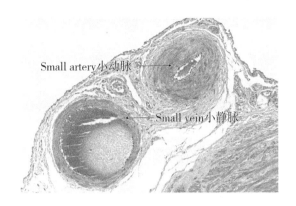

图 9 - 5　精索（HE 染色，200 ×）

Fig. 9 - 5　Spermatic cord（H & E stain，200 ×）

4. 毛细血管

➤ **材料**

人心脏，含连续毛细血管（HE 染色）。

人腺垂体，含血窦（HE 染色）。

➤ **肉眼观察**

几个细胞构成的微细管状结构。

➤ **高倍镜**

连续毛细血管：直径最小的血管，只有一层内皮细胞卷曲而成，或伴有周细胞（图 9 - 6）。

不连续毛细血管（窦状毛细血管）：窦状毛细血管（血窦）拥有不连续的内皮和基膜，窦腔很大，形状不规则（图 9 - 7）。

思考题

（1）毛细血管一般分布于何处？

（2）周细胞的作用？

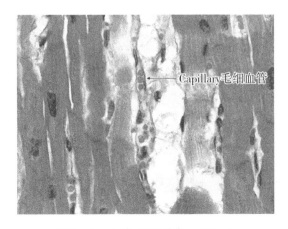

图 9 - 6　心脏（HE 染色，400 ×）

Fig. 9 - 6　Heart（H & E stain，400 ×）

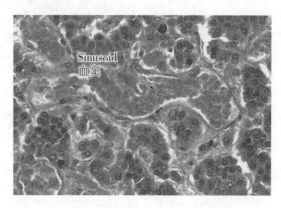

图 9 -7　腺垂体（HE 染色，400 ×）

Fig. 9 -7　Adenohypophysis（H & E stain, 400 ×）

5. 心脏

➤ **材料**

人心脏（HE 染色）。

➤ **肉眼观察**

HE 染色下，分层清晰，中间大量的红色心肌纤维构成心肌膜，心内膜和心外膜分布于两侧。

➤ **低倍镜**

心壁分为三层。最内层为心内膜，其延伸构成了心瓣膜。心内膜游离面为内皮，其下由结缔组织构成。心肌膜中富含心肌纤维，可以模糊地看到红色染色较深的阶梯状结构为闰盘。外膜由结缔组织构成，含有大量脂肪、血管以及神经组织。

➤ **高倍镜**

高倍下内膜可见浦肯野纤维（图 9 -8），浦肯野纤维为肥大的心肌纤维（图 9 -9），所起作用是传导冲动。浦肯野纤维多为单核或双核，居中，其胞质富含线粒体和糖原，染色较浅。

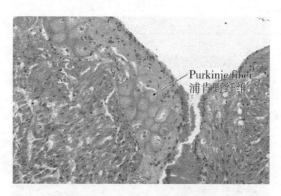

图 9 -8　心脏（HE 染色，200 ×）(1)

Fig. 9 -8　Heart（H & E stain, 200 ×）(1)

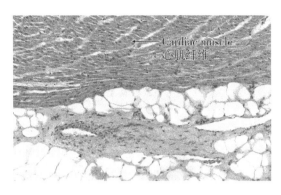

图 9-9　心脏（HE 染色，200×）（2）
Fig. 9-9　Heart（H & E stain，200×）（2）

课后作业

描述动脉和静脉的结构及功能特点。

病例教学

患者，男，52 岁，在体检中接受计算机体层成像血管造影（computed tomography angiography，CTA），其检查结果异常，显示为高血管病风险。该男子无冠心病史、无心绞痛症状，经常锻炼。转院后经进一步检测，冠状动脉钙化（coronary artery calcium，CAC）分值为 120，确诊为动脉粥样硬化。

（1）动脉粥样硬化是血管壁的哪个结构异常？

（2）这种异常对机体有何影响？

（滕藤）

Chapter 9 CIRCULATORY SYSTEM

Circulatory system is composed of the cardiovascular system and lymphatic system. The heart and a continuous system of blood vessels including arteries, veins and capillaries form the cardiovascular system.

Learning Objectives

(1) Understand the general components of the vascular wall.

(2) Be able to distinguish between arteries and veins and describe their structures.

(3) Understand the structure of the heart and its conducting system.

Pre-class Questions

(1) What are the subclassification of arteries and veins, and how have they been classified?

(2) What structures is vascular wall composed of?

Observation and Reflection

1. Large Artery（大动脉）

➤ Material

Human aorta, cross section (H & E stain, elastic stain).

➤ Gross observation

Large Artery wall is a donut-looking regular circle and clear layered after H & E staining.

➤ Low power

The large artery is an elastic artery which has a relatively thick tunica intima（内膜）bounded by endothelium（内皮）and the internal elastic membrane（内弹性膜）. The distribution of elastin in the elastic laminae which are dramatically enriched in tunica media（中膜）, is revealed as red-staining or black-staining material by the elastin stain. Tunica adventitia（外膜）consists of fibroelastic connective tissue（Fig. 9 – 1 and Fig. 9 – 2）.

➤ High power

Tunica Intima: From inside to outside, there are endothelial lining and its basement membrane, the subendothelial layer (loose connective tissue), and the internal elastic lamina. The nuclei of the endothelium protrude into the lumen of the vessel. The internal elastic lamina is less obvious, and smooth muscle cells run parallel to the long axis.

Tunica media: This layer comprises abundant circularly arranged elastic lamellae, and elastic fibers. There may also be a variable amount of smooth muscle fibers and collagen fibers.

Tunica adventitia: This layer consists of predominant fibroelastic connective tissue. Therefore, enriched adipose tissue and nerves could be observed. Like the internal elastic lamina, the external elastic lamina is not obvious too.

> **Reflection**
> (1) How can we distinguish tunica intima, tunica media and tunica adventitia?
> (2) Why is large artery also called elastic artery?

2. Medium-sized Artery (中动脉)

➢ Material

Human medium-sized artery, cross section (H & E stain, Elastin stain).

➢ Gross observation

Regular circle and clear layered after Elastic staining.

➢ Low power

By elastic staining, both the internal, external elastic laminae are clear to be observed, and the structure of three-layer is clearly distinguished.

➢ High power

The major component of the wall of the artery is spirally arranged smooth muscle fiber, also called muscular artery. If the smooth muscle cells are examined at high power, the nuclei are elongated. Due to contraction of the vessel wall, some of them appear corkscrew shaped. The nuclei are relatively euchromatic (Fig. 9 – 3 and Fig. 9 – 4).

> **Reflection**
> (1) What are differences between large artery and medium-sized artery?
> (2) Why are there structural differences between large artery and medium-sized artery?

3. Small Artery (arteriole) and Small Vein (venule) (小动脉和小静脉)

➢ Material

Human spermatic cord (H & E stain).

➢ Gross observation

Small diameter circles with fewer layers of cells.

➢ Low power

Small Artery exhibits thicker wall and small lumen whereas small vein shows thinner wall and bigger lumen.

➢ High power

Small Artery: The wall consists of endothelial cells, an internal elastic lamina opposed by one or two layers of smooth muscle cells, and a thin layer of collagen fibers. The inner elastic lamina is usually absent from small arterioles (Fig. 9 – 5).

Small vein: The wall is composed of endothelial cells, followed by one or two layers of smooth muscle cells, and very thin adventitia from inside to outside (Fig. 9 – 5).

Reflection

(1) Where are small artery and vein located?

(2) What are functions of small artery and vein?

---

4. Capillary （毛细血管）

➢ **Material**

Human heart, contain continuous capillaries (H & E stain).

Human adenohypophysis, contain sinusoidal capillaries (H & E stain).

➢ **Gross observation**

Tiny vessel formed by few cells.

➢ **High power**

Continuous capillaries: blood vessels with the smallest diameter, which may contain a few scattered pericytes (Fig. 9 – 6).

Discontinuous capillaries (Sinusoidal capillaries): Sinusoidal capillaries (or sinusoids) have a discontinuous endothelium and basement membrane. The sinusoids have large, irregular shaped lumens (Fig. 9 – 7).

Reflection

(1) Where are capillaries distributed?

(2) What is the role of pericyte?

---

5. Heart （心脏）

➢ **Material**

Human heart (H & E stain).

➢ **Gross observation**

Three layers are clearly separated by color (H & E stain), reddish layer in the middle is the myocardium, whereas the endocardium and the epicardium are by the side of myocardium.

➢ **Low power**

The cardiac wall is divided into three layers. The heart valves are extensions of the innermost layer, the endocardium. The endocardium contains a single layer of endothelium on the free surface and underlying supportive connective tissue, which includes sub-endocardium and purkinje fiber. Myocardium is the area where cardiac muscle fibers are enriched. The intercalated discs appear as red-staining step-like lines perpendicular to the long axis of the fiber. The epicardium includes a layer of simple squamous epithelium called the mesothelium and underlying supportive connective tissue.

➤ **High power**

Purkinje fibers (Fig. 9 – 8) are hypertrophied cardiac muscle fibers (Fig. 9 – 9) that are specialized for conducting an impulse rather than for contraction. They contain one or two nuclei, centrally situated in a pale staining mass of sarcoplasm that is rich in mitochondria and glycogen.

Post-class Task

Describe the structure of artery and vein and explain the differences.

Case-based Learning

A 52-year-old man was referred to our clinic for risk factor management after undergoing coronary computed tomography angiography (CTA) as part of an Executive Physical. He has no history of coronary artery disease and exercises regularly without experiencing anginal symptoms. His coronary artery calcium (CAC) score is 120. Finally, the patient was diagnosed with atherosclerosis.

(1) Which component of vascular wall will lead to atherosclerosis when it is disrupted?

(2) How does this abnormality of vascular wall effect our health?

(滕藤)

第 10 章 免疫系统

免疫系统是人体重要的防御系统，主要由淋巴器官、淋巴组织、免疫细胞和免疫活性分子组成。淋巴组织和器官分布在人体的各个部位，在血液和淋巴系统中循环的淋巴细胞是发挥免疫功能的关键成分。

学习目标
（1）掌握淋巴结的结构和功能。
（2）掌握脾的结构和功能，熟悉其与淋巴结在组织结构上的差异。
（3）掌握胸腺的结构和功能。

课前问题
（1）免疫系统的组成是什么？
（2）淋巴器官的分类是什么，分别有哪些淋巴器官？
（3）免疫细胞包括哪些，人类免疫系统最关键的免疫细胞是什么？

实验观察与思考

1. 淋巴结

➢ **材料**

人淋巴结（HE 染色）。

➢ **肉眼观察**

切片呈椭圆形或豆形，某些切片切到的凹陷处为门部。表面被覆染成粉红色的薄层是被膜，实质包括周边染成深蓝紫色的皮质，和中央浅染的髓质。

➢ **低倍镜**

被膜和小梁：被膜为淋巴结表面被覆的薄层致密结缔组织，被膜内可见带有瓣膜的输入淋巴管，门部由疏松结缔组织构成，可见较大的血管和输出淋巴管。被膜和门部的结缔组织可深入实质内形成小梁，构成淋巴结的粗支架。被膜下方和小梁周围的浅色区域为皮质淋巴窦。

实质可分为周边的皮质和中央的髓质（图 10-1）。

（1）皮质：皮质由浅层皮质、副皮质区和皮质淋巴窦三部分组成。

浅层皮质由淋巴小结和弥散淋巴组织组成。淋巴小结大小不等。发育好的淋巴小结可见生发中心，生发中心可分为明区和暗区，周围有一层染色较深，密集的小淋巴细胞，为小结帽。

副皮质区为浅层皮质深部的弥散淋巴组织，又称为胸腺依赖区。

皮质淋巴窦包括被膜下淋巴窦和小梁周窦。被膜下淋巴窦位于被膜与浅层皮质之间浅染的区域；小梁周窦位于小梁与浅层皮质之间浅染的区域。

（2）髓质：包括髓索和髓窦两部分组成。髓索是相互连接吻合的索条状淋巴组织，髓窦与皮质淋巴窦结构相同，位于髓索之间或者髓索和小梁之间。髓窦腔较宽大，互相通连成网状。

> **高倍镜**

重点观察副皮质区的毛细血管后微静脉和淋巴窦（皮质淋巴窦和髓窦）的结构。

（1）毛细血管后微静脉：在副皮质区可见高内皮毛细血管后微静脉，与一般微静脉相比，其内皮细胞为单层立方形，常见淋巴细胞跨越管壁。

（2）淋巴窦：窦壁由扁平的内皮衬里，内皮外为一层扁平的网状细胞，在镜下因为密集的淋巴组织不是很明显。窦腔内可见胞质粉红有突起的星状内皮细胞，还有淋巴细胞和巨噬细胞。

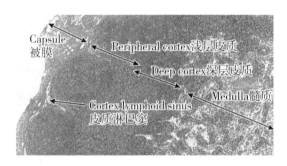

图 10 – 1　淋巴结（HE 染色，100 ×）
Fig. 10 – 1　Lymph node（H & E stain, 100 ×）

思考题

（1）淋巴结的结构不是固定不变的，当抗原刺激后体液免疫应答或是细胞免疫应答占优势时，淋巴结的结构分别可能有什么变化？

（2）淋巴结是如何滤过淋巴液的？

2．脾

> **材料**

人脾脏（HE 染色）。

> **肉眼观察**

标本边缘的粉红色部分为脾被膜，内部为脾实质。实质内散在的圆形或椭圆形深蓝紫色结构，为脾的白髓，白髓之间疏松的暗红色部分为脾的红髓。

> **低倍镜**

（1）被膜：较厚，由致密结缔组织组成，其内含有少量平滑肌，外表面被覆间皮。被膜深入实质形成小梁（图 10 –2）。

（2）白髓：散在分布脾实质内的蓝紫色区域，可见中央动脉的不同切面，由动脉周围淋巴鞘、淋巴小结（脾小体）和边缘区组成（图 10 –2）。动脉周围淋巴鞘常位于白髓一侧，是中央动脉周围的厚层弥散淋巴组织。淋巴细胞以 T 淋巴细胞为主，相当于淋巴结的副皮质区。在鞘的一侧呈蓝紫色的球团状结构为淋巴小结，又称脾小体（图 10 - 3），以 B 淋巴细胞为主，抗原刺激后可见生发中心，小结帽朝向红髓。白髓和红髓交界的区域为边缘区，界限不是很清晰，此区含有中央动脉侧枝末端膨大而成的小血窦，即边缘窦。

（3）红髓：除白髓以外周围大部分富含血细胞的区域，由脾索和脾血窦构成（图 10 - 2）。

➤ **高倍镜**

观察脾的细微结构：

（1）被膜：表面被覆的间皮及含有的平滑肌。

（2）动脉周围淋巴鞘：各种切面的中央动脉。

（3）红髓：脾索和脾窦（图 10 - 4）。脾索是富含血细胞的索条状淋巴组织，并相互连接成网。含淋巴细胞、浆细胞、巨噬细胞和大量血细胞。脾索之间的腔隙为脾窦。在脾窦的横切面，可见内皮细胞沿窦壁点状排列，胞核突出于窦腔，腔内含有血细胞。由于脾索和脾窦均有大量血细胞，有的切面不好分辨。

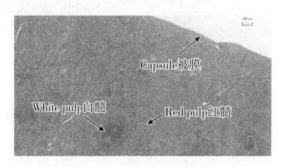

图 10 - 2　脾（HE 染色，40 ×）

Fig. 10 - 2　Spleen（H & E stain, 40 ×）

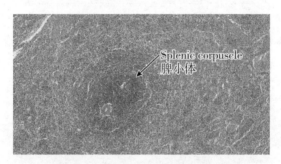

图 10 - 3　脾（HE 染色，100 ×）

Fig. 10 - 3　Spleen（H & E stain, 100 ×）

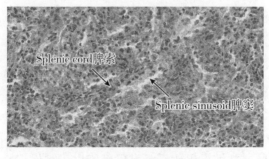

图 10 - 4　脾（HE 染色，400 ×）

Fig. 10 - 4　Spleen（H & E stain, 400 ×）

思考题

脾脏和淋巴结的结构异同点？

3. 胸腺

➤ **材料**

人胸腺（HE 染色）。

➤ **肉眼观察**

切面呈椭圆形，表面粉红色的是被膜，实质周围染成深蓝色的是皮质，中央染色浅的为髓质。

➤ **低倍镜**

胸腺表面被覆薄层结缔组织为被膜，被膜伸入实质形成小叶间隔，将实质分成多个不完全的小叶，即胸腺小叶。小叶周围染色深的是皮质，中央染色浅的是髓质，相邻小叶的髓质可相连（图 10 − 5）。皮质胸腺上皮细胞少，胸腺细胞密集，故染色呈深蓝色，而髓质胸腺上皮细胞较多，还可见胸腺小体，胸腺细胞较少，故染色较浅。

➤ **高倍镜**

胸腺小体是胸腺的特征性结构，大小不等，散在分布于胸腺髓质（图 10 − 6）。由数层至十几层胸腺上皮细胞呈同心圆排列而成。外周的上皮细胞较幼稚，可见明显的细胞核；近小体中心的上皮细胞成熟，胞核逐渐退化，小体中心的上皮细胞完全角质化，呈均质的嗜酸性结构。

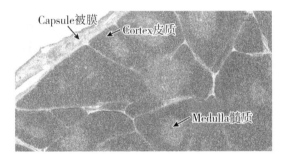

图 10 − 5　胸腺（HE 染色，40 ×）

Fig. 10 − 5　Thymus（H & E stain, 40 ×）

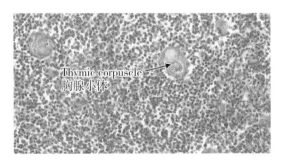

图 10 − 6　胸腺（HE 染色，400 ×）

Fig. 10 − 6　Thymus（H & E stain, 400 ×）

课后作业

（1）画一个光学显微镜下（100×）所见的淋巴结的示意图。

（2）描述胸腺的组织结构。

病例教学

一个 6 岁的男孩入院就诊，他的母亲述说他两天前被邻居的狗咬伤了。孩子的右手大拇指和食指之间被割伤，这个部位发炎，但目前正在愈合。医生的检查显示，在右肘部和腋窝的皮下有一小而无痛的肿胀包块。医生向他的母亲解释说，这些是活跃的淋巴结，是对手部感染做出反应而肿胀扩大的。试问：

（1）肿胀的原因是什么，推测其淋巴结的结构有什么变化？

（2）什么是淋巴细胞再循环？

（3）什么是单核吞噬系统？什么样的细胞构成这个系统？它对人体有什么作用？

（王艳华）

Chapter 10 IMMUNE SYSTEM

Immune system is an important defensive system in the human body, mainly composed of lymphoid organs, lymphoid tissues, immune cells and immune active molecules. Lymphoid tissues and organs distribute throughout human body, and lymphocytes circulating in the blood and lymphatic system are the key components exerting immune function.

Learning Objectives

(1) Be able to identify the microstructure of lymph node.

(2) Be able to identify the microstructure of the spleen, and be able to distinguish the structural differences between spleen and lymph node.

(3) Be able to identify the microstructure of thymus.

Pre-class Questions

(1) What is immune system composed of?

(2) What is the classification of lymphatic organs and what are the lymphatic organs respectively?

(3) Which immune cells are included? What is the most critical immune cell of human immune system?

Observation and Reflection

1. Lymph node (淋巴结)

➢ Material

Human lymph node (H & E stain).

➢ Gross observation

The tissue section of lymph node is of elliptic or lenticular morphology. The concave part in certain slices is the hilus. The thin layer coated with pink color, on the outermost surface, is the capsule. The parenchyma includes a peripheral cortex stained with dark bluish-purple, and a central medulla lightly stained.

➢ Low power

Capsule (被膜) and **trabecula** (小梁): The capsule is a thin layer of dense connective tissue covered by the surface of the lymph node. The afferent lymphatic vessel with valve can be seen in the capsule, and the hilus (门部) is composed of loose connective tissue with larger blood vessels and efferent lymphatic vessels. The connective tissue of the capsule and the hilus can penetrate into the parenchyma to form trabecula, which constitute the thick scaffold of the lymphoid nodes.

The light colored area below the capsule and around the trabecula is the cortical sinus （Fig. 10 - 1）.

The parenchyma can be divided into a peripheral cortex and a central medulla.

（1） Cortex：The cortex consists of three parts, superficial cortex, paracortical zone and cortical sinus.

The superficial cortex contains lymphoid nodules and diffused lymphoid tissue. Lymphoid nodules vary in size. The germinal center can be seen in the developed lymphoid nodules. The germinal center can be divided into bright and dark areas. There is a layer of dark and dense small lymphocytes around it, which is the nodular cap.

The paracortical zone is the diffuse lymphoid tissue deep in the superficial cortex, also known as the thymus dependent area.

Cortical sinuses include subcapsular sinuses and peritrabecular sinuses. The subcapsular sinus is the lightly stained area between the capsule and the peripheral cortex. The peritrabecular sinus is located in the lightly stained area between the trabecula and the peripheral cortex.

（2） Medulla：It consists of two parts, medullary cord and medullary sinus. The medullary cord is a cord-like lymphoid tissue that is connected and anastomosed with each other. The medullary sinuses present the same structure as the cortical sinuses and are located between the medullary cords or between the medullary cord and the trabecula. The cavity of medullary sinus is large and connected with each other into a meshwork.

➢ High power

The structures of postcapillary venules （毛细血管后微静脉） and lymphoid sinuses （cortical sinuses and medullary sinuses） in the paracortex should be carefully observed.

（1） Postcapillary venules：High endothelial venules can be seen in the paracortex. Compared with common venules, its endothelial cells are single-layer cuboidal, and lymphocytes commonly span the tube wall.

（2） Lymphoid sinuses：The wall of the sinuses is lined by a flat endothelium with a layer of flat reticular cells outside the endothelium, which is not obvious under the microscope because of the dense lymphoid tissue. In the sinus cavity, the cytoplasmic pink protrusive star-shaped endothelial cells, as well as lymphocytes and macrophages can be seen.

Reflection

（1） The structure of lymph nodes is not fixed. What might be the changes in the structure of lymph nodes when the humoral immune response or cellular immune response is dominant after antigen stimulation?

（2） How do lymph nodes filter lymph fluid?

---

2. Spleen （脾）

➢ Material

Human spleen （H & E stain）.

> ➤ Gross observation

The pink part at the edge of the specimen is the capsule, and the interior is the splenic paren-chyma. Scattered round or oval structures in dark blue can be found in the parenchyma, represen-ting the white pulp of the spleen, and dark red tissues between the **white pulp** (白髓) are the **red pulp** (红髓) of the spleen.

> ➤ Low power

(1) Capsule: It is thick, composed of dense connective tissue, containing a small amount of smooth muscle, and its outer surface is covered with mesothelium. The capsule penetrates into the parenchyma to form trabecula (脾小梁) (Fig. 10 - 2).

(2) White pulp: They are scattered in the blue-purple area of the splenic parenchyma, dif-ferent sections of the central artery can be seen, and they are composed of the periarterial lymphoid sheath (动脉周围淋巴鞘), lymphatic nodules (splenic corpuscle) (脾小体) and marginal zone (Fig. 10 - 2). The periarterial lymphatic sheath, usually located on the side of white pulp, is a thick layer of diffuse lymphatic tissue surrounding the central artery. The lymphocytes are main-ly T lymphocytes, which correspond to the paracortical region of the lymph nodes. On one side of the sheath, the bluish-purple blob-like structure is the lymphoid nodule, also known as the splenic corpuscle (Fig. 10 - 3), dominated by B lymphocytes, the germinal center can be seen after anti-gen stimulation, and the nodule cap faces the red pulp. The boundary between the white pulp and the red pulp is the marginal region, and the boundary is not very clear. This region contains a small blood sinus enlarged from the end of the lateral branches of the central artery, that is, the marginal sinus.

(3) Red pulp: Except for the white pulp, most of the surrounding areas rich in blood cells are composed of splenic cords and spleen blood sinuses (Fig. 10 - 2).

> ➤ High power

Observe the fine structure of the spleen:

(1) Capsule: The surface of spleen is covered by the mesothelium, and contains smooth mus-cle.

(2) Periarterial lymphatic sheath: Various sections of the central artery can be shown.

(3) Red pulp: It contains splenic cords (脾索) and splenic sinusoids (脾窦) (Fig. 10 - 4). The splenic cord is a long line of lymphoid tissue rich in blood cells and connected with each other to form a meshwork. It contains lymphocytes, plasma cells, macrophages and a large number of blood cells. The cavities between the splenic cords are the splenic sinusoids. In the transverse section of the splenic sinusoids, the endothelial cells are arranged discontinuously along the sinus wall, and the nucleus protrudes out of the sinus cavity. Because there are a lot of blood cells in the splenic cord and splenic sinus, sometimes the splenic cord and splenic sinusoid are difficult to be distinguished from each other.

Reflection

What are the structural similarities and differences between spleen and lymph nodes?

---

3. Thymus（胸腺）

> **Material**

Human thymus（H & E stain）.

> **Gross observation**

The section of the thymus is oval. The surface in pink is the capsule, underneath which is the parenchyma. dark blue partis the cortex, and the central area stained lightly is the medulla.

> **Low power**

The surface of the thymus is covered by a thin layer of connective tissue, which extends into the parenchyma to form lobular septa, dividing the parenchyma into several incomplete lobules. The cortex is deeply stained around the lobules, the medulla is lightly stained. And the medulla of the adjacent lobules can be connected. Cortical thymic epithelial cells are few and thymic cells are dense, so the staining is dark blue, while medullary thymic epithelial cells are more and **thymic corpuscles**（胸腺小体）are visible, meanwhile thymic cells are fewer, so the staining is lighter （Fig. 10 – 5）.

> **High power**

Thymic corpuscles are characteristic structures of the thymus, varying in size and scattering in the medulla of the thymus. It consists of several to ten layers of thymic epithelial cells arranged in concentric circles. The peripheral epithelial cells are immature with obvious nuclei. The epithelial cells near the center of the corpuscles are mature, the nuclei degenerate gradually, and the epithelial cells in the center of the corpuscles are completely keratinized, showing a homogeneous eosinophilic structure （Fig. 10 – 6）.

Post-class Task

（1）Under a light microscope （100 ×）, draw a diagram of the lymphoid node.

（2）Describe the microstructure of the thymus.

Case-based Learning

A 6-year-old boy is brought to the clinic where his mother reports that he was bitten by a neighbor's dog two days' ago. The child's right hand is lacerated between the thumb and index finger and this area is inflamed but healing. The doctor's examination reveals small but painless swellings beneath the skin inside the right elbow and arm pit and he explains to his mother that these are active lymph nodes enlarged in response to the infection in the hand.

（1）What causes the swelling? What are the changes of the lymph node's structure?

（2）What is lymphocyte recirculation?

（3）What is the mononuclear phagocytic system? What cells are made of such system? What function does it have on the body?

（王艳华）

第11章 | 内分泌系统

内分泌系统由分泌激素的内分泌细胞组成。

（1）内分泌细胞通常聚集为内分泌腺体，呈条索状，但甲状腺除外。

（2）从内分泌腺分泌的激素直接释放到血液中。

学习目标

（1）能够识别和描述甲状腺、肾上腺、垂体的微细结构。

（2）能够识别甲状旁腺的微细结构。

课前问题

（1）内分泌系统的组成有哪些？

（2）内分泌腺的一般结构特点是什么？

（3）按激素的化学性质划分，内分泌细胞主要分为哪几类，其超微结构的特点分别是什么？

实验观察与思考

1. 甲状腺

➤ **材料**

人甲状腺（HE 染色）。

➤ **肉眼观察**

一大块被染成红色的组织。

➤ **低倍镜**

甲状腺表面被覆薄层结缔组织被膜，实质内由大小不等接近圆形的滤泡组成。周边是滤泡壁，中央为滤泡腔。滤泡腔内充满红色的物质为胶质，偶见胶质脱落的滤泡。滤泡之间的结缔组织内有丰富的毛细血管，还可见成团分布的滤泡旁细胞。

➤ **高倍镜**

滤泡壁由单层立方上皮组成，细胞高度常随生理活动不同而有差异，呈现低柱状或扁平状。滤泡腔内充满红色嗜酸性均质状胶质，胶质和滤泡上皮细胞之间常见重吸收泡。在滤泡上皮细胞之间及滤泡之间的结缔组织内，可见单个或聚集成群的滤泡旁细胞，该细胞比滤泡上皮细胞稍大，细胞质着色较浅（图 11-1）。

思考题

胶质的化学成分是什么？

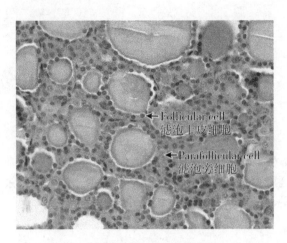

图 11 – 1　甲状腺（HE 染色，400 ×）

Fig. 11 – 1　Thyroid gland（H & E stain，400 ×）

2. 甲状旁腺

➢ **材料**

人甲状旁腺（HE 染色）。

➢ **肉眼观察**

呈现较小的、蓝紫色团块状。

➢ **低倍镜**

甲状旁腺表面被覆薄层结缔组织被膜，实质内细胞排列成团索状，可见散在分布的脂肪细胞和少量结缔组织，结缔组织内有丰富的毛细血管。

➢ **高倍镜**

实质内细胞分主细胞和嗜酸性细胞。主细胞数量最多，呈多边形，核圆，胞质着色浅而透亮；嗜酸性细胞较少，单个或成群分布，胞体较大，核小染色深，胞质嗜酸性。

思考题

在哪里能够找到甲状旁腺？

---

3. 肾上腺

➢ **材料**

人肾上腺（HE 染色）。

➢ **肉眼观察**

切面呈三角形，周围染色深的为皮质，中央染色浅的区域为髓质，其内可见较大空腔样结构为中央静脉。

➢ **低倍镜**

（1）被膜：由结缔组织组成。

（2）皮质：自外向内依次分为三个带：球状带最薄，细胞呈球团状排列，染色较深；

束状带最厚，细胞排列呈条索状，染色浅；网状带细胞成索状并互相连接成网，染色较深。

（3）髓质：细胞排列呈不规则的细胞索，可见中央静脉的切面（图11-2）。

> **高倍镜**

（1）球状带：细胞较小，核大胞浆少，细胞核着色深，因此该带偏嗜碱性。球状细胞团间有窦状毛细血管。

（2）束状带：具备最典型类固醇类内分泌细胞的特点。细胞平行排列成单行或双行的细胞索，细胞体积较大，呈多边形，细胞质染色浅，因含有较多脂滴，制片时溶解后呈泡沫状。细胞索间有丰富的窦状毛细血管。

（3）网状带：位于皮质深层，近髓质。细胞索相互吻合成网，细胞较束状带细胞小，核圆，细胞质嗜酸性，可见棕黄色的脂褐素颗粒。

（4）髓质细胞：呈多边形，胞体大，细胞排列成不规则细胞索，索间有血窦，血窦最终汇入中央静脉。经铬盐处理的标本，细胞质内可见许多黄褐色的嗜铬颗粒，胞质呈现棕黄色。髓质中偶见交感神经节细胞，胞体大而不规则，细胞质内有尼氏体，核大而圆，染色浅，核仁明显。

思考题

（1）肾上腺皮质和髓质分别分泌什么激素？

（2）肾上腺束状带细胞受哪个器官、哪个结构分泌的什么激素调控？

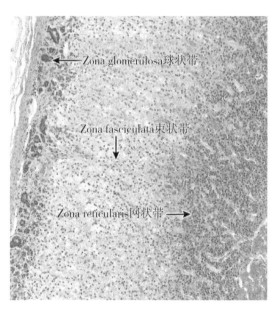

图11-2 肾上腺（HE染色，40×）
Fig. 11-2 Adrenal gland (H & E stain, 40×)

4. 垂体

> **材料**

人垂体（HE染色）。

> ➤ **肉眼观察**

标本一侧染色深的部分是远侧部，另一侧染色浅的部分是神经部，两者之间为中间部。远侧部上方为结节部。

> ➤ **低倍镜**

表面有结缔组织被膜。远侧部细胞排列成球团状和索状，细胞团索之间有丰富的血窦。中间部可见几个大小不等的滤泡，腔内充满胶质。神经部染色最浅，细胞成分少，主要是神经纤维。（图 11 - 3）

> ➤ **高倍镜**

（1）远侧部：辨认三种细胞。

A. 嗜酸性细胞：数量较多，胞体较大，为圆形或椭圆形，细胞质内含有红色嗜酸性颗粒。细胞界限清楚，核圆形，偏心性分布。

B. 嗜碱性细胞：数量少，细胞大小不等，为圆形或多边形，细胞质内含有蓝紫色嗜碱性颗粒，细胞界限清楚，核圆。

C. 嫌色细胞：数量最多，常成群存在，细胞较小，核圆形，细胞质染色浅，细胞界限不清楚（图 11 - 4）。

（2）中间部：常见大小不等的滤泡，由单层立方形滤泡上皮围成，滤泡腔内有嗜酸性或嗜碱性均质状胶质。

（3）神经部：主要由垂体细胞和无髓神经纤维组成，有丰富的毛细血管。

A. 神经纤维：数量多，有不同方向切面，为无髓神经纤维，染成粉红色。

B. 垂体细胞：即神经部的神经胶质细胞，位于神经纤维之间，细胞轮廓不清晰，仅见核呈圆形或卵圆形。

C. 赫令体：为大小不等、形状不一的均质状嗜酸性团块（图 11 - 5）。

思考题

（1）垂体远侧部内分泌细胞的功能是什么？

（2）神经部的无髓神经纤维来源于什么神经元的突起？

（3）赫令体来源于哪里，实质是什么？

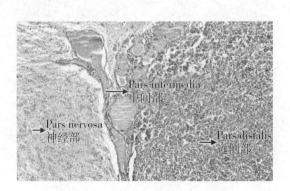

图 11 - 3　垂体（HE 染色，40 ×）
Fig. 11 - 3　Hypophysis（H & E stain, 40 ×）

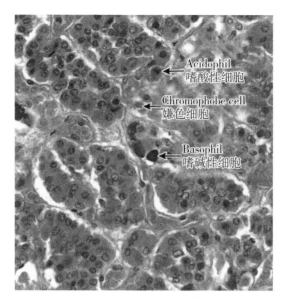

图 11 –4　垂体远侧部（HE 染色，400 ×）
Fig. 11 –4　Hypophysis（pars distalis；H & E stain，400 ×）

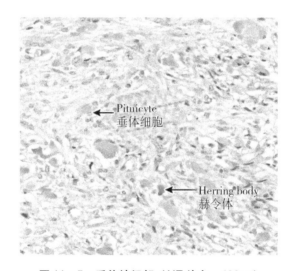

图 11 –5　垂体神经部（HE 染色，400 ×）
Fig. 11 –5　Hypophysis（pars nervosa；H & E stain，400 ×）

课后作业

画一个甲状腺滤泡。

病例教学

　　患者，男，42 岁，半年前无明显诱因出现心悸、乏力、消瘦和眼痛等多种症状。体检显示脉搏为 100 次/分，血压为 140/95 mmHg，眼睛突出。辅助检查发现血液中的 T3 和 T4 值增加。诊断为甲状腺功能亢进（甲亢）。图 11 –6 是弥漫性毒性甲状腺肿患者甲状腺的病理图片。

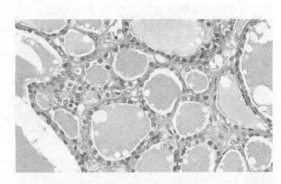

图 11-6　甲状腺功能亢进的甲状腺病理切片（HE 染色，40×）
Fig. 11-6　Hyperthyroidism（H & E stain，40×）

（1）甲亢的发病过程主要由甲状腺的哪些细胞参与？

（2）甲状腺素（T4）和三碘甲状腺原氨酸（T3）有什么生理功能？

（3）仔细观察甲状腺功能亢进的甲状腺病理图片，与正常甲状腺的结构比较，该图有什么变化？

（黄文峰，魏霞）

Chapter 11　ENDOCRINE SYSTEM

The endocrine system is made up of endocrine cells that secrete hormones.

(1) Endocrine cells usually aggregate into endocrine glands, with the exception of the thyroid gland.

(2) Hormones secreted from endocrine glands are released directly into the blood stream.

Learning goals

(1) Be able to identify and describe the microstructures of the thyroid gland, adrenal gland and the pituitary gland.

(2) Be able to identify the microstructure of parathyroid gland.

Pre-class Questions

(1) What are the main components of the endocrine system?

(2) What are the general features of endocrine gland?

(3) According to the chemical properties of endocrine hormones, what are the main types of endocrine cells and their ultrastructural characteristics?

Observation and Reflection

1. Thyroid gland (甲状腺)

➢ Material

Human thyroid (H & E stain).

➢ Gross observation

A large piece of tissue was dyed red.

➢ Low power

The surface of thyroid gland is a loose connective tissue capsule. The glandular parenchyma is composed of many thyroid **follicle** (滤泡) of different sizes. There are **colloids** (胶质) stained red in the follicular cavity, accompanied by a small amount of connective tissue and blood vessels between follicles.

➢ High power

(1) Capsule: Capsule is one layer of thin connective tissue.

(2) Follicle: Follicles of varying sizes are seen in the thyroid parenchyma. Follicular wall consists of a single layer of epithelial cells. Follicular epithelial cells are usually cubic and have cir-

cle nucleus. The follicular cavity is filled with red eosinophilic colloid.

(3) **Parafollicular cell** (滤泡旁细胞)：Single or clustered parafollicular cells with lighter cytoplasmic staining can be seen between follicular epithelial cells and between follicles, which are slightly larger than follicular cells.

(4) Connective tissue and capillaries：They are distributed among the follicles (Fig. 11 – 1).

Reflection

What are the main chemical components of colloid?

---

2. Parathyroid gland (甲状旁腺)

➢ **Material**

Human parathyroid (H & E stain).

➢ **Gross observation**

The specimen is blue-purple.

➢ **Low power**：

(1) Membrane：There is thin connective tissue.

(2) **Chief cell** (主细胞)：They are polygonal or round with circular nucleus located in the center. The cytoplasm is lightly colored, sometimes vacuolated.

(3) **Oxyphil** (嗜酸性细胞)：They are few and their cytoplasm are filled with red particles.

➢ **High power**

The chief cell is the most numerous and the cell size is small. Chief cells are polygonal or round with circular nucleus located in the center. The cytoplasm is lightly colored, sometimes vacuolated. Oxyphils with deep nucleus and eosinophilic cytoplasm are larger than the chief cells and fewer in amount and are scattered or located in clusters.

Reflection

Where is parathyroid gland located?

---

3. Adrenal gland (肾上腺)

➢ **Material**

Rat adrenal gland (H & E stain).

➢ **Gross observation**

The superficial layer of the specimen in dark red is cortex, and the central in light red is medulla.

➢ **Low power**：

(1) Membrane：There is one thin layer of connective tissue.

(2) Cortex：Cortex is located in the lower layer of the capsule. From outside to inside cortex

is divided into three zones: zona glomerulosa, zona fasciculata and zona reticularis.

(3) Medulla and central vein lie in the center (Fig. 11 – 2).

➢ High power

(1) **Zona glomerulosa** （球状带）: This is the thinnest one. It is arranged from smaller columnar or polygonal cells into a ball-like shape, with small nuclear, deep coloring, and slightly basophilia. There are sinus capillaries or a small number of connective tissues between cell groups.

(2) **Zona fasciculata** （束状带）: This band is the thickest. The cells are arranged in parallel into belts. The cells are large, polygonal and lightly stained. There are abundant sinus capillaries and a small number of connective tissues between cell cords.

(3) **Zona reticularis** （网状带）: This layer is located at the deepest cortex, close to the medulla. Cell cords anastomosis with each other into a net in shape. The cells are smaller than zona fasciculata, with circular nucleus and eosinophilic cytoplasm. It can be seen that brown yellow lipofuscin particles.

(4) Medullary cells: Polygonal and large medullary cells are located in the center of the gland, with round nucleus. There are many yellow brown pyromicular particles visible in the cytoplasm, after treated with chromium salt. Only very few sympathetic ganglia cells can be seen in the medulla.

Reflection

(1) What hormones are secreted by adrenal gland cortex and medulla?

(2) Which organ, structure, and hormone secretion regulate the adrenal fascicular zone cells?

---

4. Hypophysis （垂体）

➢ Material

Human hypophysis (H & E stain).

➢ Gross observation

The deeply stained part is the **pars distalis** （远侧部）, and the lightly stained part is the **pars nervosa** （神经部）. Between the two is the **pars intermedia** （中间部）. Above the distal part is **pars tuberalis** （结节部）.

➢ Low power

There is a connective tissue capsule outside. The cells in the distal part densely form clusters and cords, connecting each other into a network. There are rich blood sinuses between cell masses and cords. The middle part is long and narrow, having several different sizes of follicles filled with dark pink colloid. The pars nervosa is mainly made up of nerve fibers stained very light (Fig. 11 – 3).

➢ High power

(1) Pars distalis: Mainly composed of three kinds of cells and blood sinuses.

A. **Acidophils** （嗜酸性细胞）: Acidophils are rich in numbers, large, round or polygonal, with thick red eosinophilic particles in cytoplasm. The cells are well clear and the nuclei are round and centrally located.

B. **Basophils**（嗜碱性细胞）：Basophils are round or polygonal with different cells size, clear cell boundaries and round nuclei. The cytoplasm contains blue-purple basophils particles.

C. **Chromophobe cells**（嫌色细胞）：Chromophobe cells are numerous and often exist in groups, with small cell size, round nuclei, light cytoplasm and unclear cell boundary（Fig. 11 – 4）.

（2）Pars intermedia：There are some different sizes of follicles, mostly surrounded bysmall cells.

（3）Pars nervosa：Pars nervosa is mainly composed of glial cells and unmyelinated nerve fibers.

A. Never fibers：A large number of unmyelinated nerve fibers are stained in pink.

B. **Pituicytes**（垂体细胞）：Pituicytes are the neuroglias and located in between nerve fibers, with different sizes, shapes and round or oval nucleus. The cytoplasm often contains yellow brown pigment granules.

C. **Herring body**（赫令体）：Eosinophilic, homogeneous mass of different sizes.

D. Blood vessels：There are abundant sinus capillaries between thin connective tissues （Fig. 11 – 5）.

Reflection

（1）What is the function of endocrine cells in the distal pituitary gland?

（2）What neuron processes do the unmyelinated nerve fibers of the pars nervosa originate from?

（3）What is Herring body?

Post-class Task

Draw a diagram of thyroid gland follicle.

Case-based Learning

A patient, male, 42 years old, had many symptoms such as palpitation, fatigue, emaciation and eye pain six months ago without obvious causes. Physical examination showed that the pulse was 100 times/min, the blood pressure was 140/95 mmHg, and the eyes were bulging. The auxiliary examination found that the T3 and T4 values in the blood increased. The diagnosis was hyperthyroidism. The following is a pathological figure of hyperthyroidism（Fig. 11 – 6）.

（1）What kind of cells of thyroid gland are included in the hyperthyroidism process?

（2）What physiological function will thyroxine（T4）and triiodothyronine（T3）have?

（3）What are the main changes in the pathological figure of hyperthyroidism, comparing with the structure of normal thyroid gland?

（黄文峰，魏霞）

第 12 章 眼和耳

眼和耳均是人体重要的感觉器官。眼是人体的视觉器官，由眼球和眼球的附属器官组成，眼球包括眼球壁和眼球内容物，眼附属器官包括眼睑、泪腺和眼外肌等。耳是一种可通过前庭耳蜗装置中的机械感受器来感受位觉和听觉的器官。

学习目标

（1）能够识别眼球壁各层组织结构，重点掌握角膜和视网膜的结构和功能。

（2）能够识别内耳螺旋器的结构及功能。

（3）了解内耳和眼睑的结构。

课前问题

（1）眼球壁包括哪几层结构？

（2）内耳包含什么结构？

实验观察与思考

1. 眼球

➤ **材料**

人眼球矢状切面（HE 染色）。

➤ **肉眼观察**

眼球的前后部以及角膜、巩膜、虹膜、睫状体、视神经、晶状体、玻璃体、瞳孔、前后房等结构都可以清晰显示。

➤ **低倍镜**

重点观察眼球壁的结构，由外向内依次分为三层：纤维膜、血管膜和视网膜；眼球内容物包括房水、晶状体和玻璃体，房水和玻璃体在制片时已流失。

（1）纤维膜：最外层，由致密结缔组织构成，分角膜和巩膜。

A. 角膜是前方 1/6 呈透明状的、略向前突出的结构，HE 染色呈粉红色。

B. 巩膜是后方 5/6 呈白色的，镜下染色呈深红色的结构。巩膜与角膜相延续，两者交界的部位称为角膜缘。角膜边缘处常可见球结膜附于巩膜表面。

（2）血管膜：为中间富含黑素细胞和血管的疏松结缔组织构成，由前至后分为虹膜、睫状体和脉络膜。

A. 虹膜呈环形，在切片上为界于角膜和晶状体之间的两片薄膜状结构，两侧薄膜之间的缺口为瞳孔，注意分辨前后方向。

B. 睫状体切面呈三角形，连接虹膜和脉络膜，前方较宽大，并向前内侧伸出被称为睫状突的放射状突起，睫状突与晶状体之间有睫状小带相连，后方渐平坦，终止于锯齿缘。

C. 脉络膜为血管膜的后 2/3，衬于巩膜和视网膜之间，为富含黑素细胞和血管的疏松结缔组织。

（3）视网膜：位于最内层，分视部和盲部，两者以锯齿缘为界。视部即通常所称的视网膜，盲部是虹膜上皮和睫状体上皮。

> **高倍镜**

（1）角膜：由前至后依次分 5 层（图 12 - 1）。

A. 角膜上皮：为未角化的复层扁平上皮，基底面平坦。

B. 前界层：一层被染成粉红色均质状的薄膜。

C. 角膜基质：最厚，由多层胶原原纤维形成的胶原板层排列而成，可见散在分布的成纤维细胞，又称角膜细胞，无血管。

D. 后界层：结构与前界层类似，但较薄。

E. 角膜内皮：为单层扁平上皮。

（2）角膜缘：重要结构包括巩膜距、巩膜静脉窦和小梁网（图 12 - 2）。

A. 巩膜距：在角膜缘内侧，巩膜向前内侧突出的嵴状隆起。

B. 巩膜静脉窦：在巩膜距前外侧的一环形管，切面上为一被覆内皮的狭长裂隙。

C. 小梁网：位于巩膜静脉窦内侧，由小梁和小梁间隙组成，切面呈网状，小梁是胶原纤维两侧被覆内皮的细索状结构，网孔为小梁间隙。

（3）虹膜：从前向后，依次分为前缘层、虹膜基质和虹膜上皮。

A. 前缘层：由一层不连续的成纤维细胞和黑素细胞组成。

B. 虹膜基质：富含血管和黑素细胞的疏松结缔组织。

C. 虹膜上皮：前层为肌上皮细胞，包括瞳孔开大肌和瞳孔括约肌，注意两者的起止位置和方向；后层为色素上皮层，细胞呈立方形，胞质内充满色素。

（4）睫状体：切面上呈三角形，由睫状肌、基质和上皮组成。

A. 睫状肌是睫状体的主要成分，由三个方向的平滑肌纤维组成，注意肌纤维的起止点和走向。

B. 基质为富含血管和黑素细胞的疏松结缔组织。

C. 上皮分两层，外层是立方形色素上皮，内层是低柱状非色素上皮。

（5）视网膜位于眼球壁的最内层，由外到内可分有 4 层细胞层（图 12 - 3）。

A. 色素上皮层：由单层富含色素颗粒的低柱状细胞组成，细胞界限不清。

B. 视细胞层：是感光细胞视锥细胞和视杆细胞胞体聚集的部位，两者的细胞核聚集为该层，光镜下不易区分两种细胞。

C. 双极细胞层：为连接视细胞和节细胞的一层中间神经元，包括双极细胞、水平细胞等多种中间神经元，也是细胞核聚集为该层，但光镜下不易区分各种细胞。

D. 节细胞层：由一层节细胞组成，胞体较大，排列稀疏，核大浅染，轴突很长，向眼球后壁汇聚，穿出眼球壁形成视神经。

思考题

（1）从角膜的结构解释角膜透明的原因？

（2）从虹膜中瞳孔开大肌和瞳孔括约肌的结构理解它们有什么功能，由什么神经支配？

（3）巩膜静脉窦和小梁网在临床上有什么意义？

（4）从睫状体的结构，及其与晶状体的关系，思考视近远物时睫状体有什么变化？

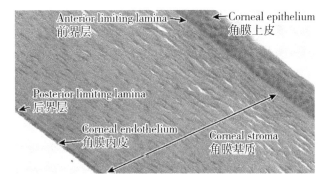

图 12 -1　角膜（HE 染色, 400 ×）

Fig. 12 -1　Cornea（H & E stain, 400 ×）

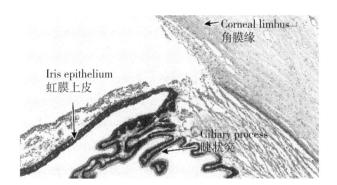

图 12 -2　角膜缘、虹膜和睫状体（HE 染色, 100 ×）

Fig. 12 -2　Corneal limbus, iris and ciliary body（H & E stain, 100 ×）

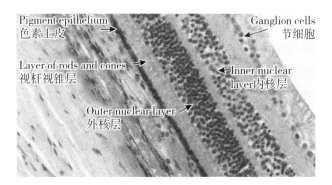

图 12 -3　视网膜（HE 染色, 400 ×）

Fig. 12 -3　Retina（H & E stain, 400 ×）

2. 眼睑

➤ 材料

人上眼睑（HE 染色）。

➤ 肉眼观察

近似长方形薄板状结构，边缘染成蓝紫色。

➤ 低倍镜

区分外侧的皮肤侧和内侧的睑结膜侧，由外向内依次分为：

（1）皮肤：表皮为薄皮，是角化的复层扁平上皮，睑缘有睫毛，根部小的皮脂腺为睑缘腺，睫毛附近有大的汗腺称睫腺（图 12 - 4）。

（2）皮下组织：疏松结缔组织。

（3）肌层：骨骼肌。

（4）睑板：呈半月形，由致密结缔组织构成，质如软骨，内含管泡状皮脂腺为睑板腺（图 12 - 4）。

（5）睑结膜：由上皮和固有层构成，上皮是复层柱状上皮，有杯状细胞；固有层为薄层结缔组织。睑结膜在结膜穹隆处移行为球结膜，变成复层扁平上皮，基底部凹凸不平。

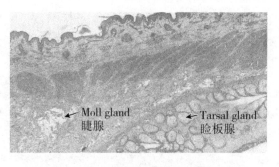

图 12 - 4　眼睑（HE 染色，40 ×）

Fig. 12 - 4　Eyelid（H & E stain，40 ×）

3. 内耳

➤ 材料

豚鼠内耳（HE 染色）。

➤ 肉眼观察

重点观察宝塔状的耳蜗结构。

➤ 低倍镜

耳蜗中间锥形红染的结构为蜗轴，两侧可见 3 ～ 4 个耳蜗管的切面，每个耳蜗管包括鼓室阶、膜蜗管和前庭阶三个部分，中间三角形的切面是膜蜗管（图 12 - 5），重点观察膜蜗管的结构。

➤ 高倍镜

（1）膜蜗管各壁的结构：

A. 顶壁：前庭膜，中间为薄层结缔组织，两侧被覆单层扁平上皮。

B. 外壁：增厚的骨膜形成螺旋韧带，被覆复层柱状上皮，内含有毛细血管，称血管纹。

C. 底壁：内侧是骨性的螺旋板，外侧是膜性螺旋板，也称基底膜。基底膜中间红染的胶原纤维为听弦，下方是单层扁平上皮，上方是螺旋器，即 Corti 器。

（2）螺旋器的结构：包括支持细胞和毛细胞（图 12 - 6）。支持细胞包括柱细胞和指细胞。

A. 柱细胞：内、外柱细胞位于基底膜，基部宽大，顶部细长，基部和顶部相互连接，形成一个三角形的内隧道。

B. 指细胞：内柱细胞内侧有 1 列内指细胞，外柱细胞外侧有 3 列外指细胞。

C. 毛细胞：内指细胞的上方托着 1 列内毛细胞，外指细胞的上方分别托着 3 列外毛细胞，内、外毛细胞的游离面有规则排列的听毛，骨性螺旋板起始处骨膜增厚形成螺旋缘。由螺旋缘伸出的盖膜，覆于螺旋器的上方，常扭曲折叠。

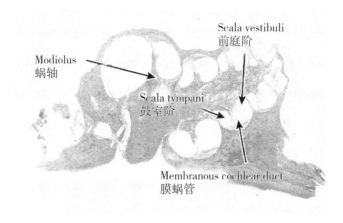

图 12 -5 内耳（HE 染色，20 ×）
Fig. 12 -5 Inner ear（H & E stain, 20 ×）

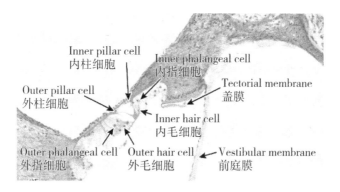

图 12 -6 耳蜗（HE 染色，200 ×）
Fig. 12 -6 Cochlea（H & E stain, 200 ×）

课后作业

（1）角膜的结构是什么？
（2）视网膜的结构是什么？

（3）螺旋器的结构是什么？

病例教学

一名 47 岁的女性患者主诉在过去的 3～4 年间视力减弱，尤其在夜间或在黑暗的地方工作越来越困难，随后眼科就诊。她在光线昏暗的房间和电影院走动都有困难。她已经放弃了晚上开车，并描述了一个从亮到暗的漫长适应期。她还说自己的白天视力"被挖了隧道"，因为她经常会走进家具里。家族史显示，她的父亲也有类似的情况。在这种疾病中，视紫红质基因的单点突变会导致信号转导的中断。

（1）该疾病影响到眼球壁的哪一层？可能受影响的细胞是什么？

（2）眼球壁的组织结构是什么？

（3）可能受影响细胞的超微结构是什么？

（王艳华）

Chapter 12　EYE AND EAR

Both eye and ear are important sensory organs in the human body. The eye is the visual organ of the human body, which is composed of the eyeball and its accessory organs. The eyeball includes the wall of the eye and the contents of the eyeball, and the accessory organs include the eyelid, lacrimal gland and extraocular muscle. The ear is an organ that senses postural balance and hearing through mechanoreceptors in the vestibular cochlear device.

Learning Objectives

(1) Be able to identify and describe the histologic structure of all layers of the ocular wall of the eyeball, especially the structure and function of the cornea and retina.

(2) Be able to identify and describe the structure of the spiral organ in the inner ear.

(3) Be able to identify the structure of the inner ear and eyelid.

Pre-class Questions

(1) What structure does the eyeball wall consist of?

(2) What structure does the inner ear contain?

Observation and Reflection

1. Eyeball（眼球）

➢ Material

Human eyeball, sagittal section (H & E stain).

➢ Gross observation

The front and back of the eyeball as well as the cornea, sclera, iris, ciliary body, optic nerve, lens, vitreous body, pupil, anterior and posterior chambers and other structures can be clearly displayed.

➢ Low power

The structure of the ocular wall can be divided into three layers: fibrous tunic, vascular tunic and retina. The eyeball contents include aqueous humor, lens and vitreous body. The vitreous body has been lost during preparation.

(1) **Fibrous tunic**（纤维膜）: It distributes in the outermost layer, which is composed of dense connective tissue, and can be divided into cornea and sclera.

A. The cornea（角膜）: Situated in anterior 1/6 of fibrous tunic, it is a transparent, slightly protruding structure, and it is pink under H & E staining.

B. The sclera（巩膜）: Situated in posterior 5/6 of fibrous tunic, it is a white structure with a deep red stain under the microscope. The sclera and cornea continue, and the junction between the two is called corneal limbus（角膜缘）. The bulbar conjunctiva is often seen attached to the sclera at the edge of the cornea.

（2）**Vascular tunic**（血管膜）: A loose connective tissue rich in melanocytes and blood vessels, can be divided into iris, ciliary body and choroid from front to back.

A. The iris（虹膜）is circular, and it contains two sheets of thin-film structures between the cornea and the lens on the section. The gap between the thin films on both sides is the pupil. Pay attention to distinguish the direction before and after.

B. The section of the ciliary body（睫状体）is triangular, connecting the iris and choroid, the front is wider, and the radial protrusion is called the ciliary process. Ciliary process is connected with the lens between the ciliary process and the lens, and the rear is gradually flat, ending in the ora serrata.

C. The choroid（脉络膜）is the part of back 2/3 of the vascular tunic, lined between the sclera and the retina, and is a loose connective tissue rich in melanocytes and blood vessels.

（3）**Retina**（视网膜）: It locates in the innermost layer, and can be divided into the pars optica retina and the pars caeca retina, and they are separated by the ora serrata. The pars optica retina is commonly called the retina, and the pars caeca retina is the iris epithelium and the ciliary epithelium.

➢ High power

（1）Cornea: It is divided into 5 layers from front to back（Fig. 12 – 1）.

A. Corneal epithelium: It is of non-keratinized laminated flat epithelium with flat basal surface.

B. Anterior limiting lamina: Such layer is dyed into pink homogeneous thin-film.

C. Corneal stroma: The thickest layer, composed of collagen plates formed by multi-layer collagen fibril, can be seen scattered in the distribution of fibroblasts. Such cells are also known as corneal cells, and no blood vessels are found in it.

D. Posterior limiting lamina: It presents similar structure with the anterior limiting lamina, but it is thinner.

E. Corneal endothelium: A single flat epithelium.

（2）Corneal limbus: As an important structure, it includes scleral spur, sinus venosus sclerae and trabecular meshwork（Fig. 12 – 2）.

A. Scleral spur: A crista-like protruding from the sclera puts forward on the medial side of the limbus of the cornea.

B. Sinus venosus sclerae: A circular tube in the anterolateral sclera, with a narrow slit covers the endothelium on the section.

C. Trabecular meshwork: It is located in the medial side of the sinus venous sclerae, and it is composed of trabecula and trabecular space, and the plane of the section is reticular. Trabecular space is a thin cable-like structure covered by endothelium on both sides of collagen fibers, and the mesh is trabecular space.

（3）Iris: From front to back, it is successively divided into the anterior border layer, the iris stroma and the iris epithelium.

A.　Anterior border layer: A discontinuous layer composed of fibroblasts and melanocytes.

B.　Iris stroma: It consists of loose connective tissue rich in blood vessels and melanocytes.

C.　Iris epithelium: The anterior layer is myoepithelial cells, including the dilator major of the pupil and the sphincter of the pupil. Note the starting and ending positions and directions of the two. The posterior layer is the pigment epithelium, the cells are cuboidal, and the cytoplasm is full of pigment.

(4) Ciliary body: It is triangular in section, composed of ciliary muscle, stroma and epithelium.

A.　The ciliary muscle is the main component of the ciliary body, composed of smooth muscle fibers in three directions. Pay attention to the start and end point and direction of the muscle fibers.

B.　The stroma is loose connective tissue rich in blood vessels and melanocytes.

C.　The epithelium is divided into two layers, the outer layer is cuboidal pigment epithelium, and the inner layer is low columnar non-pigment epithelium.

(5) The retina is located in the innermost layer of the ocular wall, and can be divided into four cell layers from the outside to the inside (Fig. 12 – 3).

A.　Pigment epithelium: It is composed of a single layer of low columnar cells rich in pigment particles, the cell boundaries are not clear.

B.　Photoreceptor cell layer: It is the site of the accumulation of light-sensitive cone cells and rod cells, and the nuclei of both are gathered for this layer, and it is not easy to distinguish between the two cells under the light microscope.

C.　Bipolar cell layer: A layer of interneurons that connects optic cells and ganglion cells, including bipolar cells, horizontal cells and other interneurons, and the nucleus is gathered as this layer, but it is not easy to distinguish various cells under the light mirror.

D.　Ganglion cell layer: It is composed of a layer of ganglion cells, the cell body is large, sparsely arranged, the nucleus is large and shallow, and the axon is very long. It converges towards the posterior wall of the eyeball and exits the ocular wall to form the optic nerve.

Reflection

(1) Can the structure of cornea explain the cause of corneal transparency?

(2) From the structure of the pupillary dilator major and the pupillary sphincter in the iris understanding what function do they have, what nerves innervate them.

(3) What is the clinical significance of scleral venous sinus and trabecular meshwork?

(4) From the structure of the ciliary body and its relationship with the lens, what is the change of the ciliary body when viewing near and far objects?

2.　Eyelid (眼睑)

➢　Materials

Human upper eyelid (H & E stain).

➤ **Gross observation**

The structure is almost rectangular and thin, and the edges are dyed blue-purple.

➤ **Low power**

The lateral cutaneous side and the medial palpebral conjunctiva side are distinguished and divided from the outside to the inside:

(1) Skin: The epidermis is a thin skin, a keratinized layered flat epithelium, the palpebral margin has eyelashes, the small sebaceous gland at the root is the palpebral margin gland, and the large sweat gland near the eyelashes is called the ciliary gland (Moll gland) (Fig. 12 –4).

(2) Subcutaneous tissue: Loose connective tissue.

(3) Muscle layer: Skeletal muscle.

(4) Tarsus: It is half-moon shaped, composed of dense connective tissue, like cartilage, and containing tubular vesicular sebaceous glands for tarsal glands (睑板腺) (Fig. 12 –4).

(5) Eyelid conjunctiva: It is composed of epithelium and lamina propria. The epithelium is a laminated columnar epithelium with goblet cells. Lamina propria is a thin layer of connective tissue. The palpebral conjunctiva can migrate into a bulbar conjunctiva at the conjunctiva fornix, and become a stratified flattened epithelium with an uneven base.

3. Inner ear (内耳)

➤ **Material**

Guinea pig inner ear (H & E stain).

➤ **Gross observation**

Focus on the pagoda shaped cochlear structure.

➤ **Low power**

The conical red-colored structure in the middle of the cochlea (耳蜗) is the cochlear modiolus (蜗轴), and 3 ~ 4 sections of cochlear duct can be seen on both sides. Each cochlear duct consists of three parts: scala tympani, scala media (membranous cochlear duct) and scala vestibuli. The section of the middle triangle is membranous cochlear duct. Pay attention to the structure of membranous cochlear duct (Fig. 12 –5).

➤ **High power**

(1) Structure of the walls of the membranous cochlear duct (膜蜗管).

A. Parietal wall: Vestibular membrane with thin connective tissue is in the center and a single flat epithelium distributes on both sides.

B. Outer wall: The thickened periosteum forms spiral ligaments and is covered by lamellar columnar epithelium, which contains capillaries and is called stria vascularis (血管纹).

C. Bottom wall: The inside is a thin sheet of osseous spiral lamina, and the outside is a membranous spiral lamina, also known as the basilar membrane. The red collagen fibers in the middle of the basilar membrane are the auditory string, the lower layer is the flat epithelium, and the upper part is the spiral organ, or Corti organ.

(2) The structure of the spiral organ (螺旋器). It includes supporting cells and hair cells, supporting cells include pillar cells and phalangeal cells (Fig. 12 –6).

A. Pillar cells: The inner and outer pillar cells are located in the basement membrane, the base is wide, the top is slender, both the base and the top are connected to each other, forming a triangular internal tunnel.

B. Phalangeal cells: there are 1 column of inner phalangeal cells inside the inner pillar cells, and 3 columns of outer phalangeal cells outside the outer pillar cells.

C. Hair cells: 1 column of inner hair cells is supported above the inner phalangeal cells, 3 columns of outer hair cells are supported above the outer phalangeal cells, the free surface of the inner and outer hair cells has a regular arrangement of trichobothrium (听毛), and the periosteum thickens at the beginning of the osseous spiral lamina to form a spiral limbus. The tectorial membrane extending from the spiral limbus covers the upper part of the spiral organ, and it is often twisted and folded.

Post-class Task

(1) What is the structure of the cornea?

(2) What is the structure of the retina?

(3) What is the structure of the spiral organ?

Case-based Learning

A 47-year-old woman is referred to an ophthalmologist after reporting increased difficulty with tasks at night or in dark places for the past 3−4 years. She has trouble walking in dimly lit rooms and the movie theater. She has given up driving at night and describes a prolonged adaptation period going from light to dark. She also describes her daylight vision as "tunneled", as she frequently walks into furniture. A family history indicates that her father had a similar condition. In this disease, a single point mutation in the rhodopsin gene leads to disruption of signal transduction.

(1) Which layer of the ocular wall in the eyeball does the disease affect? What are the cells that might be affected?

(2) What is the histological structure of this layer of the ocular wall?

(3) What is the ultrastructure of the cells that may be affected?

(王艳华)

第 13 章 | 皮肤

皮肤是人体最大的器官，由表皮和真皮组成。皮肤含有一些附属物，包括毛发、皮脂腺、汗腺和指甲等。皮肤与外部环境直接接触，可以阻止异物和病原体的入侵。皮肤中有丰富的感觉神经末梢，可以感知各种外部刺激。皮肤还具有调节体温、释放代谢物和参与维生素 D 合成的功能。

学习目标

（1）能够描述皮肤各层结构特点。
（2）能够识别和描述毛发的基本结构。

课前问题

（1）表皮是如何分层的？每一层的结构特点是什么？
（2）皮肤主要附属物有哪些？

实验观察与思考

1. 手指皮肤

➤ **材料**

人指掌皮切片（HE 染色）。

➤ **肉眼观察**

表面呈弓形，染色较深部分为表皮，下方浅红色部分为真皮和皮下组织。

➤ **低倍镜**

可见表皮、真皮和皮下组织三层（图 13 – 1）。表皮为角化复层扁平上皮，表皮浅部为角质层，较厚，着色浅红，深部为紫红色，基底部与真皮连接处成波浪状。真皮分为乳头层和网织层，乳头层由疏松结缔组织构成，向表皮基底部隆起形成真皮乳头，乳头层下方为网织层，由致密结缔组织构成。真皮下方为皮下组织，解剖学上称之为浅筋膜，由疏松结缔组织和脂肪组织构成。

➤ **高倍镜**

（1）表皮：由游离面至基底面分为五层（图 13 – 2）。

A. 角质层：位于游离面，较厚，由多层扁平的角质细胞组成，胞核消失，此层可见螺旋状走行的汗腺导管。

B. 透明层：位于角质层下方，由 2 ～ 3 层扁平细胞构成，无胞核，细胞界限不清，强嗜酸性，染成均匀粉红色。

C. 颗粒层：位于透明层下方，由 3 ～ 5 层含强嗜碱性颗粒的梭形细胞组成，染成深蓝色。

D. 棘层：位于颗粒层深部，由数层多边形细胞构成，细胞核圆形或卵圆形，细胞质丰富，弱嗜碱性。

E. 基底面：位于基膜上，由 1 层低矮柱状或立方形的基底细胞构成，细胞质嗜碱性强，染成蓝色，细胞核小，染色较深。

（2）真皮：由 1 层较厚的结缔组织构成。紧靠表皮基底层的为乳头层，含丰富毛细血管，真皮乳头内可见触觉小体（图 13－3）。乳头层下方为网织层，内含不规则胶原纤维束，可见较多血管、神经和汗腺（腺泡和导管）。真皮深部常见环层小体（图 13－4）。

思考题

（1）如何识别触觉小体和环层小体？

（2）表皮中具有活跃增生能力的细胞位于哪一层？

（3）不同人种肤色形成的原因？

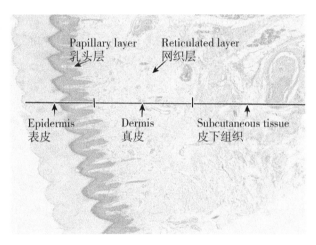

图 13 –1　手指皮（HE 染色，50 ×）

Fig. 13 –1　Finger skin（H & E stain, 50 ×）

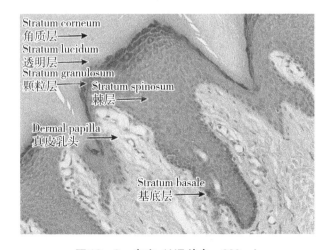

图 13 –2　表皮（HE 染色，200 ×）

Fig. 13 –2　Epidermis（H & E stain, 200 ×）

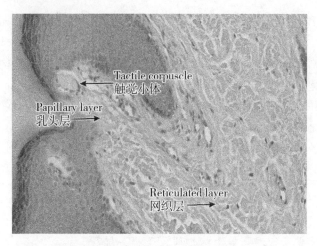

图 13 - 3　真皮（HE 染色，200×）

Fig. 13 - 3　Dermis（H & E stain, 200×）

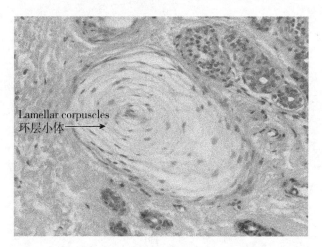

图 13 - 4　环层小体（HE 染色，200×）

Fig. 13 - 4　Lamellar corpuscles（H & E stain, 200×）

2. 头皮

➤ 材料

人头皮切片（HE 染色）。

➤ 肉眼观察

表皮薄，染色深，真皮染色略浅。

➤ 低倍镜

头皮表皮也是角化的复层扁平上皮，比指皮薄，各层细胞层数较少，不易见到透明层和颗粒层。真皮较厚，乳头层不明显。头皮中可见毛囊、毛根、立毛肌、皮脂腺等皮肤附属器。

➤ 高倍镜

（1）毛发（图 13 - 5）：暴露在皮肤外的为毛干，埋在皮肤内的为毛根。毛囊环绕毛根，分为两层，外层为结缔组织鞘，与真皮相连续，内层为上皮性鞘，是表皮向下生长的部分。毛根和毛囊上皮性鞘的下端膨大为毛球，其底面凹陷并有结缔组织突入，构成毛乳头。

（2）立毛肌（图 13-6）：一束斜行平滑肌，位于皮脂腺一侧，连接毛囊和真皮。

（3）皮脂腺（图 13-6）：位于毛囊和立毛肌之间。腺泡边缘细胞小，染色较深，腺泡中央细胞增大，脂滴增多，常呈空泡状，染色浅。

（4）汗腺（图 13-7）：单层锥体形或柱状上皮细胞围成腺泡，细胞核圆形，位于中央或近基底部，细胞质染色浅。导管由两层立方细胞构成，染色较深。

思考题

（1）皮脂腺在光镜下有何结构特点？

（2）鸡皮疙瘩形成的组织学基础是什么？

（3）导致狐臭的原因是什么？

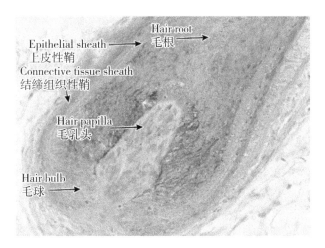

图 13-5 毛发（HE 染色，200×）

Fig. 13-5 Hair（H & E stain, 200×）

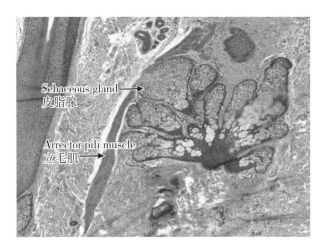

图 13-6 立毛肌和皮脂腺（HE 染色，50×）

Fig. 13-6 Arrector pili muscle and sebaceous gland（H & E stain, 50×）

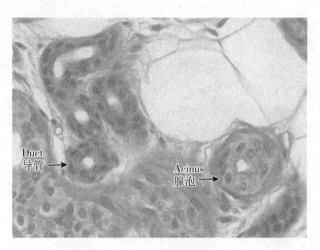

图 13 – 7　汗腺（HE 染色，400 ×）

Fig. 13 – 7　Sweat gland（H & E stain，400 ×）

课后作业

绘制高倍镜下的表皮（指皮）图。

病例教学

患者，女性，19 岁，学生。3 年前，患者前额及面颊出现小皮疹，针尖大小，有些逐渐变成小黑点。几个月后又发生红色丘疹，有的有脓头，个别有疼痛感。近几年皮疹增多并反复发作，尤其在考试期间和月经前期加重。曾外用面康净，内服四环素，均无明显效果。皮肤科检查：患者面部皮脂溢出增多，粟丘疹 30 余个。个别丘疹中央有脓疱，还有几个红色轻微凹陷性损害。患者经过去脂、角质溶解、杀菌、消炎和调节激素水平治疗，获得到满意的疗效。

（1）你生活中见到过类似病症吗？

（2）你认为该病症的组织学基础是什么？

（马百成）

Chapter 13 SKIN

Skin is the largest organ in the human body, which is composed of the epidermis and dermis. The skin contains some appendages, including hairs, sebaceous glands, sweat glands and finger nails, and so on. The skin is in direct contact with the external environment, which can block the invasion of foreign bodies and pathogens. There are abundant sensory nerve endings in the skin, which can sense various external stimuli. The skin also has the functions of regulating body temperature, releasing metabolites and participating in the synthesis of vitamin D.

Learning Objectives

(1) Be able to describe the structural characteristics of each layer of skin.

(2) Be able to identify and describe the basic structure of hair.

Pre-class Questions

(1) What layers is the epidermis (表皮) comprised of? What are the structural characteristics of each layer?

(2) What are the main appendages of skin?

Observation and Reflection

1. Finger Skin (手指皮肤)

➢ Material

Human finger skin (H & E stain).

➢ Gross observation

The surface of skin is arched, the darker area is the epidermis. Underneath the epidermis, the pink area is the dermis (真皮) and subcutaneous tissue (皮下组织).

➢ Low power

Three different layers can be seen in the section, including epidermis, dermis and subcutaneous tissue (Fig. 13 – 1). The epidermis is keratinized stratified squamous epithelium (角化复层扁平上皮). The superficial part of the epidermis is the stratum corneum, which is thick, with light red staining, and the deep part is purplish red. The junction between the epidermis and the dermis is wavy. The dermis is divided into papillary layer (乳头层) and reticulated layer (网织层). The papillary layer is composed of loose connective tissue, which bulges toward the base of the epidermis to form dermal papilla (真皮乳头). Below the papillary layer is reticulated layer, which is composed of dense connective tissue. Underneath the dermis is the subcutaneous tissue, which is anatomically called the superficial fascia (浅筋膜), and is composed of loose connective tissue and adipose tissue.

➢ **High power**

（1）Epidermis：It is divided into five layers from free surface to basal surface （Fig. 13 – 2）.

A. Stratum corneum （角质层）：It is located on the free surface, it is thick and consists of multiple layers of flat keratinocytes. The nucleus disappears. Helical sweat gland ducts can be seen in this layer.

B. Stratum lucidum （透明层）：It is located below the stratum corneum and consists of 2 – 3 layers of flat cells. The cells have no nucleus, and are strongly eosinophilic. It is stained uniformly pink. The profiles of the cells are not clear.

C. Stratum granulosum （颗粒层）：Located below the stratum lucidum, it is composed of 3 – 5 layers of spindle cells containing strongly basophilic particles, and is stained dark blue.

D. Stratum spinosum （棘层）：Located in the deep part of stratum granulosum, it is composed of several layers of polygonal cells, with round or oval nucleus and abundant palely basophilic cytoplasm.

E. Stratum basale （基底层）：It is located on the basement membrane and consists of a layer of low columnar or cuboidal basal cells. The cytoplasm is strongly basophilic and dyed blue. The nucleus is small and deeply stained.

（2）Dermis：It consists of a thick layer of connective tissue. The papillary layer is close to the basal layer of epidermis, which contains abundant capillaries. Tactile corpuscle （触觉小体） can be seen in dermal papilla （Fig. 13 – 3）. Under the papillary layer is the reticulated layer, which contains irregular collagen fiber bundles, and many blood vessels, nerves and sweat glands （acini and ducts）. Lamellar corpuscles can be observed in the deep dermis （Fig. 13 – 4）.

Reflection

（1）What are the morphological features and functions of tactile corpuscles and lamellar corpuscles?

（2）In which layer of the epidermis do the cells have active proliferative capacity?

（3）What are the histological basis for the formation of skin color of different races?

---

2. Scalp （头皮）

➢ **Material**

Human scalp （H & E stain）.

➢ **Gross observation**

The epidermis is thin and deep stained, while the dermis is lightly stained.

➢ **Low power**

The epidermis of scalp is also keratinized stratified squamous epithelium, which is thinner than that of finger skin. Each layer is thin, and it is difficult to find the stratum lucidum. The dermis is thick and the papillary layer is indistinct. Hair follicles, hair roots, arrector pili muscle, sebaceous glands and other skin appendages can be observed in the scalp.

> ➢ High power

(1) Hair (Fig. 13 – 5): The hair shaft (毛干) is exposed outside the skin and the hair root (毛根) is buried inside the skin. The hair follicle (毛囊) is surrounding the hair root and is divided into two layers. The outer layer is the connective tissue sheath, which is continuous with the dermis. The inner layer is the epithelial sheath, which is the part of the epidermis that grows downward. The lower end of the hair root and the epithelial sheath of the hair follicle expands into the hair bulb, the bottom of which is concave with connective tissue protrusion, forming a hair papilla (毛乳头).

(2) Arrector pili muscle (立毛肌) (Fig. 13 – 6): It is a bundle of oblique smooth muscle, located on the side of sebaceous gland, connecting hair follicle and dermis.

(3) Sebaceous gland (皮脂腺) (Fig. 13 – 6): It is located between the hair follicle and the arrector pili muscle. The cells at the edge of the acinus are small and deeply stained. The cells in the center of the acinus are enlarged, which have more lipid droplets, so the cells are often vacuolated and lightly stained.

(4) Sweat gland (汗腺) (Fig. 13 – 7): The acinus are composed of single-layer pyramidal or columnar epithelial cells. The nucleus is round, located in the center or near the base, and the cytoplasm is lightly stained. The duct is composed of two layers of cubic cells, which are deeply stained.

Reflection

(1) What are the structural characteristics of sebaceous glands under light microscope?

(2) What is the histological basis for the formation of goose bumps?

(3) What is the cause of bromhidrosis?

Post-class Task

Draw the epidermis of finger skin under high power lens.

Case-based Learning

Three years ago, a female student at 19 years old had rash on the forehead and cheeks with the size of the needle tip, and some of them gradually became small black spots. A few months later, red papules occurred again, some of which are purulent, and some with pain. In recent years, skin rashes have increased and recurred, especially during examinations and menstruation. She used to use facial cleanser externally, and took tetracycline orally, all of which had no obvious effect. Dermatological examination found there were increased seborrhea and more than 30 milium (粟丘疹) on the patient's face. Moreover, there are pustules in the center of individual papules, and several red slightly concave lesions (凹陷性损害). The patients were treated with degreasing, keratolysis, sterilization, anti-inflammatory and hormone regulation. She obtained satisfactory treatment results.

（1）Have you ever seen a similar disease in your life?

（2）What do you think is the histological basis of the disease?

（马百成）

第14章 | 消化管

消化道是消化系统的一部分，包括口腔、食道、胃、小肠、大肠、阑尾和肛门。

（1）消化道壁由以下四层组成：黏膜、黏膜下层、肌层和外膜。

（2）黏膜/黏膜下层的结构差异反映了消化道不同节段的功能差异。结构和功能之间的相关性是关键。

学习目标

（1）能够区分和识别消化管四层基本结构、各节段的结构差异和光镜下辨识方法。

（2）能够识别和描述食管、胃、空肠、十二指肠、回肠、结肠、阑尾的结构要点。

（3）能够分辨舌和味蕾的光镜结构。

课前问题

（1）胃液的来源在哪里？胃如何保护自身胃液免受消化？

（2）小肠到大肠，杯状细胞数量如何变化？为什么？

实验观察与思考

1. 舌

➤ **材料**

狗舌纵切面（HE 染色）。

➤ **肉眼观察**

深粉红色方形标本。

➤ **低倍镜**

由表面的舌黏膜和深部的舌肌构成。

➤ **高倍镜**

黏膜表面有未角化的复层扁平上皮，上皮下方为淡粉色固有层，上皮和固有层可构成菌状乳头，部分菌状乳头两侧可见味蕾，固有层内含有味腺（图 14-1）。

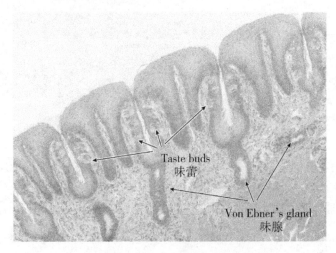

图 14 −1　舌（HE 染色，100 ×）
Fig. 14 −1　Tongue（H & E stain，100 ×）

思考题
请简述"舌"这个器官的结构判断要点。

---

2. 食管

➤ **材料**

狗食管和胃纵切面（HE 染色）。

➤ **肉眼观察**

标本近似长方形，两个长边中蓝紫色较深的一条长边，为上皮或黏膜层所在区域，该层下方标本的大部分区域嗜酸性较强。

➤ **低倍镜**

由于该标本含有两个器官，因此首先需要鉴别标本中哪个器官是食管或是胃。染色较浅的黏膜为食管黏膜，因为食管固有层为疏松结缔组织，无腺体。但是，由于胃固有层内有胃腺，故黏膜层染色较深的是胃黏膜。此外，食管的黏膜肌层不连续，而胃的黏膜肌层连续。借助上述结构差异，可以辨别食管和胃的交界处。辨别两个器官的黏膜肌层位置及四层结构的分界非常重要。

切片中，黏膜肌层下方或黏膜肌之间可见大量食管腺，腺泡周边的细胞核处染色可偏蓝。可见部分食管腺向左延伸至胃的黏膜下层。黏膜肌下方较薄的弱嗜酸性区域，为食管的黏膜下层。此层下方即为食管的肌层。肌层下方可见少量结缔组织，为食管的外膜。

➤ **高倍镜**

食管的黏膜层和黏膜下层：可见复层扁平上皮及其下方的固有层。固有层中可见食管腺导管的斜切面。固有层下方有不连续的嗜酸性黏膜肌。黏膜肌之间及其下方存在食管腺（图 14 −2）。

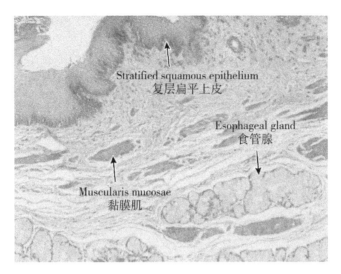

Stratified squamous epithelium
复层扁平上皮

Esophageal gland
食管腺

Muscularis mucosae
黏膜肌

图 14 -2　食管（HE 染色，100 ×）
Fig. 14 -2　Esophagus（H & E stain，100 ×）

思考题
(1) 食管和胃的纵切面能分别看出食管和胃的皱襞吗？为什么？
(2) 食管腺能够作为判断该器官是否为食管的依据吗？
(3) 食管不同区段，肌层肌纤维的变化规律是什么？

---

3. 胃

> **材料**

狗食管胃结合部纵切面（HE 染色）。

> **肉眼观察**

参见食管部分的标本描述。

> **低倍镜**

如前所述，可通过辨别切片的染色深浅和黏膜肌的形态区分食管和胃。

胃的黏膜层染色深是因为胃底腺含有主细胞和壁细胞。黏膜肌下方为黏膜下层，其嗜酸性较弱，呈淡粉红色。该层下方的结构嗜酸性显著增强，厚度增厚，为胃的肌层。部分肌层向右延伸至食管的肌层区域。肌层内斜、中环、外纵的三层结构不易区分。外膜不完整，因此间皮不可见。

> **高倍镜**

胃的黏膜层和黏膜下层：可见单层柱状上皮和胃小凹（图 14 -3）。上皮向固有层凹陷形成胃小凹。胃小凹的下方为胃底腺。胃底腺顶部和中部可见较多细胞质呈嗜酸性的壁细胞，中部和底部主细胞逐渐增多（图 14 -4）。胃底腺下方有嗜酸性较强的黏膜肌（图 14 -5）。黏膜下层为粉红色疏松结缔组织。

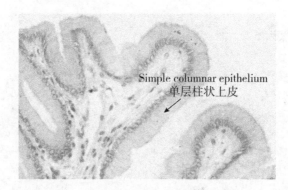

图 14 -3　胃单层柱状上皮（HE 染色，400×）

Fig. 14 -3　Simple columnar epithelium of stomach（H & E stain, 400×）

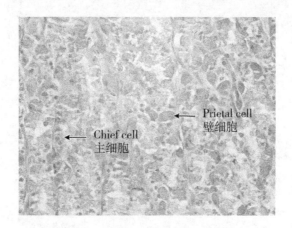

图 14 -4　胃底腺（HE 染色，400×）

Fig. 14 -4　Fundic gland（H & E stain, 400×）

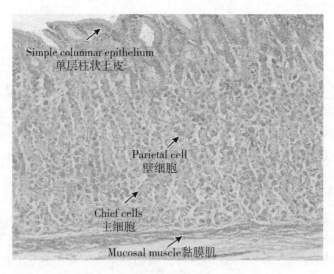

图 14 -5　胃黏膜（HE 染色，100×）

Fig. 14 -5　Gastric mucosa（H & E stain, 100×）

思考题

（1）食管和胃的纵切面能分别看出食管和胃的皱襞吗？为什么？

（2）胃的单层柱状上皮有无杯状细胞？为何此单层柱状上皮核上区看上去染色较浅？

（3）胃液对物质的化学性消化是基于哪些结构？

---

4. 十二指肠

➤ **材料**

猫十二指肠横切面（HE染色）。

➤ **肉眼观察**

壁厚腔小的椭圆形管道。

➤ **低倍镜**

管腔内小肠绒毛发达，上皮和固有层突起形成小肠绒毛。黏膜下层出现大量十二指肠腺。

➤ **高倍镜**

绒毛表面上皮细胞游离面可见纹状缘，小肠绒毛内有纵行走向的平滑肌（图14-6），可见黏膜肌层。黏膜下层有十二指肠腺（图14-7）。

思考题

（1）十二指肠腺的功能是什么？

（2）该小肠的标本为横切，能够看到小肠的环形皱襞吗？为什么？

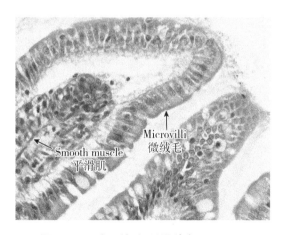

图14-6　小肠绒毛（HE染色，400×）

Fig. 14-6　Intestinal villi（H & E stain，400×）

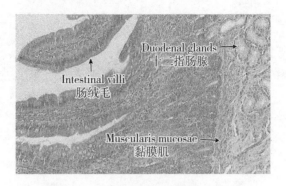

图 14 -7　十二指肠（HE 染色，200 ×）

Fig. 14 -7　Duodenum（H & E stain, 200 ×）

5. 空肠

➢ **材料**

猫空肠横切面（HE 染色）。

➢ **肉眼观察**

壁厚腔小的椭圆形管道。

➢ **低倍镜**

管腔内可见极其发达的小肠绒毛（绒毛斜切面丰富），黏膜下层较薄。

➢ **高倍镜**

黏膜下层为疏松结缔组织，无十二指肠腺和集合淋巴小结等结构（图 14 -8）。

思考题

为什么空肠是小肠各段吸收功能最强的一段？

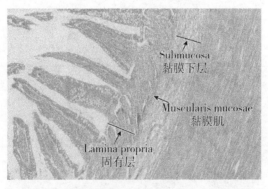

图 14 -8　空肠（HE 染色，100 ×）

Fig. 14 -8　Jejunum（H & E stain, 100 ×）

6. 回肠

➢ **材料**

猫回肠横切面（HE 染色）。

> **肉眼观察**

壁厚腔小的椭圆形管道。

> **低倍镜**

可见密集排布的小肠绒毛（绒毛斜切面较多），以及分布在黏膜下层的集合淋巴小结。

> **高倍镜**

可见固有层中若干个蓝紫色且排布连续的淋巴小结穿过黏膜肌到达黏膜下层，形成集合淋巴小结，黏膜肌在此处不连续（图 14 - 9）。

思考题

（1）光镜下，如何判断小肠绒毛的结构？

（2）如何区分小肠各段？

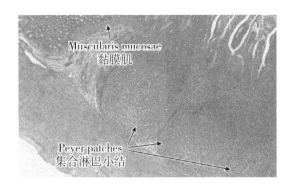

图 14 - 9　回肠（HE 染色，50 ×）

Fig. 14 - 9　Ileum（H & E stain，50 ×）

7．结肠

> **材料**

猫结肠横切面（HE 染色）。

> **肉眼观察**

皱襞明显，整体呈粉红色，腔小壁厚的圆形管道。

> **低倍镜**

表面无小肠绒毛（表面平整，无小肠绒毛各种斜切面），大肠腺长而直，腺体底部下方可见黏膜肌，黏膜肌连续（图 14 - 10）。

> **高倍镜**

大量杯状细胞密集排列，单层柱状上皮游离面无纹状缘。

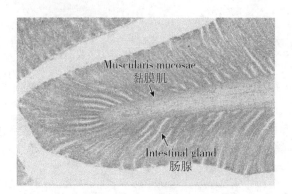

图 14 –10　空肠（HE 染色，400 ×）

Fig. 14 – 10　Colon（H & E stain，100 ×）

8. 阑尾

➤ 材料

人阑尾横切面（HE 染色）。

➤ 肉眼观察

腔大壁薄的近似圆形标本。

➤ 低倍镜

黏膜层薄，肠腺短，黏膜肌不易分辨，黏膜下层有大量淋巴组织，其中淋巴小结在阑尾的整周都存在，且淋巴小结之间存在弥散淋巴组织。

➤ 高倍镜

杯状细胞丰富，肠腺直而短，黏膜肌不连续，黏膜下层的淋巴小结大小不一，次级淋巴小结的淋巴小结帽清晰可见，小结帽朝向黏膜层（图 14 –11）。

思考题

请问阑尾发炎容易导致阑尾管腔堵塞的原因是什么？

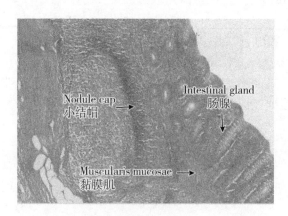

图 14 –11　阑尾（HE 染色，100 ×）

Fig. 14 – 11　Appendix（H & E stain，100 ×）

课后作业

胃和小肠内表面为了更好地吸收营养物质，因此为单层上皮而非复层上皮。那么，为何物种在进化时没有选择单层扁平上皮覆盖于胃肠内表面呢？

病例教学

患者，35 岁，女，到胃肠科门诊就诊。她有 2 个月的上腹部烧灼痛的病史，并向背部放射。两餐之间有腹胀和胃痛；服用抗酸剂后，疼痛得到了缓解；无恶心和呕吐。胃镜检查发现，胃底有一个大小为 10 mm 的单一拱形溃疡。组织病理学检查显示慢性胃炎和幽门螺杆菌感染。该患者被诊断为幽门螺杆菌相关的胃溃疡，随后进行抗幽门螺杆菌治疗。

（1）什么原因导致该患者发生胃溃疡？

（2）抗酸药为什么能够缓解胃痛？作用机制是什么？

（3）和胃相比，十二指肠既不分泌消化酶，也不产生胃酸，可是十二指肠溃疡在临床也很常见。为什么？

（葛盈盈）

Chapter 14　DIGESTIVE TRACT

Digestive tract, which is part of digestive system, includes oral cavity, esophagus, stomach, small and large intestines, vermiform appendix and anus.

(1) The wall of digestive tract consists of four following layers: mucosa, submucosa, muscularis externa, and adventitia.

(2) Structural differences of mucosa/submucosa reflect the functional differences of different segments of digestive tracts. The correlation between structure and function is the key.

Learning Objectives

(1) Distinguish and identify the four layers of digestive tract, the structural differences of each segment, and grasp the identification strategy under light microscope.

(2) Identify and describe the esophageal glands, gastric glands (chief cells and parietal cells), small intestinal villi, duodenal glands, and aggregated lymphatic nodules.

(3) Distinguish taste bud in tongue.

Pre-class Questions

(1) Where is the source of gastric juice? How does the stomach protect itself from digestion of gastric juice?

(2) How does the number of goblet cells change from small intestine to large intestine? Why is that change happening?

Observation and Reflection

1. Tongue （舌）

➢ Material

Dog tongue, longitudinal section (H & E stain).

➢ Gross observation

The sample is rectangle and stained dark red.

➢ Low power

It is composed of the lingual mucosa and lingual muscle.

➢ High power

There are nonkeratinized stratified squamous epithelium on the mucosal surface, and the pale pink lamina propria （固有层）is below the epithelium. The epithelium and lamina propria form fungiform papilla（菌状乳头）, whose top is wide and flat. Taste buds（味蕾）can be seen on both sides of some fungiform papillae. And taste gland（Von Ebner's gland）（味腺）are contained in the lamina propria（Fig. 14 – 1）.

Reflection

Please describe the structures that are critical in identifying tongue.

---

2. Esophagus（食管）

➢　**Material**

Dog gastroesophageal junction, longitudinal section（H & E stain）.

➢　**Gross observation**

The specimen is approximately rectangular. The length which is bluish-purple of the rectangle represents the location of **epithelium or mucosa**（上皮或黏膜层）, and most areas of the specimen below this layer are highly eosinophilic.

➢　**Low power**

Since this specimen contains 2 organs, the first thing is to identify which organ is either esophagus or stomach. Mucosa that was stained relatively shallow is the one of esophagus, since lamina propria of esophagus only consists of loose connective tissue without any glands. However, mucosa that was heavily stained is the one of stomach because there are gastric glands in lamina propria. Furthermore, the muscularis mucosae of the esophagus are scattered and discontinuous, while those of the stomach are continuous. According to these differences, we can identify the junction between the esophagus and the stomach. Identifying the **muscularis mucosae**（黏膜肌）of the two organs and the boundary of the four layers are very important.

In the part of esophagus, a large number of esophageal glands can be seen below or between the muscularis mucosae, which can be stained bluish at the edge of the glands. Some esophageal glands are extending to the submucosa of the stomach. The thin, weakly eosinophilic area below the muscularis mucosae is the **submucosa**（黏膜下层）of the esophagus. Below this layer is the **muscularis**（肌层）of the esophagus. A small amount of connective tissue, **adventitia**（外膜）, can be observed beneath the muscularis.

➢　**High power**

The mucosa and submucosa of the esophagus: the stratified squamous epithelium and its underlying lamina propria are observed. Below the lamina propria, there are discontinuous eosinophilic muscularis mucosae. Between and below the muscularis mucosae, there were abundant esophageal glands（Fig. 14 – 2）.

Reflection

（1）Can plica be observed in longitudinal section of the esophagus? Why?

（2）What are the microstructural features of esophagus?

（3）How are the muscle fibers in muscularis of esophagus distributed?

---

3. Stomach（胃）

➢ **Material**

Dog gastroesophageal, junction longitudinal section（H & E stain）.

➢ **Gross observation**

Please refer to the description of specimen for esophagus.

➢ **Low power**

As described above, stomach could be identified by distinguishing the staining of the mucosa and the morphology of muscularis mucosae.

That mucosa of stomach was heavily stained is due to the existence of **chief cells**（主细胞）and **parietal cells**（壁细胞）of fundic glands. Below the muscularis mucosae of the stomach is the submucosa, which is weakly eosinophilic and pale pink. Beneath this layer, the eosinophilic and thickened layer is the muscularis of the stomach. Parts of the muscularis extend to the muscularis region of the esophagus. The adventitia is incomplete, so the mesothelium is not visible.

➢ **High power**

Mucosa and submucosa of the stomach: simple columnar epithelium and **gastric pits**（胃小凹）are observed. The cells of simple columnar epithelium are called surface mucous cells（Fig. 14 –3）. The epithelium invaginates into the **lamina propria**（固有层）to form gastric pits. Below the gastric pits, there are the **fundic glands**（胃底腺）. Abundant parietal cells with eosinophilic cytoplasm are in the top and middle of the fundic gland. And chief cells mainly appear in the middle and bottom of the fundic gland（Fig. 14 –4）. There are strong eosinophilic muscularis mucosae below the lamina propria（Fig. 14 –5）. The submucosa is composed of pink loose connective tissue.

Reflection

（1）Can the epithelial types of the stomach and esophagus be reversed? Why?

（2）Does the simple columnar epithelium of the stomach have goblet cells? Why is the area above the nucleus stained lightly?

（3）What structure is the chemical digestion of substances by gastric juice based on?

---

4. Duodenum（十二指肠）

➢ **Material**

Cat duodenum, cross section（H & E stain）.

➢ **Gross observation**

An oval pipe with a small cavity and a thick wall can be seen.

➢ **Low power**

Leaf-like projections of the mucosa are **intestinal villi**（小肠绒毛）that are formed by protrusion of epithelium and lamina propria. Many duodenal glands appear in the submucosa.

➢ **High power**

The following structures can be seen: microvilli（**striated border**, 纹状缘）on the free surface of simple columnar epithelium, goblet cells in the epithelium, longitudinal section of smooth muscle fibers in intestinal villi (Fig. 14 – 6), muscularis mucosae, and duodenal glands in the submucosa (Fig. 14 – 7).

Reflection

(1) What is the function of duodenal glands?

(2) This specimen shows the cross section of duodenum. Can the **plica circulares** (环形皱襞) of duodenum be seen? Why?

5. Jejunum (空肠)

➤ Material

Cat jejunum, cross section (H & E stain).

➤ Gross observation

An oval pipe with a small cavity and a thick wall can be seen.

➤ Low power

Highly developed intestinal villi (abundant in oblique section) and the thin submucosa are seen in the lumen.

➤ High power

Paneth cells with eosinophilic granules are found at the base of the crypt. The submucosa was composed of loose connective tissue, without duodenal glands or **aggregated lymphatic nodules** (**Peyer patches**, 集合淋巴小结) (Fig. 14 – 8).

Reflection

Why is jejunum the segment that contains the strongest capacity of absorption among the small intestine?

6. Ileum (回肠)

➤ Material

Cat ileum, transverse section (H & E stain).

➤ Gross observation

An oval pipe with a small cavity and a thick wall can be seen.

➤ Low power

Densely arranged villi of the small intestine (many in oblique section), and Peyer patches distributed in the submucosal can be observed.

➤ High power

Multiple bluish violet lymphatic nodules in the lamina propria pass through the muscularis mucosae, and reach the submucosa to form the Peyer patches, where the muscularis mucosae is discontinuous（Fig. 14 - 9）.

7. Colon（结肠）

> **Material**

Cat colon, transverse section（H & E stain）.

> **Gross observation**

An oval pipe with a small cavity and a thick wall.

> **Low power**

There are no intestinal villi on the surface. The intestinal glands are long and straight, and the muscularis mucosae below the glands are continuous.

> **High power**

A large number of goblet cells were densely arranged, and the free surface of the single columnar epithelium had no striated border, intestinal glands are long and straight（Fig. 14 - 10）.

8. Appendix（阑尾）

> **Material**

Human appendix, transverse section（H & E stain）.

> **Gross observation**

The specimen is nearly round.

> **Low power**

The mucosa layer is thin, the intestinal glands are short, and the mucosal muscles are not easy to distinguish. There are a lot of lymphoid tissues in the submucosa, among which lymphatic nodules exist throughout the appendix, and there are diffuse lymphoid tissues between lymphatic nodules.

> **High power**

Goblet cells are abundant. Intestinal glands are straight and short. Muscularis mucosae are discontinuous. Lymphoid nodule in submucosa can be large or small. Cap of secondary lymphoid nodule is clearly visible, and the cap is oriented towards the mucosa（Fig. 14 - 11）.

Post-class Task

The inner surface of the stomach and small intestine is a monolayer rather than a stratified epithelium for better absorption of nutrients. So why was not simple squamous epithelium chosen during evolution?

Case-based Learning

A 35-year-old woman was referred to the gastroenterology clinic due to consistent discomfort. She reported a 2-month history of burning pain in the epigastric abdomen which radiated toward her back. She had the feeling of bloating, early fullness and stomachaches between meals. Her pain was relieved after taking antacids. She had neither nausea nor vomiting. Gastroscopy was then performed, and a single arched ulcer, 10 mm in size, was found in the gastric fundus. Histopathological examination of the lesion revealed chronic mucosal inflammation with acute inflammation and H. pylori infection. The patient was diagnosed with H. pylori-related gastric ulcer. Formal anti-H. pylori treatment was carried out.

(1) What caused gastric ulcer for the patient in the case?

(2) Why can antacid help relieve the stomachache? How does it work?

(3) Compared with the stomach, the duodenum can neither secret digestive enzyme, nor produce gastric acid, but the duodenal ulcer disease is still common clinically. Why?

(葛盈盈)

第15章 | 消化腺

主要的消化腺器官为典型的外分泌腺，也就是说，消化腺中的腺体细胞的产物通过消化管传达到效应位点。消化系统作为重要的外分泌腺功能繁杂影响大多数系统。

学习目标

（1）能够描述大唾液腺的基本结构；辨识浆液性腺泡、黏液性腺泡和混合性腺泡以及闰管和纹状管。

（2）能够识别泡心细胞，区分胰腺外分泌部和内分泌部。

（3）能够识别和描述肝小叶的结构，理解肝细胞的结构与功能联系。

课前问题

（1）外分泌腺和内分泌腺的结构功能区别是什么？

（2）相对于消化管来说，消化腺的功能是什么？

实验观察与思考

1. 腮腺

➤ **材料**

人腮腺横断面（HE染色）。

➤ **肉眼观察**

紫蓝染色的实质性器官。

➤ **低倍镜**

腮腺覆盖着一层结缔组织构成的被膜，被膜向内延伸将实质分隔成许多小叶。腮腺中存在两种导管分别为小叶间导管和纹状管。

➤ **高倍镜**

腮腺由大量的浆液性腺细胞组成，形成腺泡。浆液细胞呈锥形，核圆，底部富含粗面内质网，HE染色呈嗜碱性；顶部富含分泌性颗粒，呈嗜酸性（图15-1）。

思考题

如何区分浆液性腺细胞和黏液性腺细胞？

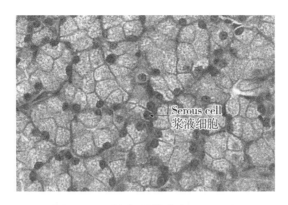

图 15 −1 腮腺（HE 染色，400 ×）

Fig. 15 −1 Parotid（H & E stain, 400 ×）

2. 下颌下腺

➢ **材料**

人下颌下腺横断面（HE 染色）。

➢ **肉眼观察**

实质性器官，小叶肉眼可见。

➢ **低倍镜**

下颌下腺含有浆液性腺泡、黏液性腺泡和混合性腺泡，所以在 HE 染色下呈明显的蓝、红色分界。浆半月可见。

➢ **高倍镜**（图 15 −2）

浆液细胞：呈管泡状排布，胞体呈极性分布，底部富含粗面内质网，HE 染色呈嗜碱性；顶部富含分泌性颗粒，呈嗜酸性。

黏液细胞：细胞呈极性分布，核扁平位于底部。胞质染色浅，呈泡沫样。

浆半月：见于混合性腺泡，少量浆液细胞位于腺泡底部，呈半月形。

思考题

浆液性腺细胞和黏液性腺细胞的结构与功能区别？

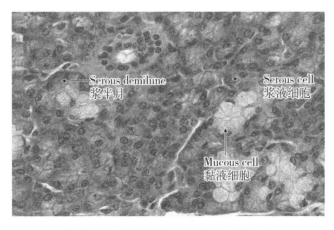

图 15 −2 下颌下腺（HE 染色，400 ×）

Fig. 15 −2 Submandibular gland（H & E stain, 400 ×）

3. 舌下腺

➤ **材料**

人舌下腺（HE 染色）。

➤ **肉眼观察**

紫蓝色染色的实质性器官。

➤ **低倍镜**

含有浆液性腺泡和黏液性腺泡。可见小叶间导管和纹状管。

➤ **高倍镜**（图 15 – 3）

浆液性腺细胞：呈管状或泡状排布，胞体呈极性分布，底部富含粗面内质网，HE 染色呈嗜碱性；顶部富含分泌性颗粒，呈嗜酸性。

黏液性腺细胞：细胞呈极性分布，核扁平位于底部。胞质染色浅，呈泡沫样。

思考题

为什么腮腺、颌下腺和舌下腺被认为是一种器官的集合？

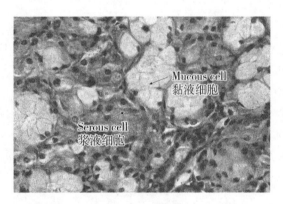

图 15 – 3　舌下腺（HE 染色，400 ×）
Fig. 15 –3　Sublingual gland（H & E stain, 400 ×）

4. 胰腺

➤ **材料**

人胰腺（HE 染色）。

➤ **肉眼观察**

组织染色呈紫蓝色。

➤ **低倍镜**

胰腺表面覆盖被膜，被膜深入实质部分将胰腺分隔为小叶。小叶内含外分泌部和内分泌部，小叶间结缔组织内血管和神经丛清晰可见。

➤ **高倍镜**

外分泌部：富含浆液性腺细胞，呈管泡状排布，胞体呈极性分布，底部富含粗面内质网，HE 染色呈嗜碱性，顶部富含分泌性颗粒，呈嗜酸性。小叶间导管可见，管壁为单层立方上皮。腺泡中心闰管的延伸部分为泡心细胞（图 15 –4）。

内分泌部（胰岛）：染色较浅，呈大小不等的细胞团。胰岛中细胞聚集分布，但 HE 染色下，不可区分不同类型细胞（图 15-5）。

思考题
（1）胰岛的作用是什么？
（2）如何区分胰腺的内分泌部和外分泌部？
（3）如何区分胰腺的外分泌部和腮腺？

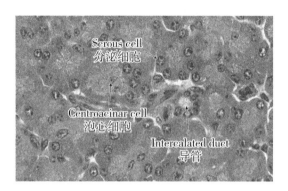

图 15-4 胰腺（H&E 染色，400×）
Fig. 15-4 Pancreas（H&E stain, 400×）

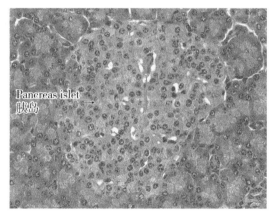

图 15-5 胰腺（HE 染色，400×）
Fig. 15-5 Pancreas（H&E stain, 400×）

5. 肝脏

➤ **材料**
人肝脏（HE 染色）。

➤ **肉眼观察**
切片染成红色。

➤ **低倍镜**
肝小叶整体染色较浅偏红，中央可见中央静脉。肝小叶四周分布的门管区染色较深呈紫蓝色。

> **高倍镜**

肝小叶：中央静脉内管壁不连续，肝细胞形成肝索呈放射状向四周分布，肝索之间有肝血窦（图 15 – 6）。肝索：由肝细胞单层排列组成，吻合链接的索状结构。可分隔肝血窦（毛细血管），肝血窦由网状纤维支撑（图 15 – 7）。

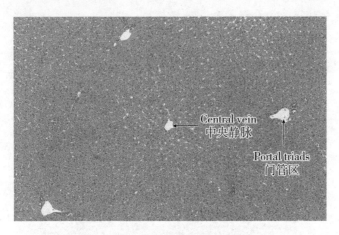

图 15 – 6　肝（HE 染色，100 ×）

Fig. 15 – 6　liver（H & E stain, 100 ×）

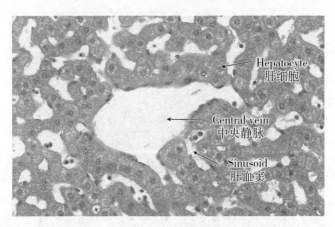

图 15 – 7　肝（HE 染色，400 ×）

Fig. 15 – 7　Liver（H & E stain, 400 ×）

门管区：分布于小叶四周，由小叶间动脉、小叶间静脉和小叶间胆管组成。小叶间动脉连接肝血窦将富含氧气的血液输送至肝脏；小叶间静脉将胃肠道提供的富含营养的血液输送至肝脏；小叶间胆管将肝细胞产生的胆汁输送至四周组织（图 15 – 8）。

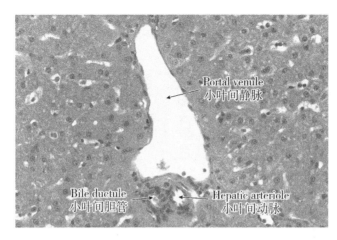

图 15 -8 肝 (HE 染色, 400 ×)
Fig. 15 -8 Liver (H & E stain, 400 ×)

课后作业

描述肝脏结构和功能。

病例教学

患者,女,19 岁,大二学生。因轻度黄疸症状就诊。患者一周前状态良好,出现类似流感症状,包括头晕,恶心,低烧和食欲不振。服用对乙酰氨基酚进行治疗,症状持续至今。早上醒来眼睛变为黄色。患者最终确诊为甲型肝炎。

(1) 甲型肝炎会对肝细胞造成何种损伤?

(2) 甲型肝炎发生后会对肝组织造成何种影响?

(滕藤)

Chapter 15　DIGESTIVE GLANDS

The major digestive glands are examples of exocrine glands, meaning the products of secretory cells are delivered via ducts to their functional site. Digestive glands perform distinct functions that impact all body systems.

Learning Objectives

(1) Be able to distinguish the microstructures of the compound of tubuloacinar glands including parotid, submandibular, and sublingual glands.

(2) Be able to identify and describe the microstructure of pancreas.

(3) Be able to identify and describe the microstructure of the liver including hepatic lobule and portal area.

Pre-class Questions

(1) What are the major structural differences between exocrine glands and endocrine?

(2) What are the roles of digestive glands in comparison to digestive tract?

Observation and Reflection

1. Parotid Gland（腮腺）

➢　Material

Human parotid, cross section (H & E stain).

➢　Gross observation

This is a parenchymatous organ stained bluish.

➢　Low power

The parotid is covered by capsule, the connective tissue that encapsulates the gland, which divides the gland into lobes. Furthermore, lobes are divided into lobules-the smallest functional unit. Two types of ducts are found within lobules, intralobular ducts and striate ducts.

➢　High power

Parotid is mainly comprised of serous cells that are arranged in acini of pyramidal serous cells. These polarized cells have rough endoplasmic reticulum at their base (basophilic) and secretion granules (eosinophilic) at their apex (Fig. 15 – 1).

2. Submandibular Gland (颌下腺)

➤ **Material**

Human submandibular gland, cross section (H & E stain).

➤ **Gross observation**

This is a parenchymatous organ with visible lobule.

➤ **Low power**

Submandibular gland contains both Serous cells and Mucous cells, therefore, submandibular gland is stained both reddish and bluish. Serous Demilune can be observed as well.

➤ **High power** (Fig. 15 −2)

Serous Cells: They are arranged in a tube or acinus. These polarized cells have rough endoplasmic reticulum at their base (basophilic) and secretion granules (eosinophilic) at their apex.

Mucous Cells: They are polarized cells with flattened nuclei at the bottom of the cells. They are very lightly stained with a "foamy" appearance (mucous has been extracted).

Serous Demilune: They are found in mixed acini. Serous cells may appear as a cap on mucous cells.

3. Sublingual gland (舌下腺)

➤ **Material**

Human sublingual gland (H & E stain).

➤ **Gross observation**

The parenchymatous organ is stained bluish.

➤ **Low power**

Sublingual gland contains both Serous Cells and Mucous Cells. Intralobular ducts and striate ducts can be observed as well.

➤ **High power** (Fig. 15 −3)

Serous cells: arranged in a tube or acinus. These polarized cells have rough endoplasmic reticulum at their base (basophilic) and secretion granules (eosinophilic) at their apex.

Mucous cells: polarized cells with flattened nuclei at the bottom of the cells. They are very lightly stained with a "foamy" appearance (mucous has been extracted).

4. Pancreas（胰腺）

➢ **Material**

Human pancreas（H & E stain）.

➢ **Gross observation**

The specimen is parenchymatous and stained bluish.

➢ **Low power**

Pancreas is divided into lobes by capsule the connective tissue. Blood vessels and nerves can be observed in pancreas as well. The whole pancreas are subdivided into two parts, exocrine and endocrine components.

➢ **High power**

Exocrine portion: Exocrine cells are arranged as acini of pyramidal serous cells. These polarized cells have rough endoplasmic reticulum at their base（basophilic）and secretion granules（eosinophilic）at their apex. Ducts start within an acinus and lead into short intercalated ducts with a simple cuboidal epithelium（Fig. 15 - 4）.

Endocrine portion: The regions stained lighter are called islets of Langerhans（Fig. 15 - 5）. Islets of Langerhans are clearly visible, however the classes of hormone producing cells are not distinguishable.

Reflection

（1）What is the role of islet of Langerhans?

（2）How can you distinguish the exocrine and endocrine components of pancreas?

5. Liver（肝）

➢ **Material**

Human liver（H & E stain）.

➢ **Gross observation**

The specimen is stained reddish. The classic liver lobule is visible but blurry.

➢ **Low power**

Individual hepatic lobules are seen as lighter areas with darker edges at low magnification. Central vein, the large venule at the center of the lobule can be used to localized the center of individual hepatic lobules.

➢ **High power**

Hepatic lobule: It is a roughly hexagonal structure with a central vein at its center and six portal triads at its periphery. However, the random direction of a section makes this classical description rarely seen in a single profile (Fig. 15 – 6).

Hepatocytes: The hepatocytes are anastomosing into cords and radiate outward from the central vein. The sinusoids run between the hepatic cords (Fig. 15 – 7).

Portal triads: At the corners of each lobule, portal triads can be found, including hepatic arterioles which supply oxygen-rich blood to sinusoids, portal venule which supply nutrient-rich blood from the gastrointestinal tract to sinusoids, and bile ductulus which drain bile from hepatocytes to the periphery (Fig. 15 – 8).

Post-class Task

Describe the structure of liver and explain the function of different structures.

Case-based Learning

A 19-years-old girl in her college sophomore who presented to her physician's office with mild jaundice. The patient reports being in good health until a week before, at which time she began having flu-like symptoms of headache, low-grade fever, nausea, loss of appetite, and malaise. She self-treated the fever with acetaminophen. The symptoms persisted. Upon awakening this morning, she noticed that her eyes were yellow. Finally, the patient was diagnosed with hepatitis A.

(1) How could the structure and function of hepatocytes affected by hepatitis A virus?

(2) What could be the pathological change of surrounding tissue of hepatocytes after hepatitis A occur?

(滕藤)

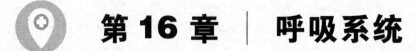

第 16 章 呼吸系统

呼吸系统在功能上分为导气部分和呼吸部分。它主要由以下器官组成：喉、气管和肺。

（1）喉：喉部会厌有助于空气流入气管，同时防止食物进入气管。喉部也能发出声音。它属于导气部分。

（2）气管：连接喉和支气管的长管。支气管将空气输送到肺部。气管是主要的导气部分。

（3）肺：气管分为支气管和细支气管，终末细支气管在肺内。呼吸部分始于呼吸性细支气管，它进一步分支为肺泡管、肺泡囊，然后是肺泡，并在那里进行气体交换。

学习目标

（1）理解呼吸系统是由一系列的导气部分（气体传导）和呼吸部分（气体交换）组成，导气部分以气管为代表，呼吸部分功能的基础则为肺泡。

（2）能够描述气管的结构特点、肺导气部、呼吸部的结构变化规律。

（3）能够在光镜下分辨肺的两个功能部，即导气部和呼吸部。

课前问题

（1）气管的各层结构与其功能有何相适应的地方？

（2）何为支气管树和肺小叶？

（3）试比较Ⅰ型和Ⅱ型肺泡上皮细胞光镜和电镜的结构与功能。

实验观察与思考

1. 喉

➤ **材料**

人喉纵断面（HE 染色）。

➤ **肉眼观察**

标本呈近似长方形，可见淡紫色弱嗜碱性的软骨片，和红色强嗜酸性的肌组织。

➤ **低倍镜**

两侧皱襞中的深沟是喉室。喉室两侧的皱襞分别是室襞和声襞。室襞里有大量腺体，声襞里有大量肌组织（图 16 - 1）。

➤ **高倍镜**

室襞：可见游离面的上皮组织为假复层纤毛柱状上皮。其下方为疏松结缔组织，含有混合性腺。

声襞：膜部覆盖有复层扁平上皮，固有层见致密结缔组织构成的声韧带。

喉室：室襞和声襞之间为喉室，上皮为假复层纤毛柱状上皮。

思考题

（1）声襞膜部黏膜表面为何为复层扁平上皮而非假复层纤毛柱状上皮？与其功能有何联系？

（2）喉部发炎时，哪里容易发生水肿？为何此处水肿可致发声改变？

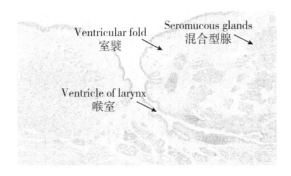

图 16 - 1　室襞（HE 染色，25 ×）

Fig. 16 - 1　Ventricular folds of the larynx（H & E stain, 25 ×）

2. 气管

> **材料**

豚鼠气管横断面（HE 染色）。

> **肉眼观察**

管壁薄，管腔大。

> **低倍镜**

黏膜和黏膜下层嗜碱性强，外膜嗜碱性较前两者弱。

> **高倍镜**

黏膜表面为假复层纤毛柱状上皮，下方为固有层，较薄；固有层下方含有大量气管腺（混合型腺），为黏膜下层所在区域。气管腺下方即为外膜，外膜可见透明软骨，及其内的同源细胞群，软骨外侧还可见脂肪组织（图 16 - 2）。

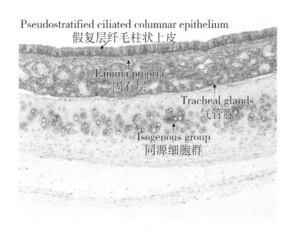

图 16 - 2　气管（HE 染色，100 ×）

Fig. 16 - 2　Trachea（H & E stain, 100 ×）

思考题

（1）在气管中，假复层纤毛柱状上皮中的纤毛和杯状细胞可发挥何种作用？

（2）与消化管相比，气管中无黏膜肌，从结构与功能的角度去分析，原因可能是什么？

（3）气管腺的作用是什么？

3．肺

➤ **材料**

人肺（HE 染色）。

➤ **肉眼观察**

内含大量浅染、微细的泡沫状结构，结构周围可见深色管道。

➤ **低倍镜**

肺的最外层有薄层结缔组织包裹，为其被膜。被膜下方大量大小不一的空泡状结构，为肺呼吸部中的肺泡、肺泡囊和肺泡管等结构。管壁厚、结构连续、深染的管道为肺的导气部。

➤ **高倍镜（导气部）**

（1）小支气管。管壁的组织结构与气管的类似，可见假复层纤毛柱状上皮，变化体现在：软骨环变为软骨片；气管腺变少，但平滑肌却相对增多，形成环形肌束（图 16 - 3）。

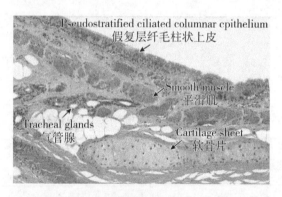

图 16 - 3　小支气管（HE 染色，100 ×）
Fig. 16 - 3　Small bronchi（H & E stain，100 ×）

（2）细支气管。管壁成分较小支气管：假复层纤毛柱状上皮变薄，向单层柱状上皮转变，甚至少量局部出现单层柱状上皮。软骨片和气管腺在图 16 - 4 中不可见。但环形平滑肌束明显，结缔组织增多。

（3）终末细支气管。管壁成分较细支气管：上皮为单层柱状上皮，软骨片和气管腺完全消失，但出现完整的环形平滑肌束，管壁薄，无结缔组织（图 16 - 5）。

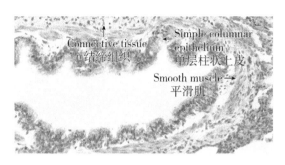

图 16 - 4　细支气管（HE 染色，200×）
Fig. 16 - 4　Bronchioles（H & E stain, 200×）

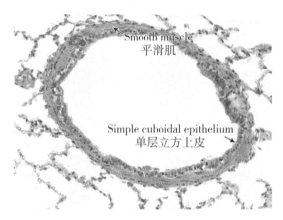

图 16 - 5　终末细支气管（HE 染色，150×）
Fig. 16 - 5　Terminal bronchioles（H & E stain, 150×）

思考题

（1）肺导气部的结构分别有哪些？

（2）肺导气部的支气管在反复分支过程中，软骨和气管腺变少，而环形平滑肌变多的原因是什么？

➢ **高倍镜（呼吸部）**

（1）呼吸性细支气管。管壁与终末细支气管相比：于肺泡处出现开口，因此管壁结构不连续；但黏膜结构类似，上皮亦为单层立方上皮（图 16 - 6）。

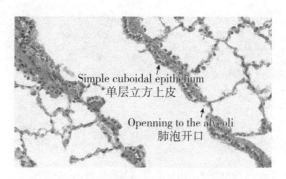

图 16 –6　呼吸性细支气管（HE 染色，200 ×）

Fig. 16 –6　Respiratory bronchioles（H & E stain, 200 ×）

（2）肺泡管。管壁与呼吸性细支气管相比：由于开口肺泡的次数增多，因此管壁极为不连续，出现结节状的膨大，膨大表面可见单层立方上皮，或单层扁平上皮。上皮深部有平滑肌纤维，呈现出嗜酸性。该特点可用辨别肺泡管还是肺泡囊。星号所在处为肺泡管管腔（图 16 –7）。

（3）肺泡囊和肺泡。多个肺泡共同开口于一侧，相邻肺泡开口处无平滑肌，无结节状膨大。可见 I 型肺泡细胞和 II 型肺泡细胞（图 16 –8）。

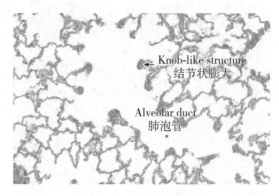

图 16 –7　肺泡管（HE 染色，100 ×）

Fig. 16 –7　Alveolar ducts（H & E stain, 100 ×）

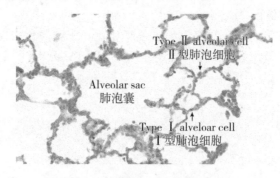

图 16 –8　肺泡囊（HE 染色，300 ×）

Fig. 16 –8　Alveolar sacs and alveoli（H & E stain, 300 ×）

思考题

（1）光镜下区分肺呼吸部和导气部的结构特征是什么？

（2）肺泡可进行气体交换的组织结构基础是什么？

（3）肺巨噬细胞可在哪些结构中找到？

（4）光镜下，Ⅰ型肺泡上皮细胞为何不易辨认？

（5）肺泡隔中含何种纤维成分较多？这种纤维有何作用？

课后作业

试比较肺内（导气部和呼吸部）管道结构反复分支过程中，上皮类型的变化。

案例讨论题

患者，男，78岁，烟龄长达55年，经常咳痰，痰多且不易咳出。2周前感冒，该症状持续加重。入院检查后发现，患者肺部有感染，脱落的气管黏膜上皮中有鳞状上皮，出现气管黏膜上皮鳞状化生现象。试分析：

（1）长期吸烟的人群痰多而不易咳出，可能是因为气管的哪些结构出现异常所致？

（2）何为气管上皮的鳞状化生？

（3）为何该患者出现气管上皮的鳞状化生？

（葛盈盈）

Chapter 16　RESPIRATORY SYSTEM

Respiratory system is divided functionally into conducting portion and respiratory portion. And it is mainly composed of the following organs: larynx, trachea, and lung.

(1) Larynx: epiglottis of larynx helps air flow into the trachea, while it prevents food from entering the trachea. And larynx also produces the voice. It belongs to conducting portion.

(2) Trachea: the long tube that connects larynx to bronchi. And bronchi send air to lungs. The trachea is the main part of conducting portion.

(3) Lung: trachea divides into bronchi and bronchioles, and terminal bronchioles inside lungs. The respiratory portion begins with respiratory bronchioles, which branch into alveolar ducts, alveolar sacs and then pulmonary alveoli, where exchange of gases takes place.

Learning Objectives

(1) Understand that the respiratory system is composed of a series of air conduction parts (gas conduction) and respiratory parts (gas exchange). The air conduction part is represented by the trachea, and the function of the respiratory part is based on the alveoli.

(2) Be able to describe the structural characteristics of the trachea, and the structural changes of the lung conducting portion and respiratory portion.

(3) Be able to distinguish the two functional parts of the lung under the light microscope, namely the conducting portion and respiratory portion.

Pre-class Questions

(1) How does the structure of each layer of the trachea adapt to its function?

(2) What are bronchial trees and pulmonary lobules?

(3) Please compare the structure and function of type I and type II alveolar cells under light microscopy and electron microscopy.

Observation and Reflection

1. Larynx（喉）

➢ Material

Human larynx, longitudinal section (H & E stain).

➢ Gross observation

The specimen is approximately oblong in shape, with red patches of strongly eosinophilic muscle tissue.

> ### Low power

The groove between the folds is **ventricle of larynx** （喉室）（Fig. 16 – 1）. The folds on both sides of the ventricle are ventricular fold and vocal fold. The ventricular fold contains abundant glands, while the vocal fold contains muscular tissue.

> ### High power

Ventricular fold （室襞）: The epithelium is pseudostratified ciliated columnar epithelium. Below the epithelium, there is loose connective tissue containing abundant seromucous glands.

Vocal fold （声襞）: The other side of the groove is membranous part of vocal fold, which is lined with nonkeratinized stratified squamous epithelium. It contains vocal ligament （dense regular connective tissue） and a thick layer of vocalis muscle （skeletal muscle）,

Ventricle of larynx: The deep groove between the ventricular fold and vocal fold is ventricle. It is covered by pseudostratified ciliated columnar epithelium.

Reflection

(1) Mucous membrane of the larynx consists mainly of respiratory epithelium, but over the **vocal folds** it becomes nonkeratinized stratified squamous epithelium. How does it relate to its function?

(2) When laryngitis occurs, where does edema easily take place? Why does edema here cause vocal changes?

---

2. Trachea （气管）

> ### Material

Guinea pig trachea, cross section （H & E stain）.

> ### Gross observation

The wall is thin, and the lumen is large.

> ### Low power

The mucosa and submucosa showed strong basophilia, while the adventitia displayed comparatively weaker basophilia.

> ### High power

The mucosal surface was lined by pseudostratified ciliated columnar epithelium. Beneath the epithelium, there is lamina propria. The lamina propria is light pink and thin. Below the lamina propria, there are abundant **tracheal glands** （气管腺, seromucous glands）, where the submucosa is located. Underneath the tracheal gland, the structure is tunica adventitia. Tunica adventitia contains hyaline cartilage, within which the isogenous groups are seen. Adipose tissue is on the lateral side of the cartilage （Fig. 16 – 2）.

Reflection

（1）What role do cilia and goblet cells in the columnar epithelium of pseudostratified cilia play in the trachea?

（2）There is no muscularis mucosae in the trachea compared with digestive tract. From the perspective of structure and function, what is the possible reason?

（3）What is the function of the tracheal gland?

3. Lung（肺）

➢ **Material**

Human lung（H & E stain）.

➢ **Gross observation**

It contains many lightly stained, fine foamy structures, with dark pipes visible around the structure.

➢ **Low power**

The outermost layer of lung is surrounded by a thin layer of connective tissue called the capsule. Abundant vacuolated structures of different sizes beneath the capsule are alveoli, alveolar sacs and alveolar tubes in the respiratory part of the lung. The tube with thick wall, continuous structure and dark staining is the air conduction part of the lung.

➢ **High power（conducting portion）**

（1）**Small bronchi**（小支气管）. The histological structure of the tube wall is similar with that of the trachea, and pseudostratified ciliated columnar epithelium can be observed. The differences are as follows：**cartilage ring**（软骨环）became **cartilage sheets**（软骨片）；Tracheal glands decreased, but smooth muscle increased relatively, forming circular muscle bundles （Fig. 16 – 3）.

（2）**Bronchioles**（细支气管）. Compared with small bronchi：the pseudostratified ciliated columnar epithelium decreases in height and turns to simple columnar epithelium. The cartilage sheets and tracheal glands are not visible in this figure （Fig. 16 – 4）. But circular smooth muscle bundles are evident, and connective tissue becomes denser.

（3）**Terminal bronchioles**（终末支气管）. Compared with bronchioles：the epithelium is simple cuboidal epithelium, and cartilage sheets and tracheal glands completely disappear. However, an intact circular smooth muscle bundle appears. The wall is thin and contains no connective tissue （Fig. 16 – 5）.

Reflection

（1）What segments does the conducting portion of lung contain?

（2）Why are there less cartilage sheets and tracheal glands, but more circular smooth muscle during repeated branching of the bronchi in the conducting potion of the lung?

> ➢　High power（**respiratory portion**）

（1）**Respiratory bronchioles**（呼吸性细支气管）. Compared with terminal bronchioles, there are a few openings to the alveoli, so the wall looks discontinuous. However, the structure of mucosa is identical, there is also simple cuboidal epithelium（Fig. 16 - 6）.

（2）**Alveolar ducts**（肺泡管）. Compared with respiratory bronchioles: due to the increasing number of the openings of alveoli, the wall of the tube is extremely discontinuous, forming knob-like structure cap the alveolar edge. And there is single cuboidal epithelium or simple squamous epithelium on the surface of the knob-like structure. Beneath the epithelium, there is acidophilic smooth muscle fibers, which could be served to discriminate between alveolar ducts and alveolar sacs（Fig. 16 - 7）.

（3）**Alveolar sacs and alveoli**（肺泡囊和肺泡）. Common space into which a cluster of alveoli open, and there was no smooth muscle or knob-like structure at the openings of adjacent alveoli. Type Ⅰ and type Ⅱ alveolar cells can be observed（Fig. 16 - 8）.

Reflection

（1）What are the structural features that distinguish the respiratory portion from the conducting portion of the lung under light microscopy?

（2）What is the histological structure that gas exchange of the alveoli bases on?

（3）Where can macrophages be found in lung?

（4）Why are type Ⅰ alveolar cells difficult to identify under light microscope?

（5）What kinds of fibers are abundant in the alveolar septum? What is the function of the fibers in the alveolar septum?

Post-class Task

Please describe the changes of epithelial types during the repeated branching of the bronchi in the lung（both conducting and respiratory portion）.

Case-based Learning

The patient was a 78-year-old male, who had been smoking for 55 years. He often coughed with phlegm, and the phlegm was hard to be coughed up. Two weeks ago, he caught a bad cold, and the symptoms worsened. After he went to hospital and received corresponding examination, it was found that he had infection in the lungs. Besides, squamous epithelium was found in the exfoliated tracheal mucosa, and squamous metaplasia of the tracheal mucosa epithelium occured. Try analyzing the following questions:

（1）People who smoke for a long time can have more sputum and the sputum is not easy to be coughed up. What pathological changes in the respiratory system would cause this symptom?

（2）What is squamous metaplasia of tracheal epithelium?

（3）What are the causes of squamous metaplasia of the tracheal epithelium?

（葛盈盈）

第17章 | 泌尿系统

泌尿系统由成对的肾脏和输尿管、膀胱和尿道组成。

（1）尿液在肾脏中形成。尿液的形成过程是一个复杂的过程，涉及过滤、吸收和分泌。除了尿液的产生，肾功能还包括调节水电解质平衡和酸碱平衡，以及代谢废物和许多生物活性物质的排泄。

（2）尿液通过输尿管进入膀胱，在此处暂时储存，然后通过尿道排出体外。输尿管、膀胱和尿道是中空器官，包含三层组织：黏膜、肌层和外膜（浆膜）。

学习目标

（1）能够识别和描述肾小体、各段肾小管及集合管的光镜结构。

（2）能够描述球旁复合体的结构，能识别致密斑的光镜结构。

（3）了解输尿管和膀胱的结构。

课前问题

（1）泌尿系统的组成是什么？肾脏的功能是什么？

（2）肾单位由什么结构组成，及其各段的分布部位？

实验观察与思考

1. 肾脏

➤ **材料**

人肾脏（HE 染色）。

➤ **肉眼观察**

切面呈锥体形，外周着色较深红色的部分是皮质，其中可见呈圆点状散在分布的肾小体；内侧着色较浅的部分为髓质（肾锥体），不含有肾小体。肾锥体旁染色深的是肾柱（图17－1）。

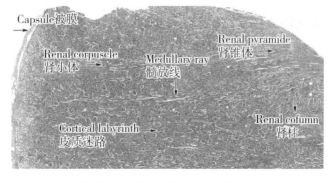

图 17 –1　肾（HE 染色，0.74 ×）

Figure 17 –1　Kidney（H & E stain, 0.74 ×）

> **低倍镜**

分辨被膜、皮质和髓质。

被膜：是包在肾表面的薄层致密结缔组织。

皮质：以弓形血管切面为界，区分皮质和髓质。皮质染色较深，由皮质迷路和髓放线构成。髓放线内有大量直行小管，由肾锥体延伸至皮质形成。皮质迷路则位于相邻髓放线之间，皮质迷路有许多散在的圆球形肾小体、着深红色的近曲小管及染色稍浅的远曲小管切面。

髓质：染色较浅，无球状肾小体，可见大量不同断面、密集平行排列的小管，主要是纵行的肾小管和集合小管。

> **高倍镜**

（1）皮质结构（图17-2）。

肾小体：肾小体由血管球和肾小囊组成。血管球位于肾小体中心的一团盘曲的毛细血管，呈现为毛细血管的各种断面，有的可见腔内的血细胞。血管球中有许多紫蓝色细胞核，核大小和染色不一致，包括毛细血管内皮细胞核、球内系膜细胞核及足细胞核，但在切片中不容易区分。血管球周围有一空白腔隙，为肾小囊腔，肾小囊壁层是一层单层扁平上皮，胞核呈扁卵圆形并突向腔面，脏层是足细胞，混杂于血管球内不易区分。

近曲小管（proximal convoluted tubule，PCT）：位于皮质迷路，在肾小体的周围，断面数量较多，管腔小且不规则，管壁厚，上皮细胞为单层立方或锥体形，细胞较大，分界不清，核圆，位于近基底部，胞质强嗜酸性，呈深红色，游离面有刷状缘。

远曲小管（distal convoluted tubule，DCT）：与近曲小管相比，其断面数量少，管腔较大而规则，管壁薄，由单层立方上皮细胞围成，细胞较小，分界较清楚，核圆，位于中央或近腔面，胞核间距较规则，胞质比近曲小管染色浅，游离面无刷状缘。有时在近肾小体血管极处，远曲小管部分上皮细胞呈柱状，并紧密排列形成致密斑。

髓放线：由三种直小管（近直小管、远直小管和集合管）构成。近直小管和远直小管分别与相应小管的曲部相似。集合管上皮细胞也是立方形，但细胞分界较明显，胞质染色更浅，透亮（图17-3）。

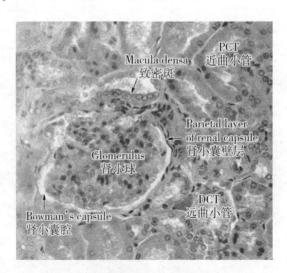

图17-2 肾皮质迷路，HE染色，400×

Figure 17-2 Renal cortical labyrinth（H & E stain，400×）

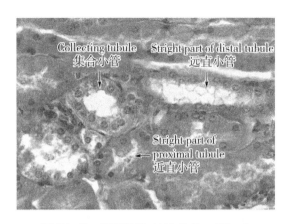

图 17－3　肾髓放线（HE 染色，400×）

Figure 17－3　Renal medullary ray（H & E stain，400×）

（2）髓质结构（图 17－4）。

细段：在近肾乳头部易找到，由单层扁平上皮围成，细胞核呈卵圆形并突向腔面。但注意与毛细血管区别，其上皮细胞比毛细血管内皮稍厚，后者腔内常见血细胞。

集合管：分布于髓放线和髓质内，管腔大而规则，管壁由单层立方或单层柱状上皮围成，细胞界线明显，胞质染色浅，部分胞质清亮，胞核圆形，位于细胞中央。

近直小管和远直小管：近直小管和远直小管分别与相应小管的曲部相似。只是近直小管管壁细胞游离面刷状缘不如近曲小管明显，其胞浆的嗜酸性染色比近直小管稍微深一点。

间质细胞：间质细胞本质上是位于肾髓质间质中的成纤维细胞，光镜下主要通过与肾髓质中直小管垂直方向的扁平形核来辨别，而其胞质因常含有脂滴而浅染。

思考题

（1）肾小体的结构与形成原尿的关系？

（2）肾小体的血管球是什么类型的毛细血管，它在滤过屏障中的作用是什么？

（3）比较肾小管各段和集合管的结构特点，并理解其主要功能。

（4）为什么肾小体周围见到近曲小管断面的数量要比远曲小管多？

（5）近曲小管管壁上皮细胞游离面的刷状缘在电镜中实质是什么结构，有什么作用？

（6）球旁复合体由什么结构组成，致密斑所在的部位是哪里？

（7）肾脏能分泌什么生物活性物质，其组织学的结构基础是什么？

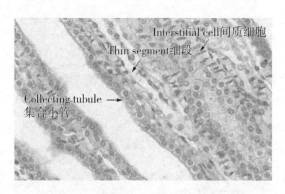

图 17－4　肾髓质（HE 染色，400×）

Figure 17－4　Renal medulla（H & E stain，400×）

2. 膀胱

➢ **材料**

兔膀胱（充盈/空虚）（HE 染色）。

➢ **肉眼观察**

组织切片呈条状，一侧不平整，表面染成紫蓝色部分为黏膜层，其下方染成粉红色的是肌层和外膜。

➢ **低倍镜**

分清膀胱壁三层：黏膜层、肌层和外膜。空虚状态的膀胱黏膜有许多皱襞；充盈状态的膀胱黏膜皱襞减少或消失（图 17－5）。

➢ **高倍镜**

黏膜层：由变移上皮和固有层组成。空虚状态，其上皮较厚，有 8 ～ 10 层细胞，表层盖细胞（伞细胞）大，呈矩形；而充盈状态，上皮变薄，较平，仅有 3 ～ 4 层细胞，盖细胞也变扁。固有层是薄层结缔组织，可见小血管各种断面。

肌层：有平滑肌构成，较厚，分内纵、中环、外纵三层。

外膜：为浆膜或纤维膜。

思考题

（1）试比较两种状态的膀胱壁形态结构有何不同？

（2）如何鉴别膀胱壁黏膜层的变移上皮与复层扁平上皮？

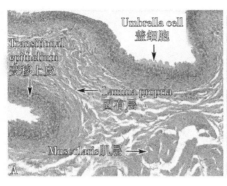
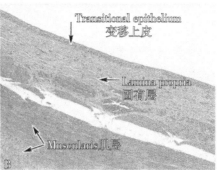

A. 空虚状态（the bladder in a relaxed status）；B. 充盈状态（the bladder in a distended state）。

图 17 - 5　膀胱（HE 染色，100 ×）

Fig. 17 - 5　Urinary bladder（H & E stain，100 ×）

3. 输尿管

➤ **材料**

人输尿管（HE 染色）。

➤ **肉眼观察**

管径很细，管腔不规则。

➤ **低倍镜**

从内向外分黏膜层、肌层和外膜三层（图 17 - 6）。

➤ **高倍镜**

黏膜层：上皮和固有层构成，上皮仍是变移上皮。

肌层：上 2/3 段为内纵和外环行两层平滑肌；下 1/3 段肌层增厚，为内纵行、中环行和外纵行三层构成。

外膜：纤维膜。

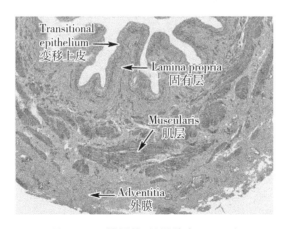

图 17 - 6　输尿管（HE 染色，40 ×）

Fig. 17 - 6　Ureter（H & E stain，40 ×）

课后作业

在高倍镜下绘制皮质迷路的结构图（包括一个肾小体及其邻近的近曲小管和远曲小管，最好有致密斑的断面），并描述它们的形态结构和特点。

病例教学

患者，男性21岁，3周前曾咽部不适，轻咳，自服药物无效。近一周因双眼睑浮肿和双下肢水肿，同时伴有尿量减少（200 ~ 500 mL/d）而入院。血压升高（160/96 mmHg），未发现肝脾肿大和腹水。常规血尿检查发现血尿，蛋白尿，不同程度的氮质血症，以及血C3和C4补体水平下降。最后该患者诊断为急性肾小球肾炎。

（1）泌尿系统的组成？各自的生理功能是什么？

（2）该患者出现水肿，尿量减少的可能原因是什么？

（3）你推测该患者肾脏可能什么微细结构受到损害（出现蛋白尿和血尿）？

（4）什么是氮质血症，该患者为何出现不同程度的氮质血症？

（张巍）

Chapter 17　URINARY SYSTEM

The urinary system consists of the paired kidneys and ureters, the bladder, and the urethra.

(1) Urine is formed in kidney. The process of urine formation is a complex process that involves filtration, absorption and secretion. Except for urine production, renal function includes regulation of the balance between water and electrolytes and the acid-base balance, and excretion of metabolic wastes, as well as excretion of many bioactive substances.

(2) Urine passes through the ureters to the bladder, where it is temporarily stored. And then released to the exterior through the urethra. The ureters, bladder, and the urethra are hollow organs, containing three layers: mucosa, muscularis and adventitia (serosa).

Learning Objectives

(1) Be able to identify and describe the microstructure and function of the renal corpuscle and the uriniferous tubule.

(2) Be able to describe the structure of juxtaglomerular complex, especially to identify the microstructure of macula densa.

(3) Be able to understand the structure of urinary bladder and ureter.

Pre-class Questions

(1) What structures is urinary system comprised of? What is the function of kidney?

(2) What components is a nephron and what is the distribution of its various segments from a kidney section?

Observation and Reflection

1.　Kidney (肾脏)

➢　Material

Human kidney, cross section (H & E stain).

➢　Gross observation

The section is conic in shape. The red outer portion is **cortex** (皮质), and the light inner portion is **medulla** (髓质) which is also called **renal pyramid** (肾锥体). Some round renal corpuscles are found scattered in renal cortex, while none can be found in renal pyramid. **Renal column** (肾柱) is deeply stained next to the renal pyramid, where the **renal corpuscle** (肾小体) is also found （Fig. 17 – 1）.

> ➤ **Low power**

Find out the **capsule** （被膜）, the cortex and the medulla.

The cortex is covered by a fibrous capsule, composed of thin dense connective tissue. **Arcuate artery** （弓形动脉） is the marker of the cortex and medulla. In cortex, the **cortical labyrinth** （皮质迷路） and **medullary rays** （髓放线） can be distinguished. The cortical labyrinth is the region where renal corpuscles and convoluted tubules, including the **proximal convoluted tubules** （近曲小管） and the **distal convoluted tubules** （远曲小管） are located, while the medullary rays are straight tubules （including the straight parts of both proximal tubules and distal tubules） which arranged parallel and grouped into a bundle. The medulla consists of straight tubules （including the straight renal tubules and collecting ducts） often oblique or longitudinal sectioned.

Then turn to the cortex again to find a good field of renal corpuscle, and observe it in high power.

> ➤ **High power**

（1） Structure of the cortex （Fig. 17 – 2）.

Renal corpuscle: The renal corpuscle is formed by **glomerulus** （血管球） and **renal capsule** （肾小囊）. Within the capsule, the glomerulus is a tightly-coiled network or tuft of anastomosing capillaries, which display various sections of capillaries. The blood cells can be seen in some of the capillary lumen. There are numerous blue nuclei of endothelial cells, **intraglomerular mesangial cells** （球内系膜细胞） and **podocytes** （足细胞） in visceral layer of the capsule, but they are not distinguishable. The glomerulus is enveloped by a double-walled epithelial capsule called the renal capsule. The **urinary space** （**Bowman's capsule**, 肾小囊腔） is between the visceral and parietal layers. The parietal layer is a simple squamous epithelium. The glomerular basement membrane is interposed between the capillary endothelium and the visceral layer of Bowman's capsule. These two layers are difficult to be distinguished from each other by light microscopy.

Proximal convoluted tubule （PCT）: Surrounding each corpuscle are many convoluted tubules. They are of two types: proximal convoluted and distal convoluted tubules. The proximal convoluted tubules are numerous, have a relatively small, uneven lumen and are composed of large broad cuboidal cells whose cytoplasm stains deeply red with eosin. **Brush borders** （刷状缘） are present.

Distal convoluted tubule （DCT）: The distal convoluted tubules are fewer and have a large regular lumen. The cells are smaller and more distinctly cuboidal, the cytoplasm stains less deeply and brush borders are absent. At one side of the distal convoluted tubule near to the **vascular pole** （血管极） of renal corpuscle, the epithelial cells become columnar from cuboidal, and are arranged tightly to form **macula densa** （致密斑）.

Medullary ray: The medullary rays include three types of tubules, **straight part of proximal tubule** （近直小管）, **straight part of distal tubule** （远直小管） and **collecting tubule** （集合管）. The straight part of proximal tubule （thick descending limb） is generally similar in structure to the convoluted parts of proximal tubule. The straight part of distal tubule （thick ascending limb） is generally similar in structure of distal convoluted tubules. Collecting tubules are distinct because of their lightly stained cuboidal cells with visible cell boundary （Fig. 17 – 3）.

（2）Structure of medulla （Fig. 17 –4）.

Thin segment（细管）: Thin segment has a thin squamous epithelial lining similar to the endothelium of capillaries. But the capillaries can be identified by the erythrocytes in their lumen.

Collecting tubule: The lining cells of collecting tubules are cuboidal or columnar, when coming across from the cortex to the medulla. Their cytoplasm is pale stained with obvious borders between adjacent cells.

Straight part of proximal and distal tubules: The structure of the straight part is generally similar as that of proximal or distal convoluted tubule, respectively, but the brush borders of epithelial cells of the straight part of proximal tubule are not obvious, and its cytoplasm staining is a little deeper than that of the straight part of distal tubule.

Interstitial cell（间质细胞）: Interstitial cells are the fibroblasts mainly located in the interstitial tissue of renal medulla. They are characterized by their flat nuclei with a vertical direction to the straight tubules in medulla. And their cytoplasm may be stained lightly because of the presence of lipid droplets.

Reflection

（1）What's the association between the structure of renal corpuscle and the formation of primary urine?

（2）What kind of capillary is the glomerulus and what's its structural features? What is its role in the filtration barrier?

（3）What's the structural difference between various renal tubules and collecting tubules? Can you relate their functions to the structures?

（4）Why are the section of the proximal convoluted tubules more frequently seen adjacent to the renal corpuscle, than that of the distal convoluted tubules?

（5）Within the epithelial cells of the proximal convoluted tubules, what's the ultra-structure of the brush border at the electron microscopic level and what's the function?

（6）What are the components of the juxtaglomerular apparatus? Where is the macula densa?

（7）What bioactive substances does the kidney secret? What are the functions of interstitial cells?

2. Urinary Bladder （膀胱）

➢ Material

Rabbit urinary bladder （in a relaxed or distended state）, cross section （H & E stain）.

➢ Gross observation

The bladder wall is in strip in shape, which is thick in the relaxed state, but thin in the distended state. The surface adjacent to the mucosa is usually irregular.

➢ Low power

The wall of the bladder is divided into three layers: the mucosa （purple-blue staining）, the muscularis (deeply pink staining) and adventitia (Fig. 17 – 5).

> **High power**

Mucosa: The mucosa is made of transitional epithelium and lamina propria. The most characteristic feature of the transitional epithelium is the presence of large umbrella cells in the superficial layer. In distended bladder the superficial cells are flat and thin.

Muscularis: The muscularis is a thick coat, mainly composed of smooth muscles. It contains 3 layers, the inner is longitudinal, while the middle is circular and the outer is longitudinal. But these 3 layers are often intermingled with each other and are difficult to be identified.

Adventitia: The adventitia is made of connective tissue (fibrosa or serosa).

Reflection

(1) What's the structural differences of the bladder's wall in a different state (a relaxed or distended state)?

(2) How to distinguish the transitional epithelium of the bladder mucosa from the stratified squamous epithelium?

---

3. Ureter (输尿管)

> **Material**

Human ureter, cross section (H & E stain).

> **Gross observation**

The ureter has a small and irregular lumen, due to the longitudinal folds of the mucosa.

> **Low power**

From inside to outside, three layers can be identified in the wall of the ureter. They are mucosa, muscularis and adventitia. We can compare it to the structure of urinary bladder wall (Fig. 17 – 6).

> **High power**

Mucosa: The mucosa consists of transitional epithelium, and lamina propria of connective tissue.

Muscularis: The muscle layer is made of smooth muscle. The smooth muscle is arranged in three layers: an inner longitudinal layer, a middle circular layer and an outer longitudinal layer. However, the outer longitudinal layer is present only at the distal end of the ureter.

Adventitia: The adventitia is made up of loose connective tissue and continuous with surround connective tissue.

Post-class Task

Draw a diagram of the structures in cortical labyrinth at a high magnification under light microscope, including the renal corpuscle, the proximal convoluted tubule, the distal convoluted tubule and macula densa.

Case-based Learning

A 21-year-old male had a feeling of pharyngeal discomfort 3 weeks ago. One week before admission, the patient had found both eyelid edema and non-concave edema in both lower limbs, associating with the decreased urine volume at the same time (200 – 500 mL/d). After admission, the patient also presented high blood pressure (160/96 mmHg) without hepatosplenomegaly (肝脾肿大) and ascites (腹水). Routine analysis showed hematuria (血尿), proteinuria (蛋白尿), variable azotemia (氮质血症) and decreased blood C3 and C4 level. Finally, the patient was diagnosed with acute glomerulonephritis (急性肾小球肾炎).

(1) what's the components and function of the urinary system?

(2) Why had this patient edema and decrease urine volume?

(3) What microstructures in the kidney might be injured in this patient (according to the hematuria and the proteinuria)?

(4) What's the azotemia? And why variable azotemia might appear in this patient?

（张巍）

第18章 | 男性生殖系统

男性生殖系统由睾丸、生殖管道、附属腺和外生殖器阴茎组成。睾丸能产生精子和分泌雄激素。生殖管道可以促进精子成熟、营养、储存和运输。附属腺包括精囊、尿道球腺和前列腺。精子以及附属腺和生殖管道的分泌物构成精液。

学习目标
（1）能够描述各级生精细胞的形态学特点。
（2）能够识别和描述支持细胞及睾丸间质细胞的结构。
（3）了解附睾、输精管、精囊、前列腺光镜结构。

课前问题
（1）生精上皮由什么构成？
（2）睾丸间质细胞的功能是什么？

实验观察与思考

1. 睾丸

➤ **材料**

人睾丸切片（HE染色）。

➤ **肉眼观察**

表面为浅粉色被膜，被膜下方有许多红色小点，即生精小管断面。

➤ **低倍镜**

睾丸表面为致密结缔组织构成的白膜。白膜下方可见大量大小不等的生精小管，生精小管上皮为复层上皮，基膜粉红色。睾丸间质位于生精小管之间，由疏松结缔组织构成，内含丰富的血管和嗜酸性强的睾丸间质细胞。靠近睾丸纵隔处为直精小管，管径小、管壁薄、管腔相对较大。睾丸网腔面内衬单层立方上皮。

➤ **高倍镜**

（1）生精上皮。生精上皮由生精细胞和支持细胞构成，其基膜外侧有肌样细胞。生精细胞分布在上皮基部至腔面，依照发育次序排列（图18-1），分别为：①精原细胞。其紧贴基膜，体积较小，细胞圆形或椭圆形，细胞核圆形染色深。②初级卵母细胞。其位于精原细胞近腔侧，为最大的生精细胞，细胞圆形，细胞核大而圆，染色深，核内染色体相互交联成丝球状。③次级精母细胞。其位于初级精母细胞近腔侧，细胞圆形，体积较小，内含小的圆形细胞核，染色深，因存在时间短，不易观察到。④精子细胞。其靠近生精小管腔面，细胞小而圆，细胞核圆形，染色深。⑤精子。其多位于管腔，头部浓缩染色很深，尾部较长。

（2）支持细胞：分布在生精细胞之间，体积大，呈锥形或不规则形，轮廓不清，含浅染的卵圆形或三角形细胞核，核仁明显。

（3）睾丸间质细胞：位于睾丸间质中，常成群分布，胞体较大，圆形或多边形，细胞核大而圆，细胞质嗜酸性强，染成粉红色（图18-2）。

思考题

（1）什么是精子发生和精子形成？

（2）精子产生后，马上就有运动能力吗？

（3）什么是血睾屏障？

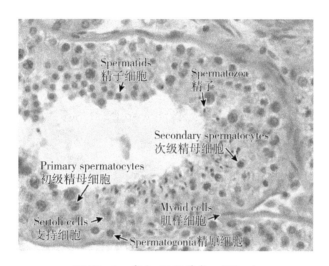

图18-1 睾丸（HE 染色，400×）

Fig. 18-1 Testis（H & E stain, 400×）

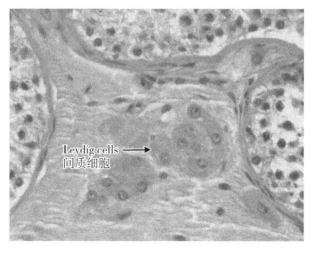

图18-2 睾丸间质细胞（HE 染色，400×）

Fig. 18-2 Leydig cells（H & E stain, 400×）

2. 精液涂片

➤ **材料**

人精液涂片（HE 染色）。

➤ **低倍镜**

外形像蝌蚪，头部三角形或椭圆形，染成蓝色，尾巴细长，染成红色。

➤ **高倍镜**

头部细胞核圆形紫色，顶部顶体浅染，尾部几乎占据整个长度，染成红色（图 18-3）

思考题

精子都有哪些畸形？

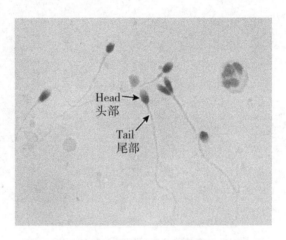

图 18-3　精液涂片（改良巴氏染色，1000×）

Fig. 18-3　Semen Smear（Modified Papanicolaou Stain，1000×）

3. 附睾

➤ **材料**

人附睾切片（HE 染色）。

➤ **肉眼观察**

结构疏松，可见许多腔室。

➤ **低倍镜**

表面被覆浆膜，由致密结缔组织和间皮构成，实质内可见两种管腔，输出小管管壁薄，管腔呈波浪状，附睾管管壁较厚，管腔较规则（图 18-4）。

➤ **高倍镜**

输出小管上皮为假复层柱状上皮，由高柱状纤毛细胞和低柱状非纤毛细胞交替排列而成，因此管腔呈波浪状，少数平滑肌包绕基膜外侧。附睾管上皮也是假复层柱状上皮，由主细胞和基细胞构成，主细胞靠近腔面，柱状，游离面有静纤毛，基细胞位于上皮深层，细胞小。基膜外有一层环形平滑肌。管腔内常见大量精子。

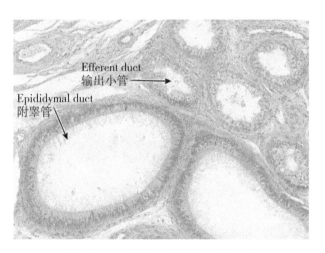

图18-4　附睾（HE染色，100×）

Fig. 18-4　Epididymis（H & E stain, 100×）

4. 输精管

➢ **材料**

人输精管切片（HE染色）。

➢ **肉眼观察**

中央管腔不规则，管壁较厚。

➢ **低倍镜**

管腔由内向外依次分为黏膜、肌层和外膜。黏膜向管腔突出形成皱襞，肌层较厚，分为内纵、中环和外纵三层，外膜为浆膜，含较多血管（图18-5）。

➢ **高倍镜**

黏膜由假复层柱状上皮和固有层构成，固有层较薄，弹性纤维丰富。中环和外纵肌层较厚。外膜由薄层结缔组织和间皮构成。

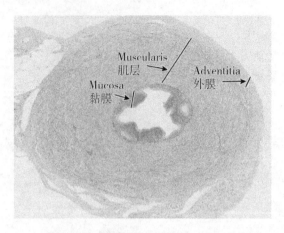

图 18 –5　输精管（HE 染色，50 ×）

Fig. 18 –5　Ductus deferens（H & E stain，50 ×）

5. 前列腺

➤ **材料**

人前列腺切片（HE 染色）。

➤ **肉眼观察**

前列腺中心为尿道，管腔不规则，周围浅染区有许多小间隙，为腺泡和导管。

➤ **低倍镜**

腺体表面为结缔组织被膜，结缔组织伸入实质形成支架，含较多平滑肌。实质内可见较多大小不等的腺泡（图 18 –6）。

➤ **高倍镜**

腺腔不规则，依据分泌功能状态，上皮可能是单层立方上皮、单层柱状上皮或假复层柱状上皮。腔内充满红色均质分泌物，有时会发现同心圆状嗜酸性致密体，称为前列腺结石。

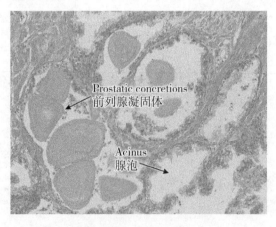

图 18 –6　前列腺（HE 染色，100 ×）

Fig. 18 –6　Prostate gland（H & E stain，100 ×）

6. 精囊

> **材料**

人精囊切片（HE 染色）。

> **低倍镜**

黏膜由假复层纤毛柱状上皮和薄层固有层构成，向腔内突出形成高大皱襞。黏膜外为薄层平滑肌和结缔组织外膜

> **高倍镜**

上皮细胞内富含分泌颗粒和黄色的脂色素（图 18 - 7）。

思考题

精囊如何为精子运动提供能量？

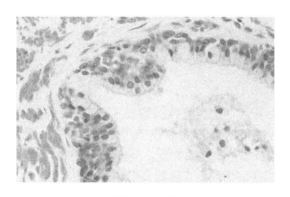

图 18 - 7　精囊（HE 染色，400 ×）

Fig. 18 - 7　Seminal vesicle（H & E stain，400 ×）

7. 阴茎

> **材料**

人阴茎切片（HE 染色）。

> **低倍镜**

可见三个粉红色圆柱形海绵状组织块，两个阴茎海绵体，一个尿道海绵体（中间空腔为尿道）（图 18 - 8）。

> **高倍镜**

海绵体被覆致密结缔组织构成的白膜，内含小梁和血窦。尿道位于尿道海绵体中央，有一个不规则的内腔。

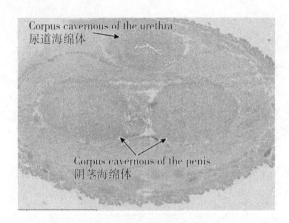

图 18 -8　阴茎（HE 染色，5.5×）
Fig. 18 -8　Penis（H & E stain，5.5×）

课后作业

绘制生精小管结构图（高倍镜下）。

病例教学

患者，男性，11 岁，学生，患流行性腮腺炎 3 天后，一侧睾丸肿痛，疼痛向同侧腹股沟、下腹部放射。体格检查：体温 39 ℃，患侧阴囊皮肤红肿，睾丸肿大，张力高，有明显的触痛。初步诊断为流行性腮腺炎性睾丸炎。经抗菌消炎治疗 7 天，症状基本消失后出院。

（1）该患者睾丸的哪些结构发生变化能够引起以上症状？

（2）结合所学组织学知识，你认为病情严重者会发生哪些后续变化？

（马百成）

Chapter 18 MALE REPRODUCTIVE SYSTEM

The male reproductive system is composed of the testes, genital ducts, accessory glands and external penis. The testis is an organ that produces spermatozoa and secretes androgen. The genital ducts can promote spermatozoa maturation, nutrition, storage and transportation. The accessory glands include seminal vesicle, bulbourethral gland and prostate gland. Spermatozoa and the secretions of both accessory glands and genital ducts are the composition of semen.

Learning Objectives

(1) Be able to describe the morphological characteristics of spermatogenic cells.

(2) Be able to identify and describe the structure of Sertoli cells and Leydig cells.

(3) Understand the structure of epididymis, vas deferens, seminal vesicle and prostate gland under light microscope.

Pre-class Questions

(1) What structures is the spermatogenic epithelium comprised of?

(2) What is the function of Leydig cells?

Observation and Reflection

1. Testes (睾丸)

➢ Material

Human testes (H & E stain).

➢ Gross observation

The superficial thin pink band surrounding the testis is the capsule (被膜). The tiny red spots underlying the capsule are cross-sections of seminiferous tubules (生精小管).

➢ Low power

The surface of the testis is the tunica albuginea (白膜) composed of dense connective tissue. A large number of seminiferous tubules of different sizes can be seen below the tunica albuginea. The epithelium of seminiferous tubules is stratified epithelium, and the basement membrane is pink. The interstitial tissue of testis (睾丸间质) lies amongst the seminiferous tubules and is composed of loose connective tissue. It contains abundant blood vessels and acidophilic Leydig cells. Near the mediastinum testis (睾丸纵隔), there are straight seminiferous tubules with small diameter and thin wall. The rete testis (睾丸网) is anastomosed together and lined with simple cuboidal epithelium.

> ➢ **High power**

（1）Spermatogenic cells

The seminiferous epithelium is composed of spermatogenic cells（生精细胞）and Sertoli cells（支持细胞），and there are myoid cells on the outside of the basement membrane. The spermatogenic cells are distributed from the base of the epithelium to the lumen, and are arranged according to the development order（Fig. 18 – 1）. They are：①Spermatogonia（精原细胞）. They are closely attached to the basement membrane. The small and round or oval cell has pale-stained cytoplasm, and a round or ovoid deeply stained nucleus. ②Primary spermatocytes（初级精母细胞）. They are the largest spermatogenic cells located near the lumen side of spermatogonia. The round cell has a large, round and deeply stained nucleus. ③Secondary spermatocytes（次级精母细胞）. They are located near the primary spermatocytes. The small and round cell contains small and round nucleus with deep staining. They are not easy to be observed because of their short life span. ④Spermatids（精子细胞）. Lying closely to the lumen of the seminiferous tubule, the cells are small and round with round deeply stained nucleus. ⑤Spermatozoa（精子）. Most of them are located in the lumen, and each spermatozoon has a condensed deeply stained head and a long tail.

（2）Sertoli cells（支持细胞）：They are distributed among spermatogenic cells. The large cell is conical or irregular with unclear outline, and contains lightly stained and oval or triangular nucleus with obvious nucleolus.

（3）Leydig cells（睾丸间质细胞）：They are located in the interstitial tissue of testis, often distributed in groups. The cell body is large, round or polygonal, and the nucleus is also large and round. The Leydig cell has strong acidophilic cytoplasm（Fig. 18 – 2）.

Reflection

（1）What is spermatogenesis and spermiogenesis?

（2）Does the spermatozoon have the ability to move immediately after spermiogenesis?

（3）What is the blood-testis barrier?

---

2. Semen Smear（精液涂片）

> ➢ **Material**

Human semen smear（H & E stain）.

> ➢ **Low power**

Spermatozoon looks like a tadpole（蝌蚪）with an oval or triangular blue head and a long, thin red tail.

> ➢ **High power**

The head consists of a condensed round and purple nucleus capped by a pale-stained acrosome（顶体）. The red tail almost occupies the whole length.（Fig. 18 – 3）

Reflection

What malformations may spermatozoa have?

3.　Epididymis（附睾）

➢　**Material**

Human epididymis（H & E stain）.

➢　**Gross observation**

The structure is loose and many chambers are visible.

➢　**Low power**

The capsule is covered with serous membrane（浆膜）, which is composed of dense connective tissue and mesothelium（间皮）. Two kinds of lumens can be seen in the parenchyma（实质）. The wall of the efferent duct（输出小管）is thin, and the lumen is wavy, while the epididymal duct（附睾管）has a thick wall and a regular cavity（Fig. 18 – 4）.

➢　**High power**

The epithelium of the efferent duct is pseudostratified columnar epithelium, which is formed by alternating high columnar ciliated cells and low columnar non-ciliated cells. Therefore, the lumen is wavy. A few smooth muscles surround the outside of the basement membrane. The epithelium of epididymal duct is also pseudostratified columnar epithelium, which is composed of principal cells（主细胞）and basal cells（基细胞）. The principal cells are close to the lumen side of epididymal duct. These cells are columnar with stereocilia（静纤毛）on the free surface. The small basal cells are located on the basal lamina of epithelium. There is a layer of circular smooth muscle outside the basement membrane. A large number of spermatozoa can be found in the lumen.

Reflection

（1）What are the functions of epididymis?

（2）How can we distinguish the epididymal duct from the efferent duct?

4.　Ductus Deferens（输精管）

➢　**Material**

Human ductus deferens（H & E stain）.

➢　**Gross observation**

The center is an irregular lumen and surrounded by a thick layer of muscle.

➢　**Low power**

The lumen is divided into mucosa（黏膜）, muscularis（肌层）and adventitia（外膜）from the inner to the outward. Mucosa protrudes into the lumen to form plica（皱襞）. The muscular layer is thick, and is divided into three layers: inner longitudinal, middle circular and outer longitudinal. The adventitia is serous membrane with many blood vessels（Fig. 18 – 5）.

➢　**High power**

The mucosa is composed of pseudostratified columnar epithelium and lamina propria. The lamina propria is thin and is abundant of elastic fibers（弹性纤维）. The middle circular and outer longitudinal muscle layers were very thick. The adventitia consists of thin layers of connective tissue and mesothelium.

5. Prostate Gland （前列腺）

➤ **Material**

Human prostate gland （H & E stain）.

➤ **Gross observation**

The center of the prostate is the urethra （尿道）with irregular lumen. There are many small spaces in the peripheral pale-stained area, which are acini and ducts.

➤ **Low power**

The surface of the prostate gland is a connective tissue capsule. The connective tissue extends into the parenchyma to form the scaffold, containing more smooth muscle. There are many acini of different sizes in the parenchyma （Fig. 18 – 6）.

➤ **High power**

The glandular cavity is irregular. According to the status of the secretory function, the epithelium may be simple cuboidal epithelium, simple columnar epithelium or pseudostratified columnar epithelium. The lumen is filled with red homogeneous secretions, and sometimes concentric round acidophilic dense bodies called prostatic concretions （前列腺凝固体）are found.

6. Seminal Vesicle （精囊）

➤ **Material**

Human seminal vesicle （H & E stain）.

➤ **Gross observation**

Several similar tubular profiles.

➤ **Low power**

The mucosa consists of pseudostratified ciliated columnar epithelium and thin lamina propria, which protrude into the cavity to form tall plica. Outside the mucosa is the muscularis which is composed of thick layers of smooth muscle. The outmost layer is the adventitia which is made up of connective tissue.

➤ **High power**

The epithelial cells are rich in secretory granules and yellowish lipofuscin （黄色脂褐素） （Fig. 18 – 7）.

7. Penis（阴茎）

➢ **Material**

Human penis（H & E stain）.

➢ **Gross observation**

Oval section.

➢ **Low power**

Three pink cylindrical masses of spongy tissue, two corpora cavernous（海绵体）of the penis and one corpus cavernous of the urethra, can be seen（the middle cavity is the urethra）（Fig. 18 – 8）.

➢ **High power**

The corpora cavernous are covered with tunica albuginea composed of dense connective tissue, which contains trabeculae and sinusoid. The urethra is located in the center of the corpus cavernous of the urethra and has an irregular internal cavity.

Post-class Task

Draw a seminiferous tubule under high power.

Case-based Learning

A 11-year-old male student suffered mumps（流行性腮腺炎）for 3 days, one side of the testis became swollen and painful. The pain radiated to the ipsilateral groin（同侧腹股沟）and lower abdomen（下腹部）. Physical examination showed the body temperature was 39 ℃, the scrotum（阴囊）skin on the affected side was red and swollen. The testis was swollen and the tension was high, in addition, there was obvious tenderness（触痛）. The initial diagnosis was mumps orchitis（腮腺炎性睾丸炎）. After 7 days of anti-bacterial and anti-inflammatory treatment, the patient was discharged（出院）after the symptoms basically disappeared.

（1）Which structural changes of the patient's testis can cause the symptoms mentioned above?

（2）Based on the histological knowledge you have learned, what follow-up changes do you think will happen when the disease becomes serious?

（马百成）

第19章 ｜ 女性生殖系统

女性生殖系统由成对的卵巢和输卵管，以及子宫、阴道和外生殖器组成。卵巢培育和产生雌性配子（卵子）以及分泌类固醇激素，从而调节女性生殖器官的生长发育。输卵管是输送卵子的管道，也是完成受精的场所。子宫是孕育胎儿的器官，也是月经发生的地方。乳腺相应的内容也编写于本章中，因为它与生殖器官的功能相关。

学习目标

（1）能够描述女性生殖系统的组成。

（2）能够识别和描述每个阶段的卵泡、黄体、子宫壁的结构和各时期子宫内膜的特点，能够描述输卵管、子宫颈、阴道和乳腺的结构特点。

（3）能够理解子宫内膜周期性变化与卵巢激素水平的联系。

课前问题

（1）女性生殖系统有哪些器官构成？

（2）子宫内膜为什么会出现周期性改变？

实验观察与思考

1. 卵巢

➤ **材料**

兔卵巢切片（HE 染色）。

➤ **肉眼观察**

卵巢的横切面呈椭圆形，周边为皮质，皮质表面光滑，皮质中可见大小不等不同发育阶段的卵泡。中央为髓质，由疏松结缔组织构成，着色较浅。

➤ **低倍镜**

区分卵巢皮质和髓质。皮质位于卵巢浅层，皮质表面为单层扁平细胞或单层立方细胞，上皮下方为致密结缔组织构成的白膜。皮质中可见大量不同形态的卵泡、闭锁卵泡、黄体和卵泡间的结缔组织。髓质着色浅，为疏松结缔组织构成。

➤ **高倍镜**

灰质位于白膜深层，由不同发育阶段的各级卵泡和黄体构成。

（1）原始卵泡：位于皮质浅层，数量最多，体积最小。由一个体积较大的初级卵母细胞和单层扁平的卵泡细胞组成。初级卵母细胞体积大，核圆形，居中，染色浅，核仁明显。卵泡细胞围绕着卵母细胞单层排列，细胞体积小，界限不清（图19-1）。

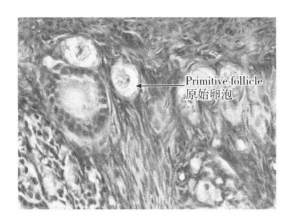

图 19 -1 原始卵泡 (HE 染色，400 ×)
Fig. 19 -1 Primitive follicle (H & E stain，400 ×)

（2）初级卵泡：体积增大，卵泡中央有一个体积较大的初级卵母细胞，卵母细胞周边有染色较红的透明带。围绕着初级卵母细胞的卵泡细胞为立方体或柱状，细胞为多层，早期也可为单层。卵泡细胞周围的结缔组织逐渐密集，形成卵泡膜（图 19 -2）。

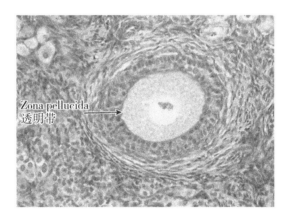

图 19 -2 初级卵泡 (HE 染色，400 ×)
Fig. 19 -2 Primary follicle (H & E stain，400 ×)

（3）次级卵泡：卵泡体积进一步增大，卵泡中出现卵泡腔，为其特有特征，围绕卵母细胞周边透明带的卵泡细胞呈放射状排列，为放射冠，细胞形态为柱状。随着卵泡腔的增大，初级卵母细胞、透明带放射冠和其周围的卵泡细胞被推挤到卵泡腔的一侧，称为卵丘。组成卵泡壁的卵泡细胞则称为颗粒层。此时包绕在卵泡周边的由结缔组织组成的卵泡膜分成为内、外两层。卵泡膜内层细胞较多，外层纤维较多（图 19 -3）。

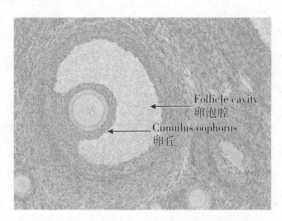

图 19 – 3　次级卵泡（HE 染色，400×）
Fig. 19 – 3　Secondary follicle（H & E stain，400×）

（4）成熟卵泡：其结构与晚期次级卵泡相似，但是成熟卵泡体积进一步增大，卵泡腔体积也增大，突出卵巢表面，颗粒细胞层变薄，通常情况下切片中不易找到成熟卵泡。

（5）闭锁卵泡：数量较多，卵巢内大部分卵泡不能发育成熟，这些卵泡可以在不同发育阶段退化，退化的卵泡为闭锁卵泡。闭锁卵泡结构特点表现为：形态结构不一致，大小不规则，呈塌陷状。卵泡细胞退化，卵母细胞核固缩，细胞形态不规则，卵泡细胞变小和分散，透明带皱缩。有些卵泡膜细胞肥大呈上皮样的细胞团，称间质腺。

思考题

（1）卵泡发育经过哪些阶段？各阶段有哪些特征？
（2）光镜下，你能找到卵丘吗？
（3）什么是闭锁卵泡？
（4）什么是透明带？
（5）透明带有哪些蛋白组成？

---

2. 黄体

➤ **材料**

兔卵巢切片（HE 染色）。

➤ **肉眼观察**

体积较大的淡红色细胞团。

➤ **低倍镜**

数量较少，由体积较大、染色浅的细胞团组成，散在分布于卵泡之间。

➤ **高倍镜**

体积大，周围有结缔组织包绕，细胞排列呈团索状或条索状，毛细血管丰富。黄体由颗粒黄体细胞和膜黄体细胞组成，颗粒黄体细胞，位于黄体中央，数量多，体积大，呈多边形，核大，圆形或者椭圆形，居中，胞质呈红色，染色浅，可见空泡状的脂滴。膜黄体细胞，位于黄体周边，数量少，体积小，胞质和核染色较深（图 19 – 4）。

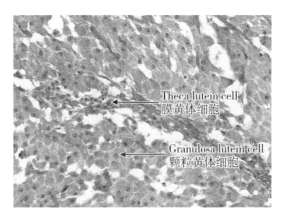

图 19-4　黄体（HE 染色，400×）

Fig. 19-4　Corpus luteum（H & E stain，400×）

3. 子宫

➢　**材料**

人子宫切片（HE 染色）。

➢　**肉眼观察**

子宫切片呈卵圆形，中央紫蓝色部分为子宫内膜，粉红色较厚的部位为肌层。

➢　**低倍镜**

辨别出子宫内膜、肌层及浆膜三层结构，但三层之间没有明显分界，重点观察内膜以及分期。

➢　**高倍镜**

（1）内膜。

A. 增生期子宫内膜：子宫内膜较厚，表面上为单层柱状上皮，上皮向固有膜凹陷形成子宫腺，子宫腺为单管腺，切片上多为横形切面和斜形切面，管腔内可见分泌物情况，固有层纤维很细，不明显，但细胞很多。此时可见到一些血管，为微型动脉横切面，即为螺旋动脉（图 19-5）。

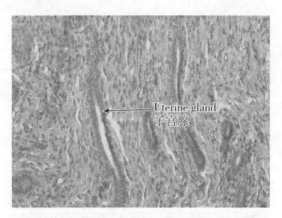

图 19 -5　增生期子宫内膜（HE 染色，400 ×）

Fig. 19 -5　Proliferative endometrium（H & E stain，400 ×）

　　B. 分泌期子宫内膜：子宫内膜最厚，子宫腺增长而弯曲，腺腔扩大，形态不一，腺细胞着色浅，在胞核上方或下方可见空泡。此外，可见体积较大的基质细胞，胞质内充满糖原和脂滴，细胞着色较浅。螺旋动脉增生弯曲，切片中螺旋动脉增多（图19 -6）。

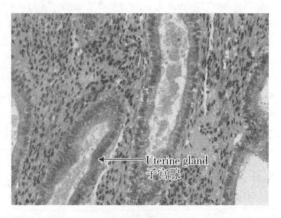

图 19 -6　分泌期子宫内膜（HE 染色，400 ×）

Fig. 19 -6　Secretory endometrium（H & E stain，400 ×）

　　C. 月经期子宫内膜：此时子宫内膜最薄，子宫腺减少，腺细胞着色浅，体积变小，基质细胞减少，体积变小（图 19 -7）。

　　（2）肌层：最厚，可见大量平滑肌束的不同切面，肌束间可见结缔组织（图 19 -8）。

　　（3）外膜：为浆膜，表面为单层扁平上皮，上皮深部为结缔组织（图 19 -8）。

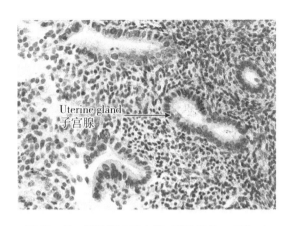

图 19 -7　月经期子宫内膜（HE 染色，400 ×）

Fig. 19 -7　Menstrual endometrium（H & E stain，400 ×）

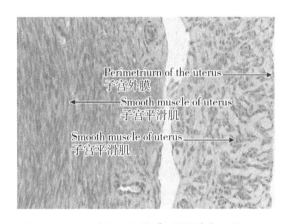

图 19 -8　子宫肌层和外膜（HE 染色，400 ×）

Fig. 19 -8　Myometrium and perimetrium of the uterus（H & E stain，400 ×）

思考题

子宫内膜分哪几个期，每个阶段的特点？

---

4. 子宫颈

➢ **材料**

人子宫颈切片（HE 染色）。

➢ **肉眼观察**

染色较深的皱褶细胞团为黏膜，黏膜深层为肌层，肌层的深部为纤维膜。

➢ **低倍镜**

区分子宫颈三层结构，即黏膜、肌层和纤维膜。黏膜为单层柱状上皮，肌层为平滑肌，平滑肌小而分散，结缔组织较多，纤维膜由结缔组织组成。

➢ **高倍镜**

黏膜上皮为单层柱状细胞，由纤毛细胞、分泌细胞和储备细胞构成。纤毛细胞为柱状，核椭圆形，细胞游离面可见染成红色的纤毛，分泌细胞胞质内可见淡染的空泡状结构，储备细胞在光镜下不易辨别。子宫颈靠近阴道部时候，细胞为复层扁平上皮。肌层为平滑肌，切片上表现为横切或斜切。纤维膜为结缔组织（图 19 - 9）。

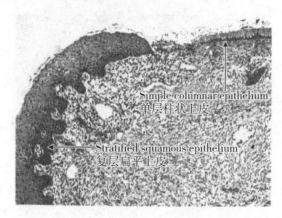

图 19 - 9　子宫颈外口（HE 染色，400 ×）
Fig. 19 - 9　The external os of cervix（H & E stain, 400 ×）

思考题
(1) 子宫颈分肌层，各层结构特点是什么？
(2) 为什么子宫颈容易发生癌变？

5. 输卵管

➤ **材料**
人输卵管切片（HE 染色）。

➤ **肉眼观察**
标本中可见环形结构，腔小而不规则，腔面染成紫色部位为黏膜，深部为肌层，最外层的结构为外膜。

➤ **低倍镜**
中央染色较深的皱襞为黏膜，由上皮和固有层组成，固有层较薄。黏膜深层为肌层，由内环形和外纵行两层平滑肌构成，内层薄，外层厚。肌层的外面为浆膜，由间皮和结缔组织构成。

➤ **高倍镜**
(1) 黏膜：由许多皱褶突入输卵管腔内，上皮为单层柱状上皮，由分泌细胞和纤毛细胞构成，纤毛细胞体积大，核椭圆形，靠近基底面，游离面有纤毛，胞质染色浅。分泌细胞体积小，核为椭圆形，胞质嗜酸性强。固有层薄，为致密结缔组织构成，血管丰富（图 19 - 10）。
(2) 肌层：由内环和外纵两层平滑肌构成，内层平滑肌被纵切，平滑肌为梭形，核呈杆状；外层平滑肌被横切，平滑肌为圆形，核呈圆形居中。
(3) 外膜：由间皮和结缔组织构成，间皮附在最外层，为单层扁平上皮。

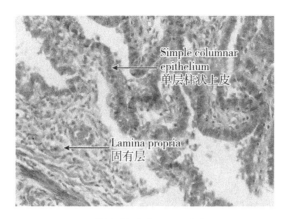

图 19 –10 输卵管黏膜（HE 染色，400 ×）

Fig. 19 –10 Mucosa of uterine tube（H & E stain，400 ×）

思考题

（1）输卵管有几层？

（2）输卵管每层的结构特点是什么？

---

6. 阴道

➤ **材料**

人阴道切片（HE 染色）。

➤ **肉眼观察**

标本一侧染成蓝色为黏膜层，其余为肌层和外膜。

➤ **低倍镜**

黏膜突起形成皱襞，由上皮和固有层构成，上皮为未角化的复层扁平上皮，固有层为结缔组织。黏膜深层为肌层，由内环形和外纵行两层平滑肌构成，两者分界不清，外面为结缔组织。

➤ **高倍镜**

（1）黏膜：上皮为未角化的复层扁平上皮，浅层由 1 ～ 2 层扁平细胞组成，核为扁平状，胞质染成红色，中间层为数层多边形细胞组成，核椭圆形居中，底层由矮柱状或立方形细胞组成，核圆形居中。固有层为含有弹性纤维和血管的结缔组织构成（图 19 –11）。

（2）肌层：由内环形和外纵形两层平滑肌构成，平滑肌为纵切时，细胞为梭形，核呈杆状，平滑肌为横切时，细胞为圆形，核呈圆形居中。

（3）外膜：由结缔组织构成。

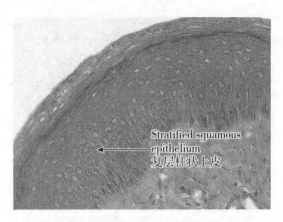

图19-11 阴道黏膜上皮（HE染色，400×）

Fig. 19-11 Vaginal mucosa epithelium（H & E stain，400×）

思考题

请问阴道壁分哪几层？各层的组织学结构有哪些特点？

---

7. 乳腺

➤ 材料

人乳腺切片（HE染色）。

➤ 肉眼观察

标本一侧染色深的结构为表皮，粉红色深部组织中形态不规则呈分叶状的结构为乳腺小叶。

静止期乳腺

➤ 低倍镜

静止期乳腺由少量的腺组织和大量的结缔组织组成，腺体和导管不发达。脂肪组织丰富。

➤ 高倍镜

在大量的结缔组织和脂肪组织中可见有少量的乳腺组织，小叶内腺泡少，腺泡上皮为单层立方形或柱状细胞，腺泡腔较小，小叶内导管和小叶间导管管腔较大，小叶内导管由单层柱状组成，小叶间导管由复层柱状上皮组成。总导管靠近皮肤时导管上皮演变为复层扁平上皮（图19-12）。

活动期乳腺

➤ 低倍镜：

活动期乳腺由大量的乳腺组织和少量的结缔组织组成，脂肪组织少。结缔组织将腺体分成许多小叶，腺泡腔大，腺泡腔内有染成紫红色的分泌物。小叶间导管管腔较大，上皮为单层柱状上皮或复层类型上皮，小叶内导管与腺泡难于区分。

➤ 高倍镜

哺乳期和妊娠期乳腺组织结构相似，结缔组织少，腺体发达，腺泡腔大，腺上皮形态可呈现高柱状、立方形或扁平状。腺泡上皮细胞为单层扁平上皮或单层立方上皮等，代表不同分泌时期的腺泡。分泌前的腺泡上皮为立方上皮，分泌后的腺泡上皮为扁平状，腔内有染成紫红色分泌物的乳汁（图 19-13）。

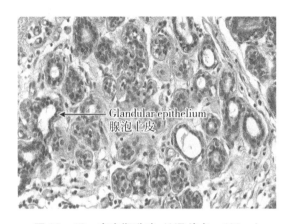

图 19-12 青春期乳腺（HE 染色，400×）

Fig. 19-12 Mammary gland during puberty（H & E stain，400×）

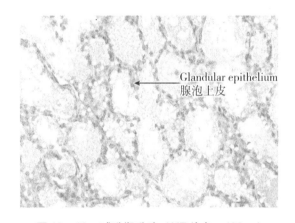

图 19-13 哺乳期乳腺（HE 染色，400×）

Fig. 19-13 Mammary gland during lactation（H & E stain，400×）

思考题

（1）乳腺分哪两个期？

（2）乳腺各期有哪些结构特点？

课后作业

绘制次级卵泡高倍镜下的结构图。

病例教学

患者，女，40 岁，平时月经周期规律，发病当日处于月经周期第 22 天。突然感觉右下腹疼痛，伴随恶心和呕吐，大小便频繁。查体：右下腹压痛反跳痛，可触及境界不清包块，移动性浊音阳性。宫颈举痛，子宫后穹隆饱满，触痛。体征为贫血貌，脉率快，血压下降。B 超提示黄体囊肿破裂。

    （1）黄体是如何形成的？黄体如何演变？

    （2）黄体囊肿破裂后该如何处理？

    （3）黄体破裂后为什么会导致血压下降？

（陈雄林）

Chapter 19　FEMALE REPRODUCTIVE SYSTEM

The female reproductive system is composed of the paired ovaries and uterine tubes, the uterus, the vagina, and the external genitalia. The ovary cultivates and produces female gametes and secretes steroid hormones, which regulate the growth and development of female reproductive organs. The uterine tubes carry female gametes and is the place for fertilization. The uterus is the organ that breeds the fetus and the place where menstruation occurs. The mammary gland is also included in this chapter because of its relationship with the function of reproductive organs.

Learning Objectives

(1) Be able to describe the composition of female reproductive system.

(2) Be able to identify and describe the structures of follicles, corpus luteum and uterine wall and the characteristics of endometrium at each stage, as well as the structural characteristics of fallopian tubes, cervix, vagina and mammary gland.

(3) Be able to understand the relationship between endometrial periodic changes and ovarian hormone levels.

Pre-class Questions

(1) What are the components of the female reproductive system?

(2) Why does the endometrium periodically change?

Observation and Reflection

1. Ovary（卵巢）

➢ Material

Rabbit ovary, section（H & E stain）.

➢ Gross observation

The transverse section of the ovary is oval, and the peripheral part is **cortex**（皮质）. The cortex surface is smooth, and the follicles of different development stages can be seen in the cortex. The central part is **medulla**（髓质）, which is composed of loose connective tissue with light staining.

➢ Low power

The cortex and medulla of ovary can be distinguished using low power microscope. The cortex is located in the superficial layer of the ovary. The surface of the cortex is a single layer of squamous cells or a single layer of cuboidal cells. Below the epithelium is the tunica albuginea（白膜）which is composed of dense connective tissue. A large number of follicles, corpus luteum（黄体）and connective tissue between follicles can be seen in the cortex. The medulla is lightly stained and consists of loose connective tissue.

  ➢ High power

The cortex is located in the deep layer of the tunica albuginea and consists of follicles at different stages of development and corpus luteum（黄体）.

（1）Primitive follicle（原始卵泡）：Primitive follicles locate in the superficial cortex, with the largest number and the smallest volume. It consists of a large primary oocyte（初级卵母细胞）and a single layer of flat follicular cells. The primary oocyte is large in size, round in nucleus, located in the middle, and lightly stained with obvious nucleolus. Follicular cells are arranged in a single layer around the oocyte with small size and unclear boundaries（Fig. 19－1）.

（2）Primary follicle（初级卵泡）：The volume of the primary follicle increases. There is a large primary oocyte in the center of the follicle, and the zona pellucida（透明带）is located between follicular cells and oocytes and is stained eosinophilic. At the early stage, the follicular cells surrounding the primary oocyte are cuboidal or columnar in monolayer. Later, the follicular cells are arranged in multilayers. The connective tissue around the follicle cells becomes gradually dense and forming a follicular theca（卵泡膜）（Fig. 19－2）.

（3）Secondary follicle（次级卵泡）：The follicle further increases in volume. And the unique feature is that the follicular cavity（卵泡腔）appears in the secondary follicle. The follicular cells around the zona pellucida are columnar and arranged in a radial manner to form the corona radiata（放射冠）. When the follicular cavity gets enlarged, the primary oocytes, zona pellucida, corona radiata and the follicular cells around them are pushed to one side of the follicle cavity to form a hillock called the cumulus oophorus（卵丘）. The follicular cells that make up the wall of the follicle are called the granulosa layer（颗粒层）. At this time, the follicular theca surrounding the follicle is divided into inner and outer layers. There are more cells in the inner layer of the follicular theca and more fibers in the outer layer（Fig. 19－3）.

（4）Mature follicle（成熟卵泡）：Its structure is similar to that of the late secondary follicle with further increased size. The volume of the follicular cavity also increases, and the granular layer becomes thinner. It bulges out on the surface of the ovary. It is not easy to find mature follicles in sections.

（5）Atretic follicle（闭锁卵泡）：There are many follicles in the ovary, most of which can not develop and mature. These follicles may degenerate at different stages of development, and the degenerated follicles are atretic follicles. The structural characteristics of atretic follicles are as follows. The morphological structure is inconsistent, the size is irregular, and the follicles collapse. Follicular cells degenerate and become smaller or dispersed. The oocyte exhibits nucleus pyknosis, and the zona pellucida shrinks. Some theca cells are hypertrophic and epithelioid, forming interstitial glands（间质腺）.

2. Corpus luteum (黄体)

➤ **Material**

Rabbit ovary, section (H & E stain).

➤ **Gross observation**

The corpus luteum is a large reddish cell mass.

➤ **Low power**

The number of corpus luteum is small, and it is composed of large cells with light staining and scattering among follicles.

➤ **High power**

The corpus luteum is large and rich in capillaries and surrounded by connective tissue. The cells in the corpus luteum are arranged in cords or in bands. The corpus luteum is composed of granulosa lutein cells (颗粒黄体细胞) and theca lutein cells (膜黄体细胞). The granulosa lutein cells are located in the center of the corpus luteum. The granular lutein cells is polygonal and large in size. Its nucleus is large and round or oval, which is located in the center of the cell. The cytoplasm is red, lightly stained, with lipid droplets inside. The theca lutein cells are locating around the corpus luteum. They are small in number and size, and their cytoplasm and nucleus are deeply stained (Fig. 19 – 4).

3. Uterus (子宫)

➤ **Material**

Human uterus, section (H & E stain).

➤ **Gross observation**

The uterus was oval in shape. The purple blue part in the center of the uterus is endometrium of uterus, and the pink thicker part around the uterus is myometrium.

➤ **Low power**

Three layers of the uterus including endometrium (内膜), myometrium (肌层) and perimetrium（外膜）are identified under low power lens, but there is no obvious boundary between the layers. Endometrium in different phases is the main object of observation.

➤ High power

(1) Endometrium.

A. Proliferative phase（增生期）. In the proliferative phase, the endometrium is thick with a layer of single columnar epithelium. The epithelium depresses to the lamina propria（固有层）and forms uterine gland（子宫腺）. The uterine glandis a single tubular gland. We can find the transverse and oblique sections of uterine glands on the slice. Secretions can be seen in the lumen of the uterine gland. The lamina propria is thin with abundant cells. At this time, the cross section of the arteriole named spiral artery（螺旋动脉）can be seen（Fig. 19 – 5）.

B. Secretory phase（分泌期）. During the secretory phase, the endometrium is the thickest, the uterine glands grow and bend, and the glandular cavities expand and vary in shape. Uterine gland cells are lightly stained, and vacuoles can be seen above or below the nucleus. In addition, large stromal cells are seen, and the cytoplasm is full of glycogen and lipid droplets, and the cells are lightly stained. The spiral arteries are proliferating and curved, and more spiral arteries can be seen in the section（Fig. 19 – 6）.

C. Menstrual phase（月经期）. At this time, the endometrium in the menstrual phase is the thinnest, the number of uterine glands decreases, the glandular cells are lightly stained, and the size of glandular cells becomes smaller. The number of stromal cells decreased, and the size of stromal cells became smaller. Many fragments of the epithelium and stroma, abundant blood and neutrophils can be seen in the endometrium（Fig. 19 – 7）.

(2) Myometrium. The myometrium of the uterus is the thickest. A large number of different sections of smooth muscle bundles can be seen, and the connective tissue can be seen between muscle bundles（Fig. 19 – 8）.

(3) Perimetrium. The perimetrium of the uterus is serosa, which is composed of a single layer of simple squamous epithelium on the surface and connective tissue underneath the epithelium（Fig. 19 – 8）.

Reflection

What is menstrual cycle and what are the characteristics of endometrium in each phase of menstrual cycle?

---

4. Cervix（子宫颈）

➤ Material

Human cervix, section（H & E stain）.

➤ Gross observation

The deeply stained and pleated part of the cervix is the mucosa（黏膜）, underneath the mucosa is the muscularis, and the outmost layer is the fibrosa（纤维膜）.

> **Low power**

At low power the three layers structure of the cervix are composed of mucosa, muscularis and fibrosa. The mucosa of the endocervix is composed of simple columnar epithelium and lamina propria, and the muscularis consists of smooth muscles. The smooth muscle is small and fractional. The fibrosa is composed of connective tissue. At the external os of cervix, there is an abrupt junction between the columnar epithelium of the endocervix and the stratified squamous epithelium of the exocervix.

> **High power**

The cervical mucosa of endocervix is lined by simple columnar epithelium composed of ciliated cells, secretory cells and reserve cells. Ciliated cells are columnar in shape and elliptical in nucleus. The supra-nuclear areas of secretory cells are lightly stained. Reserve cells are not easily identified under light microscope. The exocervix is covered by stratified squamous epithelium. The muscularis is composed of smooth muscles. The fibrosa is composed of connective tissue (Fig. 19 –9).

Reflection

(1) How many layers does the cervix have and what are the structural characteristics of each layer?

(2) Why are the women prone to cervical cancer?

---

5. Uterine tube (输卵管)

> **Material**

Human uterine tube, section (H & E stain).

> **Gross observation**

In the specimen we can see a circular structure with a small and irregular cavity. The inner surface part of the cavity which is dyed purple is mucosa, the deep part is muscularis, and the outermost structure is adventitia.

> **Low power**

The deeply stained folds in the center of the uterine tube are made up of mucosa, which are composed of epithelium and lamina propria. The lamina propria is thin. Below the mucosa is the muscularis which is composed of two layers of smooth muscle including the inner circular and the outer longitudinal layers. The inner layer is thin and the outer layer is thick. Outside of the muscularis is serosa which consists of mesothelium and connective tissue.

> **High power**

(1) Mucosa. The mucosa forms many folds that stretch into the oviduct cavity. Mucosa is lined by simple columnar epithelium which is composed of secretory cells and ciliated cells. The ciliated cells are large in size, with oval nuclei, and the nuclei are close to the basal surface. There are many cilia on the free surface of the ciliated cells, and the cytoplasm is lightly stained. The secretory cells are small in size, oval in nucleus and strongly eosinophilic in cytoplasm. The lamina propria is thin and composed of dense connective tissue and rich in blood vessels (Fig. 19 – 10).

（2）Muscularis. The muscularis is composed of two layers of smooth muscle including the inner ring and the outer longitudinal one. The inner smooth muscle is longitudinally cut, therefore the smooth muscle is spindle shaped and the nucleus is rod-shaped. The outer smooth muscle is transversely cut, so that the smooth muscle is round and the nucleus is round in the center.

（3）Adventitia. The adventitia is composed of mesothelium（间皮）and connective tissue. The mesothelium is simple squamous epithelium.

Reflection

（1）How many layers does uterine tube have?

（2）What are the structural characteristics of each layer of uterine tube?

---

6. Vagina（阴道）

➤ **Material**

Human vagina, section（H & E stain）.

➤ **Gross observation**

One side of the specimen stained blue is the mucosa, and the rest is the muscularis and adventitia.

➤ **Low power**

Vaginal mucosa forms folds, which is composed of epithelium（上皮）and lamina propria. The epithelium is non-keratinized stratified squamous epithelium, and lamina propria consists of connective tissue. The deep layer below the mucosa is the muscularis, which is composed of two layers of smooth muscle: the inner ring and the outer longitudinal. The boundary between the two layers of smooth muscle is unclear, and the adventitia is composed of connective tissue.

➤ **High power**

（1）Mucosa. Mucosal epithelium is non-keratinized stratified squamous epithelium. The superficial layer is composed of 1 – 2 layers of squamous cells. The nucleus is flat, and the cytoplasm is red. The middle layer is composed of several layers of polygonal cells. The nucleus is oval in the middle. The bottom layer is composed of short columnar or cuboidal cells, and the nucleus is round in the middle. The lamina propria（固有层）consists of connective tissue containing elastic fibers and blood vessels（Fig. 19 – 11）.

（2）Muscularis. The Muscularis is composed of two layers of smooth muscle including the inner ring and the outer longitudinal.

（3）Adventitia. The adventitia is composed of connective tissue.

Reflection

（1）How many layers does the vaginal wall have?

（2）What are the characteristics of the histological structure at each level of the vaginal wall?

7.　Mammary gland （乳腺）

➢　**Material**

Human breast, section （H & E stain）.

➢　**Gross observation**

The deeply stained structure on one side of the specimen is epidermis, and the irregular lobulated structure in the deep pink tissue is mammary lobule.

Inactive mammary gland （静止期乳腺）

➢　**Low power**

The inactive mammary gland is composed of a small amount of glandular tissue and a large amount of connective tissue. There are few glands and ducts, but rich adipose tissue.

➢　**High power**

A small number of mammary glands and a lot of connective tissue and adipose tissue can be seen. There are just a few mammary glands in the lobule. The acinus is composed of simple cuboidal or columnar cells. The cavity of acinus is small, and the duct and duct lumen in the lobule are large. The intralobular duct is composed of simple columnar epithelium, and the interlobular duct is covered by multiple columnar epithelium. When the common duct is close to the skin, the duct epithelium transitions into stratified squamous epithelium （Fig. 19 – 12）.

Active mammary gland （活动期乳腺）

➢　**Low power**

Mammary gland during pregnancy and lactation consists of much more mammary gland tissue, a small amount of connective tissue and less adipose tissue than inactive gland. The gland is divided into many lobules by the connective tissue. The acinar cavity is large, and there are purple red secretions in the acinar cavity. The interlobular duct is large, which is simple columnar epithelium or stratified epithelium. It is difficult to distinguish the duct and acinus in the lobule.

➢　**High power**

Active mammary gland during pregnancy and lactation are similar, with less connective tissue than inactive gland. The mammary gland tissue is abundant, the acinar cavity is large, and the shape of the glandular epithelium can be high columnar, cuboidal, or squamous.

The glandular epithelium is simple cuboidal or squamous, which represents the acinus at different secretory phases. The glandular epithelium before secretion is cuboidal, while the glandular epithelium after secretion is squamous, and there is milk stained purplish red in the cavity （Fig. 19 – 13）.

Reflection

（1）Does the microstructure of mammary gland change during the menstrual cycle?

（2）What are the structural characteristics of the mammary gland in each phase?

Post-class Task

Draw a structural diagram of the secondary follicle under a high-power microscope.

Case-based Learning

The patient, female, 40 years old, has regular menstrual cycle, and the day of onset is on the 22nd day of the menstrual cycle. The patient suddenly felt pain in her right lower abdomen, accompanied by nausea and vomiting, and frequent urination and defecation. Physical examination showed that there was tenderness and rebound pain in the right lower abdomen, the palpable boundary was unclear, and the mobile dullness was positive. The cervix is painful, and the posterior vault of the uterus is full and tender. The physical signs are anemia, rapid pulse rate and decreased blood pressure. The ultrasound showed rupture of corpus luteum cyst.

（1）How is the corpus luteum formed? How does the corpus luteum evolve?

（2）How can we treat the patient with ruptured corpus luteum cyst?

（3）Why does the rupture of corpus luteum lead to the decrease of blood pressure?

（陈雄林）

第 20 章 | 胚胎学绪论

胚胎学研究从生殖细胞的起源到出生前的发生过程。

产前分为三个阶段：受精后的前 2 周为胚前期，第 3～8 周为胚期，第 9 周至出生前为胎儿期。

学习目标

（1）了解胚胎学的主要领域。

（2）理解胚胎学和其他医学课程之间的关系。

（3）理解胚胎学实验课的一些基本要求。

课前问题

胚胎学实验课前，你会做哪些准备？

胚胎学主要领域和研究方法

胚胎学的各个领域，通常是相互重叠和合并的，已经被几代胚胎学家所探索。

1. 描述胚胎学

描述胚胎学对多细胞生物个体发育的不同阶段的形态进行描述。用来研究和描述胚胎结构和生殖的常用方法有解剖、观察和批判性分析。许多杰出的科学家，例如，Reinier De Graaf（1641—1673）、Kaspar Friedrich Wolff（1733—1794）、Karl Ernst von Baer（1792—1876）和 Edouard Van Beneden（1845—1910），在描述胚胎学的发展中发挥了决定性作用。

2. 进化胚胎学

进化胚胎学研究和比较各种物种的发育阶段，为进化和生命的系统发育树提供证据。Johann Meckel，Etienne Serres，Karl Ernst von Baer，Louis Agassiz，Ernst Haeckel 是这个领域的杰出先驱。

3. 实验胚胎学

实验胚胎学旨在利用化学和物理学的规律来解释发育事件的机制。W. Roux（1850—1924）被认为是实验胚胎学的创始人。

4. 分子胚胎学

分子胚胎学研究在发育过程中调控胚胎细胞生长和形态发生的分子、遗传和细胞学机制。这个领域开始于 20 世纪 50 年代。自从 James Watson 和 Francis Crick 在 1953 年揭示了 DNA 结构后，分子胚胎学与分子生物学和遗传学深度融合。许多胚胎学家利用胚胎学、分子生物学和遗传学的方法，揭示了发育过程中基因型与表型的关系。1952 年，Rita Levi-Montalcini（1909—2012）和 Stanley Cohen 利用鸡胚胎发现了生长因子。1957 年，Edward B.

Lewis 在果蝇和小鼠胚胎中发现了基因在染色体上的排布与体节的顺序呈现共线性的规律。1962 年，John B. Gurdon 利用一个肠道细胞的细胞核和一个无核的卵子培育了蝌蚪，这表明细胞的特化是可逆的。1963 年，童第周的团队利用核移植技术获得了克隆鱼。1980 年，Christiane Nüsslein-Volhard 和 Eric Wieschaus 确定了控制果蝇胚胎节段的 15 个不同的基因。1989 年，Mario R. Capecchi、Martin J. Evans 和 Oliver Smithies 首次利用同源重组技术对胚胎干细胞的目的基因进行失活产生了基因剔除小鼠。1996 年，Keith Campbell 和 Ian Wilmut 利用一个成年体细胞核移植获得克隆羊 Dolly。2006 年，Shinya Yamanaka 通过引入 4 个转录因子，将成熟体细胞重编程成为诱导多能干细胞（iPS）。

5. 临床胚胎学

临床胚胎学的重点是研究生殖科学、不孕不育、体外受精和胚胎的健康发育。这个领域出现了大量里程碑式的成就。例如，在 20 世纪 50 年代，Gregory Pincus（1903—1967）开发了节育药。1959 年，张民觉（Min Chueh Chang, 1908—1991）是第一个通过体外受精获得哺乳动物（兔子）的人，他开辟了辅助生殖的道路。1969 年，Robert Edwards（1925—2010）和 Patrick Steptoe（1913—1988）成功地在体外使人类卵子受精。1978 年，第一个试管婴儿 Louise Brown 诞生了。

6. 畸形学

畸形学是一个跨学科的领域，关注出生缺陷的原因、病理和机制。畸形学开始于 19 世纪。20 世纪 40 年代发现致畸物可导致胎儿畸形。1941 年，Norman Gregg 确定了由德国麻疹引起的孕妇风疹可导致胎儿出现白内障、心脏畸形和耳聋三联征。20 世纪 60 年代，沙利度胺（反应停）被发现是导致大量新生儿畸形的原因。近年来，随着分子生物学、毒理学、动物实验科学和遗传学的进步，该领域在不断扩展。

胚胎学的意义

1. 胚胎学与其他医学科学学科的关系

胚胎学解释了组织学和解剖学结构的发展过程，以及解剖结构变异的原因。胚胎学的学习可为学习发育生物学和出生缺陷的病理生理学做好准备。

2. 胚胎学与临床医学之间的关系

胚胎学是桥梁学科，理解胚胎发育过程，为产科、生殖医学、胎儿医学、围产医学、儿科和外科之间架起了桥梁。全球每年至少有 790 万新生儿有出生缺陷（Christianson, Howson, and Modell, 2006）。更好地理解胚胎学为改善产前诊断和治疗、提高体外受精 - 胚胎移植技术，即提高试管婴儿的成功率和预防出生缺陷奠定基础。

胚胎学实验的基本要求

1. 从静态形态学到动态胚胎学

与组织学和大体解剖学中研究的静态形态结构不同，胚胎学研究的是发育过程中形态学变化的动态事件。因此，发育过程中，形态（what）、时间（when），地点（where），机制（why），怎样变化（how）很重要。

2. 联系和比较

首先，将胚胎的结构与成人的解剖结构进行比较，能够更好地理解人体的发育和器官的发生。第二，联系和比较不同时期的胚胎解剖结构，发育是跨越空间和时间的动态过程。第三，将功能与结构联系起来，因为胚胎的发育不仅表现为结构的不断变化，也表现为功能的不断变化。最后，要理解出生缺陷是如何发生的，需要比较异常发育与正常发育的解剖学、遗传学和分子机制。

3. 将二维图片与多维胚胎联系

在讲座和实验课上使用的图片和照片大多是二维的。然而，胚胎发育是多维的，包含了时间和立体结构的变化。因此，将不同解剖断面的二维结构整合为不同时期胚胎的立体结构是很重要的。可以利用胚胎模型、动画和橡皮泥来帮助理解。

4. 绘图和标注

绘图和标注对于胚胎学实验与组织学实验课来说一样重要。通过绘图和标记，可以更好地理解结构的基本特征和解剖学细节。

5. 基于案例的学习（CBL）

基于案例的学习（case-based learning，CBL）侧重于培养合作、探索和解决临床问题的能力，有助于在真实的临床案例中整合和应用理论知识。本教材中的案例均来自已发表的论文中的真实临床案例。

课后作业

检索一个你感兴趣的胚胎学家的故事。

案例讨论题

童第周（1902 年 5 月 28 日—1979 年 3 月 30 日），中国胚胎学家，被誉为"中国的克隆技术之父"。他在 1963 年克隆了世界上第一条克隆鱼。童第周从事水生动物和实验胚胎学研究，长期担任中国科学院海洋研究所主任。童第周和他的团队通过使用尼罗蓝染色给文昌鱼胚胎卵裂球着色，绘制了从受精卵到 32 细胞期的文昌鱼胚胎的发育图。他们还通过胚层移植实验观察胚胎中不同胚层的发育潜能。20 世纪 60 年代初，他开始了对克隆的研究。他们将金鱼胚胎中提取的细胞核注射到去核的金鱼卵子中，克隆细胞长成了鱼的胚胎，并发育成幼年金鱼，这是世界上第一个克隆鱼。1963 年，童第周在《科学通报》上发表了中文论文《鱼类细胞核移植》。

（1）请找到更多关于童第周的故事。

（2）什么是克隆？克隆和受精的区别是什么？

（3）什么是卵裂球？

（谢小薰，岳晓阳）

Chapter 20 INTRODUCTION TO EMBRYOLOGY

Embryology is a branch of science that studies the development from the origin of the germ cells until birth.

Prenatal period is divided into 3 stages: the first 2 weeks after fertilization is the germinal period, the period from the 3rd to the 8th week is the embryonic period, and the time from the 9th week until birth is the fetal period.

Learning Objectives

(1) Be able to understand the main fields of embryology.

(2) Be able to understand the relation between embryology and other medical disciplines.

(3) Be able to understand some basic requirements for embryology lab.

Pre-class Questions

What would you do to get yourself prepared for embryology lab class?

Main Fields and Methods of Embryology

Various fields of embryology, which usually overlap and merge with one another, have been explored by generations of embryologist.

1. Descriptive Embryology

Descriptive embryology deals with the morphological description of different stages in the ontogenetic development of multicellular organisms. Dissections, observations and critical analysis were used to study and describe the embryo structure and procreation. Many scientists, for example, Reinier De Graaf (1641 – 1673), Kaspar Friedrich Wolff (1733 – 1794), Karl Ernst von Baer (1792 – 1876), and Edouard Van Beneden (1845 – 1910), played determining roles in the development of descriptive embryology.

2. Evolutionary Embryology

Evolutionary embryology studies and compares developmental stages of various species and provided evidence for evolution and phylogenetic tree of life. Johann Meckel, Etienne Serres, Karl Ernst von Baer, Louis Agassiz, Ernst Haeckel were prominent forerunners in this field.

3. Experimental Embryology

Experimental embryology aims to use the laws of chemistry and physics to explain mechanism in the developmental events. W. Roux (1850 – 1924) is generally considered the founder of experimental embryology.

4. Molecular Embryology

Molecular embryology studies the molecular, genetic and cellular mechanisms that regulates embryonic cell growth and morphogenesis during development. This field started in 1950s. Since James Watson and Francis Crick revealed DNA structure in 1953, molecular embryology merges deeply with molecular biology and genetics. Many embryologists endeavored to reveal genotype-phenotype relation during development using arsenal of embryologic, molecular biological, and genetical approaches. In 1952, Rita Levi-Montalcini (1909 – 2012) and Stanley Cohen found the growth factor using chick embryo. In 1957, Edward B. Lewis discovered the principle of collinearity in Drosophila and mouse embryos. In 1962, John B. Gurdon produced tadpoles using nuclei from a mature intestinal cell and an enucleated egg, which showed that the specialization of cells is reversible. Dizhou Tong, a Chinese scientist, and his team injected the nucleus from a goldfish blastocyst into an enucleated egg and obtained a goldfish in 1963. In 1980, Christiane Nüsslein-Volhard and Eric Wieschaus identified 15 different genes which controlled segmentation of Drosophila embryo. In 1989, Mario R. Capecchi, Martin J. Evans, and Oliver Smithies were the first to generate knockout mice using homologous recombination in embryo stem cells. In 1996, Dolly, the Sheep was cloned through transplanted nuclear from an adult somatic cell into an enucleated egg by Keith Campbell and Ian Wilmut. In 2006, Shinya Yamanaka reprogrammed mature cells to become induced pluripotent stem (iPS) cells by introducing 4 transcription factors.

5. Clinical Embryology

Clinical embryology focuses on the study of reproductive science, infertility, in vitro fertilization and the healthy development of the embryos. Several milestones were achieved by prominent scientists. For example, in 1950s, Gregory Pincus (1903 – 1967) developed birth control pill. In 1959, Min Chueh Chang (张民觉, 1908 – 1991), a China-born scientist, was the first to obtain a mammal (a rabbit) by in vitro fertilization, opening the way to assisted reproduction. In 1969, Robert Edwards (1925 – 2010) and Patrick Steptoe (1913 – 1988) succeeded fertilizing human egg in vitro. They brought the first test tube baby, Louise Brown, to the world in 1978.

6. Teratology

Tetralogy is an interdisciplinary field which concerns with causes, pathology, and mechanisms of birth defects. Teratology began in the 19th century. Teratogens were found to cause malformation in 1940s. In 1941, Norman Gregg established a cause-and-effect relation between maternal rubella caused by German measles and the triad of cataracts, heart malformations, and deafness. In 1960s, Thalidomide, a medication used to treat a number of cancers, graft-versus-host disease, and skin conditions, was found to be the cause of the largest medical tragedy of birth defect in history. In recent years, the field has expanded with the advancements in molecular biology, toxicology, animal laboratory science, and genetics.

Significance of Embryology

1. Relation between embryology and medical related disciplines

Embryology builds an understanding of the developmental process of histological and anatomical structures, and it explains the causes of variations of these structures. The knowledge of the embryology is able to provide a foundation for further studying developmental biology and pathophysiology of birth defects.

2. Relation between embryology and clinical medicine

Embryology bridges the gap between prenatal development and obstetrics, reproductive medicine, fetal medicine, perinatal medicine, pediatrics, and surgery. It has been reported that at least 7.9 million neonates globally are born with birth defects every year (Christianson, Howson, and Modell, 2006). A better understanding of embryology paves the way for improving prenatal diagnoses and treatments, increasing in vitro fertilization-embryo transfer (IVF-ET) success rate, and preventing birth defects.

Basic Requirements for Embryology Lab

1. Static Morphology vs Dynamic Embryology

In contrast to static morphology studied in histology and gross anatomy, embryology deals with the dynamic events of morphological change during development. It is important to remember "what, when, where, why, how" for explaining the major events related to embryogenesis and organogenesis.

2. Connection and Comparison

First, compare the structure of an embryo with the adult anatomy so that you can better understand the development of human body and the organization of organs. Second, connect and compare the anatomic structures of an embryo at different time period as development takes place across space and time. Third, connect the functions with structures since embryological development appears as continuous changes in not only the structures but also the functions. Last, in order to discover how birth defect takes place, it is important to compare the anatomic, genetical and molecular mechanism of abnormal development with those of normal development.

3. Relating 2-dimensional Diagram to Multidimensional Embryo

The diagrams and photographs used in the lectures and lab class are mostly 2-dimensional. However, embryo development is multidimensional, and embryo structures transform rapidly. Thus, it is important to integrate diagrams from different sectional planes into 3-dimensional view of embryo at different time period. Embryo models, animation and playdough can be helpful.

4. Drawing and Labelling

Drawing diagrams and labeling in embryology lab are as important as in histology lab class. By drawing and labeling, you can better understand the basic features of characteristic structures.

5. Case-based Learning (CBL)

CBL is a method focusing on cultivation of your collaboration, exploration and clinical problem-solving skills. It helps integrate and apply the theoretical knowledge to the real-life clinical cases. Cases in this textbook are revised from published paper.

Post-class Task

Searching more stories about an embryologist you are interested in.

Case-based Learning

Dizhou Tong (May 28, 1902 to March 30, 1979), a Chinese embryologist, is regarded as "the father of China's clone technology". He cloned the first fish in the world in 1963. Tong studied aquatic animals and experimental embryology in China and served as director of the Institute of Oceanology, Chinese Academy of Sciences. Tong and his colleagues created a developmental map from zygote to 32-cell embryo of the amphioxus (文昌鱼) by using Nile Blue stain to color amphioxus embryos and to track the blastomeres. They also tested the developmental potency of different germ layers in embryos. He started his research on clone in the early 1960s. Tong and his team injected the nucleus taken from a goldfish blastocyst into a goldfish egg whose nucleus was removed. The clone cell grew into a fish embryo and developed into juvenile goldfish, the first cloned fish in the world. Tong published a paper "Nuclear Transplantation of Fish" in Chinese in Chinese Science Bulletin in 1963.

(1) Could you find more stories about Dizhou Tong?

(2) What is clone? What is the difference between clone and fertilization?

(3) What is a blastomere?

(谢小薰, 岳晓阳)

第 21 章 ｜ 胚胎学总论

学习目标

（1）能够识别合子、卵裂球、桑葚胚和胚泡。
（2）能够描述植入的过程，内细胞团的转化及二胚层胚盘的形成。
（3）能够识别原条。
（4）能够描述三个胚层的形成和演变。
（5）能够识别胎膜的结构。
（6）能够描述胎盘的结构。

课前问题

（1）何为受精？
（2）何为桑椹胚？
（3）合子是如何发育形成胚泡的？何为植入？
（4）胚泡是由什么构成的？这些结构将会发育为什么？
（5）请简述中胚层的形成。
（6）将简述三胚层胚盘的形成。

实验材料

大体标本，胚胎模型，仿真视频。

实验观察与思考

1. 第 1 至第 14 天

➤ **受精卵、胚泡与二胚层胚盘**

图 21 - 1 分别展示了卵裂发生时受精卵的形态变化、胚泡的结构、二胚层胚盘的形成和胚外体腔的发育。

➤ **植入**

胚泡的着床过程如图 21 - 2 所示，各阶段会出现其特征性结构。

思考题

（1）受精卵是如何变成胚泡的？

（2）胚泡是由哪些结构构成的？这些结构最后会演变为什么？

（3）绒毛干的类型有多少种？它们的结构差异是什么？

（4）植入后子宫内膜发生了什么变化？着床后子宫内膜可分为多少部分？

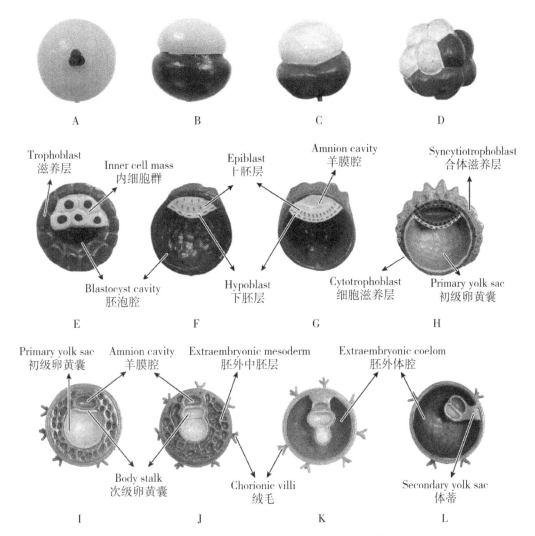

A：合子（Zygote）；B：二细胞期（Zygote of 2-cell stage）；C：三细胞期（Zygote of 3-cell stage）
D：桑葚胚（Morula）；E：胚泡（Blastocyst）；F～L：二胚层胚盘（Bilaminar embryonic disc）。

图 21-1　卵裂以及胚泡和胚盘的发育

Fig. 21-1　Cleavage and development of blastocyst and blastoderm

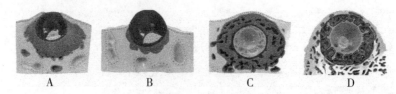

A：7天（7 days）；B：8天（8 days）；C：9天（9 days）；D：14天（14 days）。

图 21 - 2　受精后不同时间点胚泡在子宫内膜的植入

Fig. 21 - 2　Implantation of blastocyte into uterus at different timepoint after fertilization

2. 第 3 周

三胚层胚盘的结构如图 21 - 3 所示。

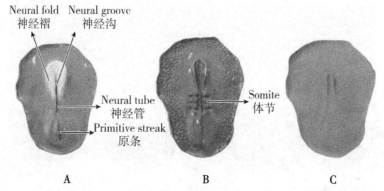

A：上胚层（Epiblast）；B：中胚层（Mesoderm）；C：下胚层（Endoderm）。

图 21 - 3　三胚层胚盘的形成

Fig. 21 - 3　Trilaminar embryonic disc

思考题

（1）中胚层是如何产生的？脊索、神经管和躯体分别是如何形成的？

（2）肠上皮和间皮分别从哪个胚层发育而来？为什么？

（3）哪些胚层可以分别分化成皮肤的表皮和真皮层？

---

3. 第 4 至第 8 周

胚体外部和内部所有主要的结构都是在第 4 周到第 8 周期间发育的。在这段时期结束时，主要的器官和相关系统已经开始发育。随着组织和器官的形成，胚体的形状也在改变。到了第八周，胚胎已经形成了明显的人类外观。由于组织和器官在这段时间内迅速发育，胚胎暴露于致畸物会导致严重的出生缺陷。致畸物是药物和病毒等物质，会导致或增加出生缺陷的发生率。

图 21 - 4 至图 21 - 8 展示了这一时期胚胎几个主要结构的形成。

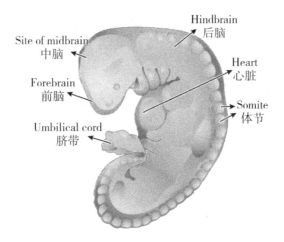

图 21 - 4　胚胎约 28 天时的侧面观（第 4 周）

Fig. 21 - 4　Embryo is shown as lateral view, roughly 28 days（4th week）

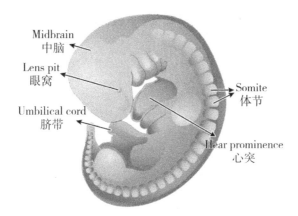

图 21 - 5　胚胎约 32 天时的侧面观（第 5 周）

Fig. 21 - 5　Embryo is shown as lateral view, roughly 32 days（5th week）

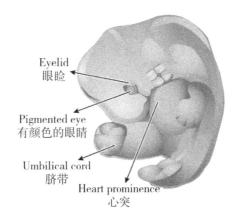

图 21 - 6　胚胎约 42 天时的侧面观（第 6 周）

Fig. 21 - 6　Embryo is shown as lateral view, roughly 42 days（6th week）

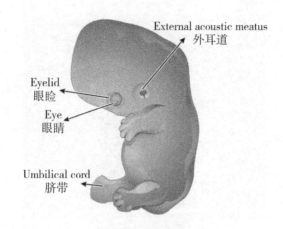

图 21 -7　胚胎约 48 天时的侧面观（第 7 周）

Fig. 21 -7　Embryo is shown as lateral view，roughly 48 days（7th week）

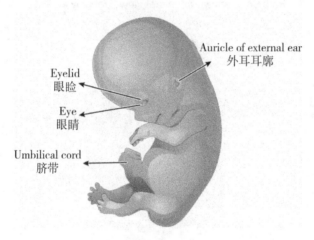

图 21 -8　胚胎约 56 天时的侧面观（第 8 周）

Fig. 21 -8　Embryo is shown as lateral view at，roughly 56 days（8th week）

思考题

在胚体各个系统当中，哪个系统的发育最早，为什么？

---

4. 胎膜和胎盘

胚泡着床后，根据子宫内膜和胚体的位置关系，子宫内膜被分成 3 部分，即壁蜕膜，包蜕膜和底蜕膜（图 21 -9）。同时，由于不同位置的绒毛膜所获的营养也不同，绒毛膜相应的发育成 2 种类型，平滑绒毛膜和丛密绒毛膜（图 21 -9）。

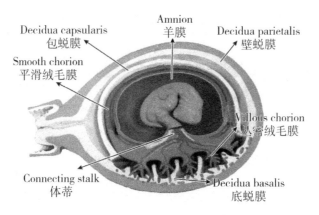

图 21-9 人胚胎及其胎膜

Fig. 21-9 Human embryo and its fetal membrane

思考题

（1）胎膜由哪几部分构成？各部分会发育或演变为何结构？

（2）胎盘由哪几个部分构成？各自的功能是什么？

（3）胎儿血和母体血能否混合？在胚胎发育的早期和晚期，胎儿和母体分别如何进行物质交换？

课后作业

请列表归纳三胚层胚盘各胚层的分化结局。

案例讨论题

一名 19 岁的女孩多年来一直营养不良。有一天，她惊讶地发现自己怀孕了。然而，女孩害怕告诉父母怀孕的事，没有找医生做进一步的检查。直到快要分娩时，女孩才前往医院。孩子出生后，被诊断为脊髓脊膜膨出。试分析：

（1）胚胎发育过程中脊髓脊膜膨出的原因是什么？

（2）什么样的人群，其后代容易出现这种畸形？

（3）预防脊髓脊膜膨出的措施是什么？

（葛盈盈）

Chapter 21　GENERAL EMBRYOLOGY

Human development begins when a spermatozoon fertilized an oocyte. Embryonic early development refers to the first 8 weeks since the fertilization occurs（containing pre-embryonic 2 weeks as well as embryonic 3 ～ 8 weeks）. The first 2 weeks includes that the embryo moves to the uterus where implantation takes place. And the 3 ～ 8 weeks contains events like differentiation that occurs to establish organ systems, while week 8 to week 38 is a period of growth and enlargement（fetal phase）. Human embryo development is a continuous process involving in complicated changes in embryonic morphology. Because the early embryo of human is hard to obtain, embryonic models and videos are provided for you to grasp the dynamic changes of embryo development.

Learning Objectives

（1）Be able to identify zygote, blastomere, morula, and blastocyst.

（2）Be able to describe process of transplantation, and the transformation of inner cell mass and the formation of bilaminar blastoderm.

（3）Be able to identify the primitive streak and trilaminar germ disc.

（4）Be able to describe the main derivation of trilaminar blastoderm.

（5）Be able to identify the fetal membranes.

（6）Be able to identify the structure of the placenta.

Pre-class Questions

（1）What is fertilization?

（2）What is morula?

（3）How does a zygote develop into blastocyst? What is implantation?

（4）What is blastocyst composed of? What will these structures develop into?

（5）Please describe the development of mesoderm.

（6）Please describe the formation of trilaminar germ disc.

Materials

Gross specimens, embryo models, and simulation videos.

Observation and Reflection（Models）

1. Day 1 ～ 14（第 1 至第 14 天）

➢ Zygote（合子），Blastocyst（胚泡）and bilaminar blastoderm（二胚层胚盘）

The morphological changes of zygote when cleavage occurs, the structure of blastocyst, the formation of bilaminar blastoderm, and the development of extraembryonic coelom have been demonstrated in Fig. 21 – 1 respectively.

➢ Implantation（植入）

The implantation of blastocyte has been illustrated by Fig. 21 – 2. Characteristic structures were developed at different stages. Briefly, seven days after fertilization, the blastocyst invades the endometrium and begins to implant（Fig. 21 – 2A）. Eight days after fertilization, the amniotic cavity has been built within the epiblast. Syncytiotrophoblasts grow and invade blood vessels of endometrium（Fig. 21 –2B）. Nine days after fertilization, the embryo has completely implanted inside the uterine endometrium. Lacunae appear in the syncytiotrophoblasts, which completely envelop the embryo（Fig. 21 –2C）. Fourteen days after fertilization, secondary yolk sac and exocoelomic cavity have formed（Fig. 21 –2D）.

Reflection

（1）How does a fertilized egg become a blastocyst?

（2）What is blastocyst consisted of? What would these structures eventually evolve into?

（3）How many types of chorionic villi are there? What are the structure differences among them?

（4）What is implantation? Please briefly describe the timepoint, location, and process of implantation.

（5）What happens to the endometrium after implantation? How many parts of the endometrium could be divided into after implantation?

2. 3rd week（第 3 周）

Structures of **trilaminar embryonic disc**（三胚层胚盘）have been demonstrated by Fig. 21 –3.

Reflection

（1）How does mesoderm occur? How do notochord, neural tube and somite form respectively?

（2）From which germ layers respectively do intestinal epithelium and mesothelium develop? Why?

（3）Which germ layers can differentiate into the epidermis and dermis of the skin respectively?

3. 4th to 8th week（第 4 至第 8 周）

All major exterior and interior structures are developed during 4th to 8th week. By the end of this time, the major organ systems have begun to develop. As tissues and organs form, the embryo's shape changes. When it comes to the eighth week, the embryo has built up an obviously human appearance.

Fig. 21 – 4 to Fig. 21 – 8 display several main structure developments of embryo during this period.

Reflection

Of all the organ systems in the embryo, which develops the earliest, and why?

4. Fetal membrane and placenta（胎膜和胎盘）

After implantation occurred, according to the positional relationship between endometrium and the embryo, the endometrium was divided into 3 parts, namely decidua parietalis, decidua capsularis and decidua basalis（Fig. 21 – 9）. Meanwhile, chorions that located differently received different amount of nutrition, so they developed into 2 types accordingly, smooth chorion and villous chorion（Fig. 21 – 9）.

Reflection

(1) What is fetal membrane composed of? What will each part develop into?

(2) How many parts do placenta include? What is the function for each part?

(3) Does the fetal blood mix with the maternal blood? How does mother and fetus exchange substances at early and late stages of the fetal development respectively?

Post-class Task

Please list a table and summarize the differentiation of the three germ layers of trilaminar embryonic disc.

Case-based Learning

A 19-year-old girl had been suffered from malnutrition for years. One day, she was surprised to find out she was pregnant. However, the girl was afraid of telling her parents about the pregnancy and didn't go to a doctor for further examination. She only went to hospital until it's time to deliver. By the time the baby was born, it was diagnosed with menigomyelocele（脊髓脊膜膨出）.

(1) What could be the cause of menigomyelocele during embryonic development?

(2) What kind of people's offspring are prone to such malformation?

(3) What is the preventive measure of menigomyelocele?

（葛盈盈）

第22章 | 颜面的发生

颜面的发育大多与咽弓的发育有关。咽弓是人体早期发育阶段较为复杂的结构。颜面的发生一般会经历几个阶段，从颜面结构的融合，到第一咽弓周围软骨组织膜内钙化形成下颌主体，再到腭架的形成、提拉、融合等等。每个阶段都包含了多种分子机制。颜面的先天畸形是人类最频发的先天遗传疾病之一，因此颜面的发生过程极为重要。

学习目标

（1）能够理解颜面的发生和三个咽弓的关系。
（2）能够理解腭的发育过程。
（3）能够了解不同颜面发生畸形。

课前问题

（1）颜面的各个组成部分是如何发生的？
（2）颜面的各个组成部分发生的时间节点是何时？

实验材料

大体标本，切片，胚胎模型，仿真视频。

实验观察与思考

1. 咽器

肉芽状的咽弓对称分布于胚体两侧，咽弓之间有咽裂。口腔在这个发育阶段由上颌突和下颌突包围。可见到刚刚发育成形的鼻板（图22-1）。

思考题

咽弓是从何发育而来的？

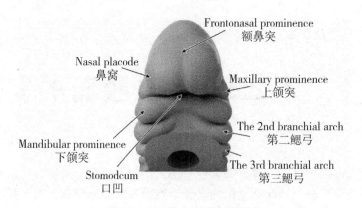

图 22 - 1　28 天人类胚胎示意

Fig. 22 - 1　Schematic 28 days human embryo

2. 颜面的发生

胚胎发育第 4 周：第一咽弓发育成为上颌突和下颌突。额鼻突在这一阶段开始生长以覆盖前脑的腹侧部位，鼻板由额鼻突的前侧部发育而成（图 22 - 2A）。

胚胎发育第 5 周：在这一阶段，原始耳郭于下颌突和舌骨弓之间形成，围绕着第一咽沟。耳郭由耳丘发育而来而外耳道则发生自第一咽沟。上颌突与内侧鼻突二者融合形成鼻中线、上唇以及主腭（图 22 - 2B）。

胚胎发育第 6 周：上颌突和外侧鼻突融合形成鼻泪沟，并继而形成鼻子和脸颊（图 22 - 2C）。

胚胎发育第 7 周：两侧的上颌突、内侧鼻突和外侧鼻突相互融合，形成连续性的上颌和上唇，以分隔口腔和鼻腔（图 22 - 2D）。

思考题

什么是组织融合？为什么组织融合对于颜面发生很重要？

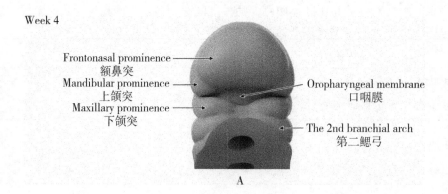

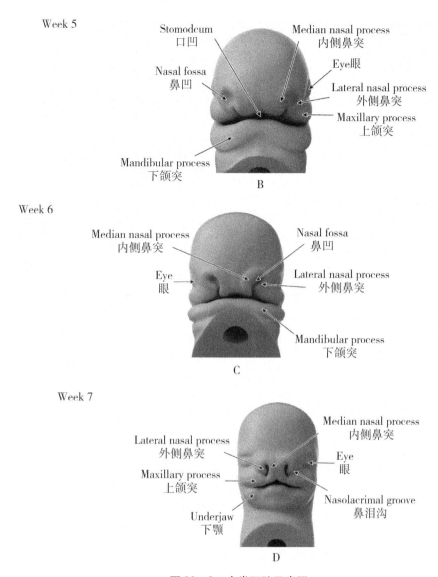

图 22 -2　人类胚胎示意图
Fig. 22 -2　Schematic human embryo

3. 腭的发生

水平切面：硬腭的发育始于上颌突内侧，上颌突内侧向外生长形成腭架，腭架垂直向下生长至舌的两侧（图 22 -3A），然后向上提拉并相对生长（图 22 -3B）。两侧腭架相对生长并从中间向两侧融合并形成完整的硬腭（图 22 -3C）。

横截面：腭架（图 22 -4A）垂直向下生长与舌的两侧（图 22 -4B）。

思考题

相对于颜面其他结构的发生，硬腭的发生有什么特点？

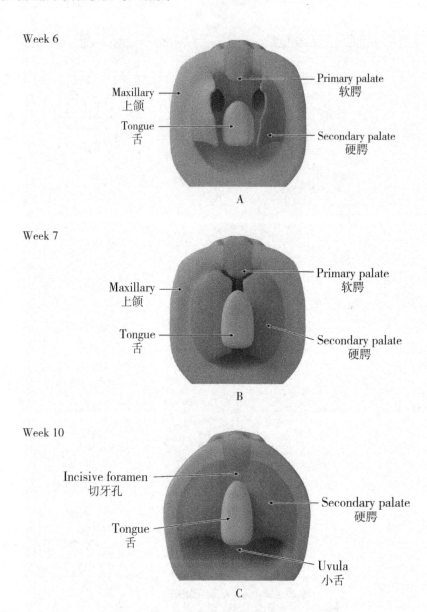

Week 6

Maxillary
上颌

Tongue
舌

Primary palate
软腭

Secondary palate
硬腭

A

Week 7

Maxillary
上颌

Tongue
舌

Primary palate
软腭

Secondary palate
硬腭

B

Week 10

Incisive foramen
切牙孔

Tongue
舌

Secondary palate
硬腭

Uvula
小舌

C

图 22 -3　人类胚胎硬腭示
Fig. 22 -3　Schematic secondary palate，human embryo

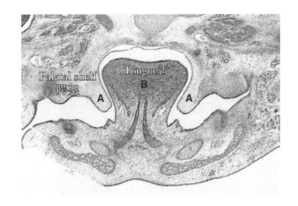

A：腭架（Palatal shelf）；B：舌（Tongue）。

图 22 - 4 人类胚胎继发腭冠状切片（马松染色，100 ×）

Fig. 22 - 4 Secondary palate, human embryo

(cross section, Masson's trichrome stain, 100 ×)

4. 颜面先天畸形

（1）皮埃尔罗宾序列症：常见下颌发育不良，舌后坠，腭裂的临床表征。

（2）Apert 综合征：发生颅缝早闭，前额高而突出，颅骨后部平坦。面部扁平或凹陷。

（3）唇腭裂（图 22 - 5）：①单侧唇裂伴随鼻孔内裂；②双侧唇裂；③腭裂；④唇裂。

（4）颜面畸形（图 22 - 6）：特征包括鼻根宽、耳朵低、眼睛及眉毛向下倾斜。

思考题

结合硬腭的发育过程，尝试分析不同唇腭裂的病因？

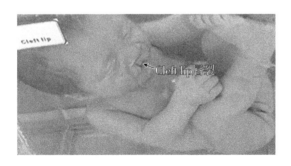

图 22 - 5 唇裂，人类胚胎

Fig. 22 - 5 Cleft lip, human embryo

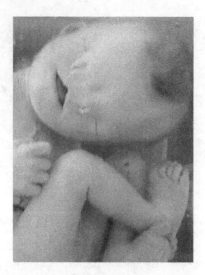

图 22 - 6　颜面多发性畸形，人类胚胎
Fig. 22 - 6　Multiple facial dysmorphia，human embryo

课后作业

描述颜面的发生过程。

案例讨论题

一个 1 岁的女婴，出现了神经发育迟缓、肝脏肿大、双侧听力损失和视觉问题。眼科检查显示为视中隔发育不良。颅脑磁共振成像（magnetic resonance imaging，MRI）显示皮质下和脑室周围深部白质有非特异性胶质增生。

（1）导致这种临床表现的原因可能是什么？
（2）是否存在潜在的颅面畸形？

（滕藤）

Chapter 22   FORMATION OF FACE

Craniofacial development is mostly related to derivatives of the pharyngeal arches, which is a complex process during human early developing stage. From the merging of mesenchymal facial processes, to the intramembranous calcification around the cartilage of the first pharyngeal arch to form the body of the mandible, to the hydration of palatal shelves to produce shelf elevation necessary for the formation of the definitive palate, many different mechanisms are involved. Craniofacial development is clinically important since craniofacial anomalies are amongst the most common congenital anomalies found in man.

Learning Objectives

(1) Be able to understand the relationship of facial development and three pairs of pharyngeal arches.

(2) Be able to understand the process of palate development.

(3) Be able to understand the facial abnormalities.

Pre-class Questions

(1) How are different facial components generated?

(2) What are the time points of generations of different facial components?

Materials

Gross specimens, sections, embryo models, and simulation videos.

Observation and Reflection

1. Pharyngeal apparatus (咽器)

Buds-like pharyngeal arches are symmetrically distributed by the side of embryo body. Between pharyngeal arches there are pharyngeal clefts. Oral cavity is initiating at this stage surrounded by maxillary prominence and mandibular prominence. Nasal placodes are visible (Fig. 22 – 1).

> **Reflection**
>
> Where are pharyngeal arches derived from?

2. Formation of the face（颜面的发生）

（1）**4th developmental week**：The 1st pharyngeal arch gives rise to the maxillary and mandibular prominences. The frontonasal prominence（FNP）grows to cover the ventral part of the forebrain. Nasal placodes develop on the frontolateral aspects of the FNP.（Fig. 22 –2A）

（2）**5th developmental week**：The formation of the primordial ear auricles around the first pharyngeal groove, at the interface between the mandibular prominences and the hyoid arches. The auricular hillocks give rise to the auricle while the external acoustic meatus arises from the first pharyngeal groove. The maxillary prominence will merge with the medial nasal prominences, and cause their fusion. The fused medial nasal prominences will form the midline of the nose and that of the upper lip, as well as the primary palate.（Fig. 22 –2B）

（3）**6th developmental week**：The maxillary and lateral nasal prominences will fuse with the nasolacrimal groove and result in continuity between the nose and cheek.（Fig. 22 –2C）

（4）**7th developmental week**：Two maxillary nasal prominences are fused with the median and lateral nasal prominences. The merge between the maxillary and medial nasal prominences creates continuity between the upper jaw and lip, and results in partition of the nasal cavity from the oral cavity.（Fig. 22 –2D）

> **Reflection**
>
> What is tissue fusion? Why tissue fusion is crucial during face formation?

3. Formation of the palate（腭的发生）

（1）**Horizontal section**：Outgrowths that initiate from the medial edges of the maxillary prominences form the shelves of the secondary palates. These palatal shelves grow downward beside the tongue（Fig. 22 – 3A）. Palatal shelves keep on growing towards to each other and contact from middle to anterior and posterior respectively（Fig. 22 – 3B）. Tissue fusion leads to a continuous formation of palate（Fig. 22 –3C）.

（2）**Cross section**：Palatal shelves（Fig. 22 –4A）grow vertically and symmetrically by the side of developing tongue（Fig. 22 –4B）.

> **Reflection**
>
> What are the differences between the development of other facial components and palate development?

4. Abnormalies of face and palate（颜面先天畸形）

➢ Gross observation

（1）**Pierre Robin sequence**：The very small mandible keeps the tongue from dropping out of the palatal shelves, and results in cleft palate.

(2) **Apert syndrome**: It is an autosomal dominant inherited disease caused by genetic muta-tion of fibroblast growth factor receptor-2 (FGFR2). Craniosynostosis occurs, a high, prominent forehead with a flat back of the skull. A flat or concave face may develop.

(3) **Cleft lip and/or palate**: Upper lip and/or secondary palate midline cleft. (Fig. 22 – 5)

(4) **Facial dysmorphia**: Features including broad nasal root, low set ears, downward slant-ing eyes, downward slanting eyebrows. (Fig. 22 – 6)

Reflection

How do all types of cleft palate occurr?

Post-class Task

Describe the facial developing process.

Case-based Learning

A one-year-old girl presented with neurodevelopmental delay, hepatomegaly, bilateral hearing loss, and visual problems. Ophthalmologic examination suggested septo-optic dysplasia. Cranial magnetic resonance imaging (MRI) showed nonspecific gliosis at subcortical and periventricular deep white matter.

(1) What could be the reason that leads to this clinical manifestation?

(2) Is there any craniofacial deformation underlying?

(滕藤)

第23章 | 心血管系统的发生

学习目标

（1）能够描述心管的发生及心脏外形的演变过程。

（2）能够识别心内膜垫、第一房间隔、第二房间隔、第一房间孔、第二房间孔、卵圆孔、室间隔肌部、室间隔膜部、室间孔，并描述心脏内部的分隔过程。

（3）能够结合心脏发生的相关知识解释常见先天性心脏病的成因。

课前问题

（1）成体心脏的正常位置、外形和内部结构是怎样的？

（2）心脏壁由什么组织构成？

（3）原始心管是如何形成的？头褶和侧褶会导致心管与围心腔的相对位置及数量发生怎样的变化？

实验材料

大体标本，胚胎模型，仿真视频。

实验观察与思考

1. 心脏外形的演变

随着胚胎的发育，当左、右心管合并成一条心管时，心脏外形便开始发生变化。先是心管自头端向尾端先后出现4个膨大：心球、心室、心房和静脉窦，其中心球的远侧份（头端）较细长，称为动脉干；静脉窦末端则分为左右两个角。之后，心管呈弯曲状生长，心球和心室部弯曲形成"U"形（球室襻）；心房和静脉窦发生位移，进而使心脏呈"S"形。心房向左右方向扩展，膨出于心球的两侧。心房扩大，房室沟加深。此时心脏已初具成体心脏的外形。图23-1模型显示了心脏外形的演变过程，可分别从腹面观（图左侧）和背面观（图右侧）观察动脉干、心球、心室、心房和静脉窦各段，尤其注意各段相互位置的变化。

思考题

（1）心管为何会出现膨大？

（2）原始心脏可区分为几部分？其头端和尾端分别与什么血管相连？

（3）心管为何弯曲生长？原始心房、心室位置和外形发生什么变化？

（4）原始心房为何不能向前后方向扩展？

（5）心管各段将最终演变为成体心脏的哪些结构？

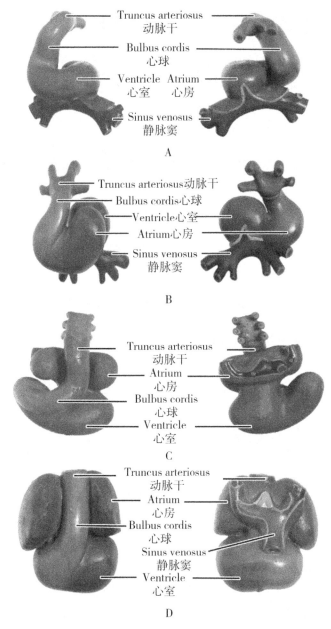

图 23 - 1 心脏外形的演变

Fig. 23 - 1 The evolution process of heart shape

2. 心脏内部的分隔

> **房室管的分隔**

心房与心室之间的狭窄管道为房室管，在房室管的背、腹侧壁正中可分别形成背、腹心内膜垫。两个心内膜垫相对生长并融合，将房室管分成左、右房室管。从图23-2的心脏冠状切面模型，可观察到心内膜垫发育形态变化及分隔后的房室管。

> **心房的分隔**

心房之间的间隔称为房间隔。第一房间隔由心房头端背侧壁正中发出，并向心内膜垫方向生长，其游离缘与心内膜垫之间暂留一孔为第一房间孔（图23-2A，3A）。当第一房间隔与心内膜垫完全融合时，第一房间孔随之被封闭。但在第一房间孔封闭之前，第一房间隔的上部出现第二房间孔（图23-2B，3B）。第二房间隔位于第一房间隔的右侧，由心房头端腹侧壁正中发出，并向心内膜垫方向生长，与心内膜垫之间形成卵圆孔（图23-2B，3C）。卵圆孔被第一房间隔从左侧所覆盖，形成卵圆孔瓣膜（图23-3C，3D）。最终，原始心房被第一房间隔和第二房间隔分隔成左心房和右心房（图23-2C）。

> **心室的分隔**

心室之间的间隔称为室间隔。室间隔由肌部和膜部组成。由心室底壁形成的肌性纵隔为肌部，其向心内膜垫方向生长，与心内膜垫之间的孔为室间孔（图23-2B）。室间孔被室间隔膜部封闭之后（图23-2C，4C），原始心室被分隔成左心室和右心室。

> **动脉干和心球的分隔**

动脉干和心球的内膜组织增厚分别形成一对心球嵴和动脉干嵴（图23-4A，4B），相应的嵴对向生长，并在中线处融合，形成螺旋状走形的主动脉肺动脉隔（图23-4C），此隔将动脉干和心球分隔成主动脉和肺动脉。

思考题

（1）心房的分隔为何需要2个房间隔？

（2）卵圆孔和第二房间孔的位置关系如何？

（3）卵圆孔在胎儿血液循环中有何作用？在出生后有何变化？

（4）室间隔膜部是怎样形成的？

（5）肺动脉和主动脉是怎样形成的？二者的位置关系如何？

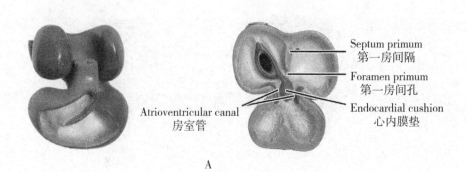

Septum primum
第一房间隔

Foramen primum
第一房间孔

Endocardial cushion
心内膜垫

Atrioventricular canal
房室管

A

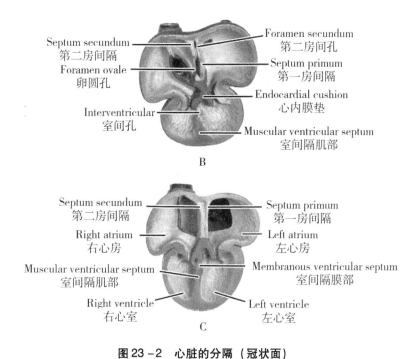

图 23-2 心脏的分隔（冠状面）

Fig. 23-2 Partitioning of the heart (coronal view)

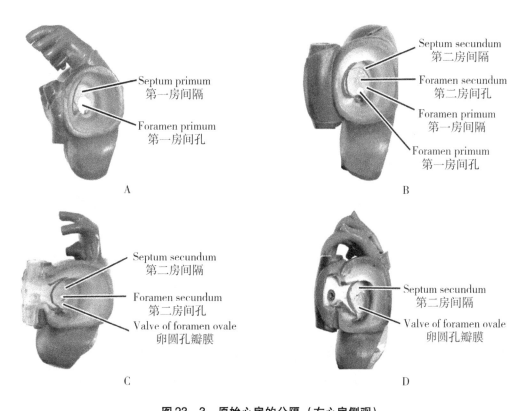

图 23-3 原始心房的分隔（右心房侧观）

Fig. 23-3 Partitioning of the primitive atrium (right atrial view)

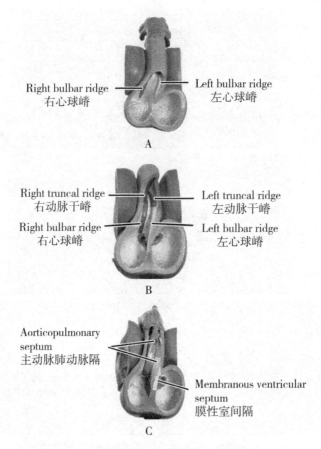

Right bulbar ridge
右心球嵴

Left bulbar ridge
左心球嵴

A

Right truncal ridge
右动脉干嵴

Left truncal ridge
左动脉干嵴

Right bulbar ridge
右心球嵴

Left bulbar ridge
左心球嵴

B

Aorticopulmonary
septum
主动脉肺动脉隔

Membranous ventricular
septum
膜性室间隔

C

图 23 - 4   动脉干和心球的分隔（冠状面）

Fig. 23 - 4   Partitioning of truncus arteriosus and bulbus cordis（coronary views）

3. 常见畸形

➤ **动脉导管未闭**

较多见，病因可能与出生后动脉导管壁的平滑肌不收缩，致使主动脉和肺动脉仍保持相通有关（图 23 - 5A）。

➤ **室间隔缺损**

常见室间隔膜部缺损，多伴有心球嵴的分隔异常（图 23 - 5B）。

➤ **房间隔缺损**

最常见的为卵圆孔未闭，可致左右心房相通（图 23 - 5C）。

➤ **法洛四联症**

较严重，可见肺动脉狭窄、主动脉骑跨、室间隔缺损和右心室肥大四种缺陷并存（图 23 - 5D）。

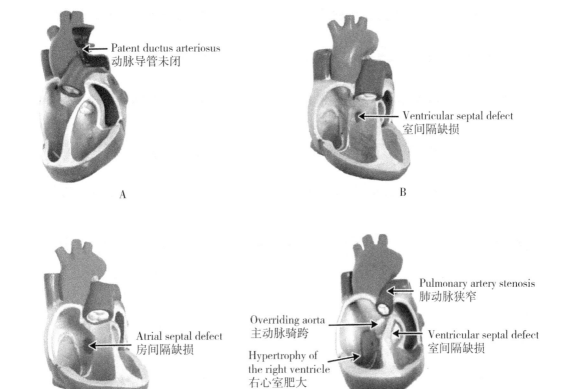

图 23 - 5 心脏发育异常

Fig. 25 - 5 Abnormal development of the heart

思考题

(1) 卵圆孔未闭的可能原因有哪些?

(2) 房间隔缺损和室间隔缺损会导致血流动力学怎样改变?

(3) 法洛四联症的主要成因是什么?

(4) 何谓主动脉骑跨?其有何后果?

课后作业

请绘制胎儿血液循环流程图,并与出生后的血液循环进行对比。

病例教学

患儿,女,3岁,因"哭闹后呼吸急促,抽搐2小时"而急诊入院。患儿出生后5个月便发现喜好安静、脸色和口唇易发紫,吃奶和哭闹时加重。体格检查:生长发育迟缓,嘴唇青紫明显,胸骨左缘2-3肋间可闻及喷射样收缩期杂音;心电图:电轴右偏;超声心动图:主动脉内径增宽,骑跨于室间隔上,肺动脉狭窄,右心室肥厚。最终,患儿被确诊为法洛四联症。

（1）何为法洛四联症？该疾病的成因是什么？

（2）患儿为何会出现上述症状和体征？

（3）如何防治法洛四联症？

（张庆梅）

Chapter 23   DEVELOPMENT OF CARDIOVASCULAR SYSTEM

The cardiovascular system is the first system to form and begin function in the embryo. This development is necessary to meet the oxygen and nutrient needs of rapidly growing embryo.

(1) Primitive cardiovascular system, which originates from extraembryonic blood islands and intraembryonic mesenchyme, consists of bilaterally symmetrical cardiac tubes, arteries and veins.

(2) The heart develops from the heart tube. The heart tube was originally a straight tube, which later forms the adult heart shape due to unequal and curved growth. More importantly, the interior of the heart is partitioned into a four-atrioventricular heart by endocardial cushion and septa.

(3) The fetal circulation, which involves the umbilical arteries, umbilical vein, venous duct, ductus arteriosus and oval foramen, is distinctly different from the postnatal circulation.

(4) Abnormal development of cardiovascular system will lead to congenital malformations, such as patent ductus arteriosus, ventricular septal defect, atrial septal defect, tetralogy of Fallot and so on.

Learning Objectives

(1) Be able to describe the occurrence of heart tube and the evolution of heart shape.

(2) Be able to identify the endocardial cushion, septum primum, septum secundum, foramen primum, foramen secundum, foramen ovale, muscular ventricular septum, membranous ventricular septum and interventricular foramen. And be able to describe the process of primitive heart partitioning.

(3) Be able to explain the causes of common congenital heart disease in combination with the relevant knowledge of heart occurrence.

Pre-class Questions

(1) Where is your heart located? What is the shape and internal structure of an adult heart?

(2) What tissue makes up the walls of the heart?

(3) How was the primitive heart tube formed? What is the effect of the cephalic and lateral folds on the relative position and number of the cardiac tube and pericardial chambers?

Materials

Gross specimens, embryo models, and simulation videos.

Observation and Reflection

1. Formation of heart shape（心脏外形的演变）

With the development of the embryo, the left and right heart tubes migrate together and fuse into one. The single heart tube quickly differentiates into four dilatations from head to tail: bulbus cordis（心球）, ventricle（心室）, atrium（心房）and venosus sinus（静脉窦）. The elongated distal part of the bulbus cordis is called truncus arteriosus（动脉干）, and the end of the venous sinus is divided into left and right horns. Then, the bulboventricular portion of cardiac tube grow quickly and fold into a "U"-shaped bulboventricular loop（球室袢）. The atria and venous sinuses are further displaced and the heart shifts into an "S" shape. Lastly, the atrium expands to the left and right, and is located on the two sides of the bulbus cordis. The atria are continuously enlarged and the atrioventricular groove（房室沟）is deepened. Now, the heart has begun to take the shape of an adult heart. Fig. 23 – 1 shows the evolution process of heart shape. The segments of heart tube including truncus arteriosus, bulbus cordis, ventricle, atrium and sinus venosus can be observed from the ventral (left) and dorsal (right) views. Note the changes in the relative positions of the segments.

> **Reflection**
>
> (1) Why is the heart tube enlarged?
>
> (2) What are the 5 regions of the primitive heart tube? What blood vessels are connected to its head and tail respectively?
>
> (3) Why does the heart tube bend to grow? What happens to the position and shape of primitive atrium and ventricle?
>
> (4) Why can't the primitive atrium expand forward and backward?
>
> (5) What structures of the adult heart will each segment of the cardiac tube eventually evolve into?

2. Partitioning of primordial heart（心脏内部的分隔）

➢ **Partitioning of atrioventricular canal（房室管的分隔）**

The narrow canal between primordial atrium and primordial ventricle is called the atrioventricular canal. The endocardial cushions（心内膜垫）form in the middle of the dorsal and ventral walls of the atrioventricular canal, respectively. When the two endocardial cushions grow toward each other and fuse, the atrioventricular canal is divided into left and right atrioventricular canals. In the coronal section of the heart model shown in Fig. 23 – 2, the morphologic changes of the endocardial cushion development and the atrioventricular canals after partitioning can be observed.

> ➤ Partitioning of primordial atrium（心房的分隔）

The septum between the atria is called the atrial septum（房间隔）. The septum primum（第一房间隔）arises from the middle dorsal wall of the atrial head and grows towards the endocardial cushions. As this septum grows, a temporary opening, the foramen primum（第一房间孔）, is formed between the lower edge of the septum primum and the endocardial cushions（Fig. 23 –2A, Fig. 23 –3A）. When the septum primum is completely fused to the endocardial cushion, the foramen primum is closed. However, Before the foramen primum disappears, perforations appear in the upper part of the septum primum and coalesce to produce the foramen secundum（第二房间孔）（Fig. 23 –2B, Fig. 23 –3B）. Later, the septum secundum（第二房间隔）, which locates the right of the septum primum, emerges from the middle ventral wall of the atrial head and forms the foramen ovale（卵圆孔）with the endocardial cushion（卵圆孔瓣膜）（Fig. 23 –2B, Fig. 23 –3C）. The foramen ovale is covered by the septum primum from the left and forms the valve of foramen ovale（Fig. 23 –3C, Fig. 23 –3D）. Finally, the primordial atrium is divided into left and right atrium by the septum primum and septum secundum（Fig. 23 –2C）.

> ➤ Partitioning of primordial ventricle（心室的分隔）

The septum between the ventricle is called the ventricular septum（室间隔）, which consists of muscular and membranous ventricular septum（室间隔肌部和室间隔膜部）. Muscular ventricular septum is derived from the muscular mediastinum created by the base wall of the ventricle. The foramen between the muscular ventricular septum and the endocardial cushion is called interventricular foramen（室间孔）（Fig. 23 –2B）. When the interventricular foramen is ultimately closed by the membranous ventricular septum（Fig. 23 –2C, Fig. 23 –4C）, the primordial ventricle is divided into left and right ventricles.

> ➤ Partitioning of the truncus arteriosus and bulbus cordis（动脉干和心球的分隔）

The subendocardial tissue in the bulbus cordis and bulbus cordis thickens into a pair of truncal and bulbar ridges, respectively（Fig. 23 –4A, Fig. 23 –4B）. They grow in opposite directions and fuse at the midline to form a spiral aorticopulmonary septum（主动脉肺动脉隔）（Fig. 23 –4C）, which separates the truncus arteriosus and bulbus cordis into the aorta and pulmonary artery.

Reflection

（1）Why does the partitioning of the primordial atrium require two atrial septa?

（2）What is the positional relationship between the foramen ovale and foramensecundum?

（3）What is the role of the foramen ovale in fetal circulation? What happens after birth?

（4）How is the membranous ventricular septum formed?

（5）How are the pulmonary arteries and aorta formed? What is the positional relationship between the two?

---

3. Anomalies of the cardiovascular system（心血管系统畸形）

> ➤ Patent ductus arteriosus（动脉导管未闭）

Patent ductus arteriosus may be caused by the failure of smooth muscle contraction of ductus arteriosus after birth, so that the aorta and pulmonary artery remain connected（Fig. 23 – 5A）.

> ➤ Ventricular septal defect（室间隔缺损）

Membranous ventricular septum defects are common. It is usually accompanied by septal Abnormalities of the bulbar ridged（Fig. 23 – 5B）.

> ➤ Atrial septal defect（房间隔缺损）

The most common type of atrial septal defect is a patent foramen ovale, which connects the left and right atria（Fig. 23 – 5C）.

> ➤ Tetralogy of Fallot（法洛四联症）

Tetralogy of Fallot is a combination of four defects, which are pulmonary artery stenosis（肺动脉狭窄）, overriding aorta（主动脉骑跨）, ventricular septal defect, and hypertrophy of the right ventricle（右心室肥大）（Fig. 23 – 5D）.

Reflection

(1) What are the possible causes of patent foramen ovale?

(2) How do atrial septal defects and ventricular septal defects change hemodynamics?

(3) What is the main cause of tetralogy of Fallot?

(4) What is an overriding aorta? What are the consequences of the overriding aorta?

Post-class Task

Please draw the flow chart of fetal blood circulation and compare the blood circulation after birth.

Case-based Learning

A 3-year-old female patient was admitted to the emergency department with shortness of breath and convulsions（抽搐）for 2 h after crying. She has been quiet and easy to have purple faces and lips, especially during feeding or crying, since 5 months after birth. Physical examination showed the child with growth retardation（发育迟缓）, lip cyanosis（发绀，又称紫绀）and systolic ejection murmur（喷射样收缩期杂音）that was heard best at the second and third left intercostal space. Electrocardiogram found right axis deviation（电轴右偏）. Echocardiogram explored widened aortic straddling the interventricular septum, pulmonary artery stenosis and hypertrophy of the right ventricle. Eventually, the patient was diagnosed with tetralogy of Fallot.

(1) What is tetralogy of Fallot? What is the cause of the disease?

(2) Why do the child patient have the symptoms and signs described above?

(3) How to prevent and treat the tetralogy of Fallot?

（张庆梅）

第24章 | 消化系统和呼吸系统的发生

第4周，内胚层形成原始消化管。原始消化管由前到后分为前肠、中肠和后肠。前肠的头端由口咽膜封闭，后肠的尾端由泄殖腔膜封闭。

原始消化管的内胚层形成消化管（除头端和末端外）的上皮和腺体，肝脏和胰腺，以及下呼吸道的器官的上皮和腺体。脏壁中胚层发育成消化道和下呼吸道器官的肌组织和结缔组织。

学习目标

（1）能够识别原始消化管及其演化的结构。
（2）能够描述消化管的发生过程。
（3）能够描述肝脏和胰腺的发生过程。
（4）能够描述呼吸系统的发生过程。
（5）能够识别和描述常见的消化系统和呼吸系统先天性畸形。

课前问题

（1）消化道和消化腺之间的解剖关系是什么？
（2）消化道和呼吸道之间的解剖关系是什么？

实验材料

大体标本，胚胎模型，仿真视频。

实验观察与思考

1. 消化管的发生

1）原始消化管识别

原始消化管的3个部分：①前肠，从口咽膜至肝脏出芽处；②中肠，从肝脏出芽处尾侧开始，至横结肠右三分之二末端；③后肠，从横结肠的左三分之一到泄殖腔膜（图24-1）。

> **思考题**
> 前肠、中肠、后肠分别发育为哪些器官？

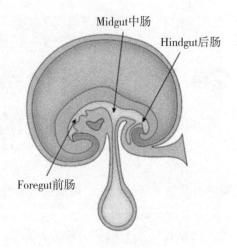

图 24 - 1　原始消化管
Fig. 24 - 1　Primordial gut

2）前肠

➤ **食管的发生**

第 4 周，可识别前肠腹侧壁的喉气管憩室（图 24 - 2）。气管食管嵴融合形成气管食管隔（图 24 - 3）。气管食管隔的背侧是食管。

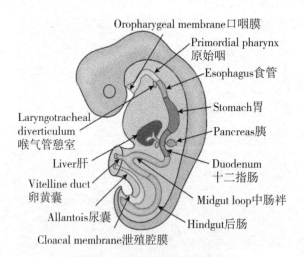

图 24 - 2　原始消化管的演变
Fig. 24 - 2　Derivatives of primordial gut

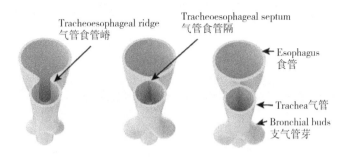

图 24 – 3　气管食管隔的发生

Fig. 24 –3　Development of tracheoesophageal septum

第 7 周，食管上皮细胞增生，食管管腔闭锁。第 8 周，食管管腔再通。

➤ **胃的发生**

第 4 周，胃的原基形成，最初位于中轴线上。胃的背侧缘比其腹侧缘生长得快。

旋转：从头端观察，胃沿纵轴顺时针方向旋转 90°，因此，背侧缘在右侧，腹侧缘在左侧。同时，胃也围绕胚体的前后轴旋转，幽门向右上方移动，而贲门向左移动（图 24 – 4）。

网膜囊：胃通过背侧系膜连接到背侧体壁，通过腹侧系膜连接到腹侧体壁。胃沿纵轴旋转将背侧系膜拉向左侧，在胃后形成一个空间，称为网膜囊，又称小腹膜腔。

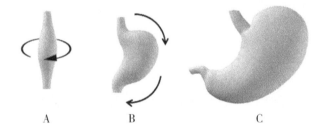

A：沿长轴旋转（Rotation along longitudinal axis）；B：沿前后轴旋转（Rotation around anteroposterior axis）；

C：胃的位置（Final position of stomach）。

图 24 – 4　胃的发生

Fig. 24 –4　Development of stomach

思考题

（1）胃在发生过程中是如何旋转的？

（2）请从胚胎发生的角度解释为什么胃前壁受左迷走神经支配，胃后壁受右迷走神经支配。

➤ **十二指肠的发生**

第 4 周，前肠尾部、中肠头端和相关的脏壁中胚层发展成十二指肠。

C 形环：十二指肠迅速生长，形成一个 C 形环，向腹侧突出（图 24 –5A）。

旋转：当胃旋转的时候，十二指肠环向右旋转（图 24 –5B）。

闭锁和再通：第 5 周，十二指肠的管腔暂时闭锁。第 8 周末，十二指肠重新通畅。

思考题
在发生过程中，十二指肠的旋转和胃的旋转方向有何相似之处？

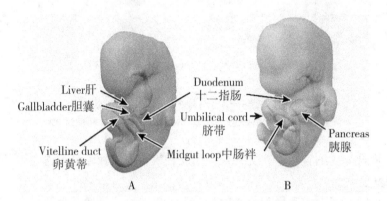

A：6周人胚（At 6 weeks）；B：7周人胚（At 7 weeks）。

图 24 –5　前肠和中肠的发生

Fig. 24 –5　Development of foregut and midgut

> **肠系膜的发生**

肠系膜来源于中胚层间充质。

背侧肠系膜：将前肠的末端、中肠和后肠的主要部分悬挂在腹壁上。识别背侧肠系膜的各部分，包括胃背系膜（大网膜）、十二指肠背系膜、空肠和回肠区域的肠系膜，以及结肠背系膜（图 24 –6A）。

识别胃和背侧腹膜之间的网膜囊（图 24 –6B），以及网膜囊与腹腔相通的网膜孔（图 24 –6C）。网膜囊由胃背系膜随着胃大弯向左旋转形成。

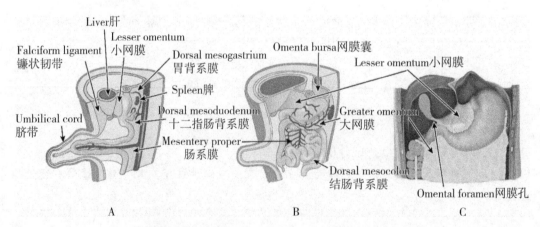

A：6周人胚（At 6 weeks）；B：12周人胚（At 12 weeks）；
C：出生后肠系膜（Definitive mesentery after birth）。

图 24 –6　肠系膜的发生

Fig. 24 –6　Development of mesentery

随着十二指肠的旋转，十二指肠背系膜被拉向右侧并与邻近的腹膜融合，只有邻近幽门处的小部分十二指肠背系膜保留下来。因此，十二指肠的大部分位于腹膜后。

腹侧肠系膜：识别食管末端、胃和十二指肠上部区域的腹侧肠系膜。肝脏在腹侧肠系膜的两层间生长，将腹侧肠系膜分隔为小网膜和镰状韧带。

思考题

网膜囊的解剖标志有哪些？

3）中肠

中肠通过卵黄管与卵黄囊相连，通过肠系膜悬挂在背侧体壁上。中肠形成胆管开口远侧的小肠、盲肠、阑尾、升结肠和横结肠近三分之二的部分。中肠由肠系膜上动脉供应。

➤ **生理性脐疝**

第6周，中肠弯曲形成中肠袢并伸入脐带近端的胚外体腔，形成生理性脐疝（图24 - 7）。识别连接在中肠环顶部的卵黄管。

➤ **中肠袢的旋转**

随着胃和十二指肠的旋转，脐带内的中肠袢围绕肠系膜上动脉的轴线逆时针旋转90°（腹侧观）（图24 - 7A）。因此，中肠袢的头支在右侧，尾支在左侧（图24 - 5B，7B）。在旋转过程中，头肢生长形成小肠袢。

➤ **小肠袢的回缩和进一步旋转**

第10周，小肠首先返回腹腔内，同时进一步发生180°的逆时针旋转（图24 - 7C）。最后，盲肠回到腹腔。

思考题

从腹侧观，中肠袢一共逆时针旋转了多少度？

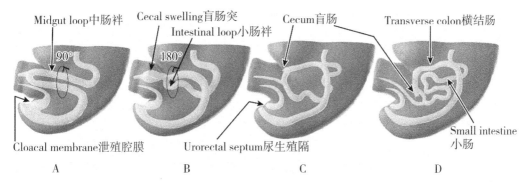

A：6 周（At 6 weeks）；B：7 周（At 7 weeks）；C：10 周（At 10 weeks）；D：11 周（At 11 weeks）。

图24 - 7　中肠和后肠的发生

Fig. 24 - 7　Development of midgut and hindgut

4）后肠

后肠形成横结肠、降结肠、乙状结肠、直肠的远端三分之一，以及肛管的上部，还有膀胱和尿道。后肠由肠系膜下动脉供应。

> **直肠的发生**

泄殖腔是后肠的末端。尿囊开口于后肠。识别尿囊和后肠之间的尿直肠隔（图24 - 7C）。尿直肠隔将泄殖腔分为背侧的直肠和肛门，腹侧的泌尿生殖窦。

> **肛管的发生**

肛管以齿状线为界，上三分之二来自后肠，下三分之一来自外胚层（图24 - 8）。

第7周末，泄殖腔膜破裂，形成肛门和泌尿生殖窦的开口。

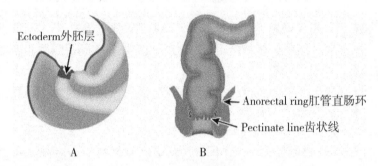

A：肛管的发生（Development of anal canal）；B：肛管的结构（Definitive structure of anal canal）。

图24 - 8 肛管的发生

Fig. 24 - 8 Development of anal canal

2. 消化腺的发生

1）肝脏和胆道系统的发生

第4周，肝憩室形成，位于前肠的远端和腹侧，胃腹系膜中。肝憩室的头端发育成肝脏，而较小的尾端则形成胆囊（图24 - 5A）。肝憩室与前肠的连接处发展为胆管。第12周，肝细胞开始分泌胆汁。

2）胰腺的发生

两个胰芽：前肠末端出现一个背胰芽和一个腹胰芽。背胰芽在背侧肠系膜，腹胰芽在胆管附近（图24 - 5A）。

旋转：当十二指肠向右旋转时，腹胰芽向背侧移动，位于背侧芽的后方（图24 - 5B）。

融合：背胰和腹胰融合形成胰腺。腹胰形成钩突和胰头的一部分。背胰导管的远端部分和整个腹胰导管形成胰腺主导管。背胰导管的近端部分有时作为副胰管持续存在。

思考题

（1）哪些器官是腹膜后位？哪些器官是腹膜间位？哪些器官是腹膜内位？请联系肠系膜的发生进行分析。

（2）在消化系统的发生过程中，哪些器官发生了旋转？哪些器官发生了闭锁和再通？

---

3. 呼吸系统的发生

1) 喉气管憩室

第4周的胚胎，原始咽的尾端腹侧出现喉气管沟。喉气管沟演化形成喉气管憩室（图24-2）。喉气管憩室的内胚层发育成喉、气管、支气管和肺的上皮和腺体。

2) 气管食管隔

第5周的胚胎，气管食管隔将前肠分为腹侧的气管和支气管芽，以及背侧的食管（图24-3）。气管通过喉口与咽相通（图24-9A）。

3) 喉的发生

在喉的发育过程中，喉腔暂时湮没，随后重新再通。喉部的上皮细胞和腺体来自内胚层，而软骨和肌肉则来自第四和第六鳃弓。

识别位于第三和第六咽弓腹侧末端的咽下突（图24-9A）。咽下突的尾侧是会厌突，发育成会厌（图24-9B、9C）。

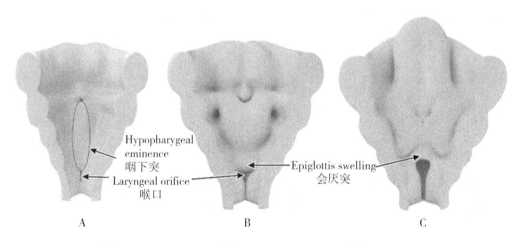

A：4周（At 4 weeks）；B：5周（At 5 weeks）；C：5个月（At 5 months）。

图24-9 喉的发生

Fig. 24-9 Development of larynx

4) 气管、主支气管和肺的发生

第4周的胚胎，气管和肺芽形成（图24-10A）。肺芽长入心包腹膜管。心包腹膜管的中胚层形成胸膜。

第5周，左右主支气管和叶支气管形成（图24-10B）。

第7周，段支气管形成（图24-10C）。

第8周，段支气管进一步形成分支（图24-10D）。

第6个月末，大约有17级支气管分支形成。

出生后还有6～7个分支形成。

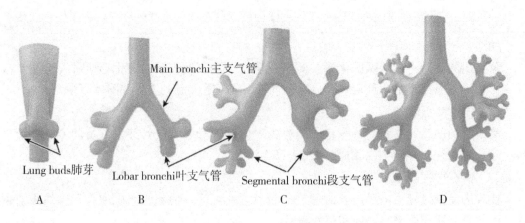

A：第4周（At 4 weeks）；B：第5周（At 5 weeks）；
C：第7周（At 7 weeks）；D：第8周（At 8 weeks）。

图24 – 10　气管、主支气管和肺的发生

Fig. 24 –10　Development of trachea, main bronchi and lungs

5）肺的成熟

肺的成熟分为四个阶段：假腺期、小管期、终末囊泡期和肺泡期。比较每个阶段的形态学特征。

假腺期：胚胎第6～16周，肺的导气部形成，但呼吸部还未形成（图24 –11A）。

小管期：胚胎第16～26周，呼吸性支气管和肺泡管开始形成（图24 –11B）。肺组织内血管丰富。第24周，Ⅱ型肺泡细胞开始发生，并产生表面活性物质。

终末囊泡期：胚胎第26～32周，更多的终末囊泡（原始肺泡）形成。毛细血管与终末囊泡密切接触（图24 –11C）。

肺泡期：胚胎第32周至出生后10年，终末囊泡发展为肺泡（图24 –11D）。毛细血管和肺泡间形成非常薄的气血屏障。约六分之五的肺泡在出生后形成。

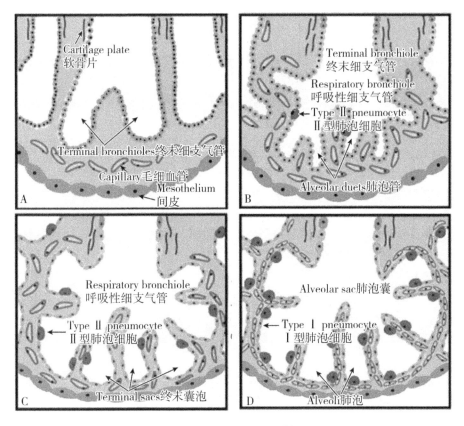

A：假腺期（Pseudoglandular stage）；B：小管期（Canalicular stage）；
C：终末囊泡期（Terminal sac stage）；D：肺泡期（Alveolar stage）。

图 24 −11　肺的成熟

Fig. 24 −11　Maturation of lungs

思考题

（1）左肺和右肺分别有多少支叶支气管和段支气管？

（2）为什么第 24 ～ 26 周出生的早产儿易患新生儿呼吸窘迫综合征（neonatal respiratory distress syndrome，NRDS）？

---

4. 常见的消化系统和呼吸系统先天性畸形

1）食管闭锁和气管食管瘘

食管闭锁指食道的上半段形成盲端。气管食道瘘是食道的下段与气管间形成瘘管。食管闭锁和气管食道瘘常同时发生（图 24 −12）。

思考题

胚胎发生过程中，什么结构分隔了气管和食管？

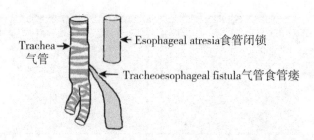

图 24 - 12　食管闭锁和气管食管瘘

Fig. 24 - 12　Esophageal atresia and tracheoesophageal fistula

2）麦克尔憩室

小部分卵黄管持续存在，在回肠处形成一个憩室，即麦克尔憩室或回肠憩室（图 24 - 13A）。麦克尔憩室通常没有临床症状。

3）脐瘘和卵黄管囊肿

脐瘘，又称卵黄管瘘，是脐部和回肠之间的卵黄管未闭锁形成（图 24 - 13B）。

卵黄管囊肿是卵黄管的两端闭锁而中间部分未闭锁形成（图 24 - 13C）。

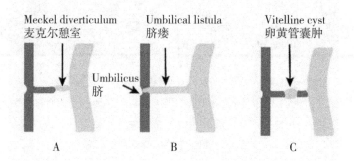

A：麦克尔憩室（Meckel diverticulum）；B：脐瘘（Umbilical fistula）；

C：卵黄管囊肿（Vitelline cyst）。

图 24 - 13　卵黄管发育异常

Fig. 24 - 13　Vitelline duct abnormalities

4）脐疝和腹裂

脐疝是腹部脏器通过扩大的脐环疝出。疝出器官有羊膜包裹，可能有肝脏、小肠、大肠、胃、脾脏或胆囊。

腹裂是腹腔脏器从脐部一侧的体壁疝出（图 24 - 14）。疝出脏器没有被腹膜或羊膜覆盖。

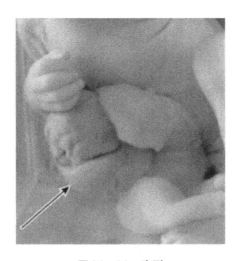

图 24 - 14　腹裂

Fig. 24 - 14　Gastroschisis

5）直肠尿道瘘和直肠阴道瘘

直肠尿道瘘（图 24 - 15A）和直肠阴道瘘（图 24 - 15B）由尿直肠隔的形成异常引起。

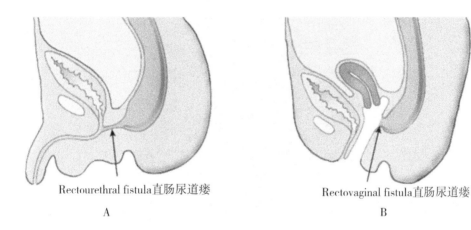

Rectourethral fistula 直肠尿道瘘　　　　　　Rectovaginal fistula 直肠尿道瘘

A　　　　　　　　　　　　　　　　　B

图 24 - 15　尿直肠隔发育异常

Fig. 24 - 15　Urorectal septum abnormalities

6）肛门闭锁

肛门闭锁是肛膜未破裂所致（图 24 - 16）。

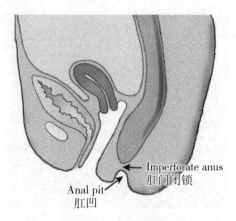

图24-16　肛门闭锁
Fig. 24-16　Imperforate anus

7）先天性巨结肠

先天性巨结肠是由于肠壁缺乏副交感神经节所致（图24-17）。

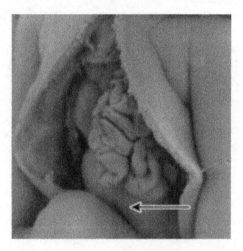

图24-17　先天性巨结肠
Fig. 24-17　Congenital megacolon

课后作业

绘制原始消化管的模式图。

病例教学

一名28岁的女性，孕1产0，妊娠38周时来医院分娩，之前未做过产前超声检查。第一产程13 h，第二产程15 min。产妇经阴道分娩生下一个男婴，体重2.5 kg。男婴患有脐疝，肠、肝和脾疝出，呼吸不畅，哭声不大，出生后有紫绀，给氧后好转。未发现其他严重的先天性畸形。出生7 h后，男婴接受了手术治疗，手术切除了羊膜囊、脾脏和约30%的肝脏，其他疝出器官回置入腹腔内。

（1）生理性脐疝和先天性脐疝之间的区别是什么？

（2）脐疝可能对呼吸有什么影响？

（3）先天性脐疝的发生机制是什么？

（周雯）

Chapter 24　DEVELOPMENT OF DIGESTIVE AND RESPIRATORY SYSTEM

During the 4th week, the **primordial gut**（原始消化管）forms as endoderm is incorporated into the embryo. The primordial gut is divided into 3 parts: **foregut**（前肠）, **midgut**（中肠）, and **hindgut**（后肠）. The foregut is closed at its cranial end by the oropharyngeal membrane, and the hindgut is closed at its caudal end by the cloacal membrane.

The endoderm of the primordial gut forms the epithelia and glands of the digestive tract, except for the cranial and caudal parts. The endoderm of the primordial gut also gives rise to liver and pancreas, as well as the epithelium of the lower respiratory organs and the tracheobronchial glands. The splanchnic mesoderm develops into the muscular and connective tissues of the digestive tract and lower respiratory organs.

Learning Objectives

(1) Be able to identify the three sections of primordial gut and its derivatives.

(2) Be able to illustrate the timeline and developmental process of digestive tracts.

(3) Be able to illustrate the developmental process of liver and pancreas.

(4) Be able to illustrate the timeline and developmental process of respiratory system.

(5) Be able to identify common congenital malformations of the digestive and respiratory systems and explain their mechanisms of occurrence.

Pre-class Questions

(1) What are anatomic relationship between digestive tracts and digestive glands prenatally and postnatally?

(2) What are anatomic relationship between digestive tracts and respiratory tracts prenatally and postnatally?

Materials

Gross specimens, embryo models, simulation videos.

Observation and Reflection

1.　Development of digestive tract

1）Primordial gut

Primordial gut consists of three parts（Fig. 24 – 1，Fig. 24 – 2）：①**foregut**，beginning from the oropharyngeal membrane to the liver bud；②**midgut**，beginning caudal to the liver bud and extending to the end of the proximal two-thirds of the transverse colon；③**hindgut**，extending from the left third of the transverse colon to the cloacal membrane.

The part of foregut from the oropharyngeal membrane to the respiratory diverticulum is called **primordial pharynx**.

Reflection

What organs develop from foregut，midgut，and hindgut?

2）Foregut

➤　Development of esophagus

In 4-week embryo，the **laryngotracheal diverticulum**（喉气管憩室）develops at the ventral wall of the foregut（Fig. 24 – 2）. The **tracheoesophageal ridges**（气管食管嵴）fuse to form the **tracheoesophageal septum**（气管食管隔）（Fig. 24 – 3）. It divides the foregut into trachea and bronchial buds anteriorly，and esophagus posteriorly.

During the 7th week，the epithelium proliferates and temporarily obliterates the lumen of the esophagus. By the 8th week，recanalization of the esophagus occurs.

➤　Development of stomach

In the 4th week，the **primordial stomach** forms. It is initially oriented in the median plane. The dorsal border（greater curvature）of the stomach grows faster than its ventral border（lesser curvature）.

Rotation：The stomach rotates 90° in a clockwise direction（viewed from the cranial end）along its longitudinal axis，so that the greater curvature is on the left and lesser curvature on the right. The stomach also rotates around an anteroposterior axis，so that the pylorus moves to the right，and the cardia moves to the left（Fig. 24 – 4）.

Reflection

（1）How does the primordial stomach rotate during the embryonic development?

（2）Please explain why the anterior and posterior wall of the definitive stomach are supplied by the left and right vagus nerve respectively from embryologic perspective.

➤　Development of duodenum

In the 4th week，the duodenum develops from the portions of both foregut and midgut，and the associated splanchnic mesoderm.

C-shaped loop: The duodenum grows rapidly, forming a C-shaped loop that projects ventrally (Fig. 24 –5A).

Rotation: While the stomach rotates, the duodenal loop rotates to the right (Fig. 24 –5B).

Obliteration and recanalization: In the 5th week, the lumen of the duodenum becomes temporarily obliterated. By the end of 8th week, the duodenum recanalizes.

Reflection

How is duodenal rotation similar to the gastric rotation during the embryonic development?

> ➢ **Development of mesentery**

The mesenteries are double layers of peritoneum derived from the mesenchyme.

Dorsal mesentery（背肠系膜）：It suspends the caudal part of the foregut, the midgut, and a major part of the hindgut from the abdominal wall. The dorsal mesentery includes the dorsal mesogastrium（胃背系膜）, the dorsal mesoduodenum（十二指肠背系膜）, the mesentery proper（肠系膜）in the region of the jejunum and ileum, and the dorsal mesocolon（结肠背系膜）(Fig. 24 –6A).

The **omental bursa**（lesser peritoneal sac, 网膜囊）is between the stomach and dorsal mesogastrium（Fig. 24 –6B）, and is formed by rotation of dorsal mesogastrium to the left with the greater curvature of stomach. The omental bursa communicates with the greater peritoneal sac through the omental foramen（Fig. 24 –6C）.

As duodenum rotates, dorsal mesoduodenum is pulled to the right and fuses with the adjacent peritoneum. Only a small portion of the dorsal mesoduodenum in the region of the pylorus retains. Therefore, most part of duodenum is fixed retroperitoneally.

Ventral mesentery（腹肠系膜）：The ventral mesentery is in the region of the caudal part of the esophagus, the stomach, and the upper part of the duodenum. The ventral mesentery is divided into the lesser omentum（小网膜）and the falciform ligament（镰状韧带）by the growth of liver between its two layers.

Reflection

Can you list the anatomical landmarks of omental bursa?

---

3) Midgut

The midgut connects with the yolk sac by the vitelline duct and is suspended from dorsal wall by mesentery. The midgut forms the small intestine distal to the opening of the bile duct, cecum, appendix, ascending colon, and the proximal two-thirds of the transverse colon. The midgut is supplied by the superior mesenteric artery.

> ➤ Physiological herniation

In the 6th week, **physiologic umbilical herniation** （生理性脐疝）occurs as the midgut loop develops and projects into the extraembryonic coelom in the proximal part of the umbilical cord (Fig. 24 – 7). The vitelline duct attaches on the apex of the midgut loop (Fig. 24 – 5).

> ➤ Rotation of midgut loop

As the stomach and duodenum rotate, the midgut loop in the umbilical cord rotates 90° counterclockwise (viewed from the ventral side) around the axis of the superior mesenteric artery (Fig. 24 – 7A). As a result, the cranial limb of the midgut loop is on the right and the caudal limb is on the left (Fig. 24 – 5B, 7B). During rotation, the cranial limb elongates and forms **intestinal loops** （小肠祥）.

> ➤ Retraction of intestinal loops and further rotation

In the 10th week, the intestines return to the abdomen. The small intestine returns first and another 180° counterclockwise rotation occurs (Fig. 24 – 7C). Lastly, the cecum returns to the abdominal cavity.

Reflection

If viewed from the ventral side, how many degrees does the midgut loop rotate counterclockwise altogether?

---

4) Hindgut

The hindgut gives rise to the distal third of the transverse colon, descending colon, sigmoid, rectum, and the upper part of the anal canal. The hindgut also forms the bladder and urethra. The hindgut is supplied by the inferior mesenteric artery.

> ➤ Development of rectum

The expanded terminal part of the hindgut is called **cloaca** （泄殖腔）. **Urorectal septum** （尿直肠隔）is between the allantois and hindgut (Fig. 24 – 7C). The urorectal septum divides the cloaca dorsally into rectum and anal canal, and ventrally into urogenital sinus.

> ➤ Development of anal canal

The upper two-thirds of the anal canal is derived from the hindgut, and the lower one-third is derived from ectoderm. The **pectinate line** （齿状线）delimits the transition between the endodermal and ectodermal regions of the anal canal (Fig. 24 – 8).

At the end of the 7th week, the cloacal membrane ruptures, creating the opening for the anus and the urogenital sinus.

2. Development of digestive glands

1) Development of Liver and Biliary Apparatus

In the 4-week embryo, the **hepatic diverticulum** （肝憩室）forms, located in the ventral mesogastrium. The hepatic diverticulum develops into the liver and the gallbladder (Fig. 24 – 5A). The connection between the hepatic diverticulum and the foregut develops into bile duct. In the 12th week, hepatic cells begin to secret bile.

2）**Development of pancreas**

Two pancreatic buds: The pancreas is derived from a dorsal bud and a ventral bud （Fig. 24 – 5A）.

Rotation: As the duodenum rotates to the right, the ventral pancreatic bud moves dorsally and lies posterior to the dorsal bud （Fig. 24 – 5B）.

Fusion: The dorsal bud and ventral bud fuse to form pancreas. The distal part of the dorsal pancreatic duct and the entire ventral pancreatic duct form the main pancreatic duct. The proximal part of the dorsal pancreatic duct may persist as the accessory pancreatic duct.

Reflection

（1）What organs are retroperitoneal? What organs are intraperitoneal?

（2）During the development of digestive system, what organs undergo rotation, what organs have obliteration and recanalization?

---

3. Development of respiratory system

1）laryngotracheal diverticulum （喉气管憩室）

In 4-week embryo, there is the **laryngotracheal groove** （喉气管沟） in the floor of the caudal end of the primordial pharynx. Soon, laryngotracheal groove evaginates to form the **laryngotracheal diverticulum** （Fig. 24 – 2）.

2）tracheoesophageal septum （气管食管隔）

In 5-week embryo, the **tracheoesophageal septum** develops （Fig. 24 – 3）. The trachea communicates with the pharynx through the **laryngeal orifice** （喉口）（Fig. 24 – 9A）.

3）Development of larynx

Laryngeal lumen temporarily obliterates and later recanalizes.

The **hypopharyngeal eminence** （咽下突） forms at the ventral parts of the 3rd and 4th pharyngeal arches （Fig. 24 – 9A）. The caudal part of hypopharyngeal eminence is called **epiglottis swelling** （会厌突） which develops into the epiglottis （Fig. 24 – 9B, 9C）.

4）Development of trachea, main bronchi and lungs

In 4-week embryo, the trachea and two lung buds develope from laryngotracheal diverticulum （Fig. 24 – 10A）. The lung buds grow into the pericardioperitoneal canals.

In 5-week embryo, the right and left main bronchi, and the secondary bronchi （lobar bronchi） form （Fig. 24 – 10B）.

In 7-week embryo, the segmental bronchi form （Fig. 24 – 10C）.

In 8-week embryo, the segmental bronchi give branches （Fig. 24 – 10D）.

At the end of the 6th month, approximately 17 generations of bronchial branches form. An additional 6 – 7 subdivisions form postnatally.

（5）Maturation of lungs

Pseudoglandular stage（假腺期）：In 6 – 16 weeks of embryo, the conducting portion of lungs forms, but the respiratory portion is not present（Fig. 24 – 11A）.

Canalicular stage（小管期）：In 16 – 26 weeks of embryo, the respiratory bronchioles and bronchial ducts begin to form（Fig. 24 – 11B）. The lung tissue is well vascularized. Type Ⅱ pneumocytes develop at approximately 24 weeks and start to produce surfactant.

Terminal sac stage（终末囊泡期）：In 26 – 32 weeks of embryo, more terminal sacs（primordial alveoli）form. Capillaries closely contact with terminal sacs（Fig. 24 – 11C）.

Alveolar stage（肺泡期）：From 32 weeks of embryo till 10 years postnatally, terminal sacs develop into alveoli（Fig. 24 – 11D）. Capillaries bulge into the alveoli to form very thin blood-air barrier. Approximately five-sixth of the adult number of alveoli form after birth.

Reflection

（1）How many lobar bronchi and segmental bronchi are on the left lung and on the right lung respectively?

（2）Why would premature neonates born at 24 to 26 weeks of gestation suffer from neonatal respiratory distress syndrome（NRDS）?

---

4. Anomalies of digestive system and respiratory system

1）Esophageal atresia（食管闭锁）and tracheoesophageal fistula（气管食管瘘）

Esophageal atresia is a malformation that the upper portion of the esophagus ending in a blind pouch. Tracheoesophageal fistula is an anomaly that the lower segment of the esophagus forms a fistula with the trachea. Esophageal atresia and tracheoesophageal fistulas often occur together（Fig. 24 – 12）.

Reflection

What structure divides the esophagus and trachea?

2）Meckel diverticulum（麦克尔憩室）

A small portion of the vitelline duct persists, forming an out pocketing of the ileum, Meckel diverticulum or ileal diverticulum（Fig. 24 – 13A）. This diverticulum is usually asymptomatic.

3）Umbilical fistula（脐瘘）and vitelline cyst（卵黄管囊肿）

Umbilical fistula, also called as vitelline fistula, is formed by patent vitelline duct over its entire length between the umbilicus and the intestinal tract（Fig. 24 – 13B）.

Vitelline cyst is formed by patent middle portion of vitelline duct with both ends of the vitelline duct transforming into fibrous cords（Fig. 24 – 13C）.

4）Omphalocele（脐疝）and gastroschisis（腹裂）

Omphalocele is herniation of abdominal viscera through an enlarged umbilical ring. The viscera, which may include liver, small and large intestines, stomach, spleen, or gallbladder, are covered by amnion.

Gastroschisis refers to herniation of abdominal viscera out of the body wall lateral to the umbilicus (Fig. 24 – 14). The viscera are not covered by peritoneum or amnion.

5) Rectourethral fistula（直肠尿道瘘）and rectovaginal fistula（直肠阴道瘘）

Rectourethral fistula (Fig. 24 – 15A) and rectovaginal fistula (Fig. 24 – 15B) are caused by abnormalities in formation of the urorectal septum.

6) Imperforate anus（肛门闭锁）

Imperforate anus is an abnormality that the anal membrane fails to breakdown (Fig. 24 – 16).

7) Congenital megacolon（先天性巨结肠）

Congenital megacolon is due to an absence of parasympathetic ganglia in the bowel wall (Fig. 24 – 17).

Post-class Task

Draw a diagram of primordial gut.

Case-based Learning

A 28-year-old woman, gravid 1, para 0, presented to the hospital at 38 weeks period of gestation. The first stage of labor lasted 13 hours and the second stage lasted 15 minutes. She had not have any antenatal ultrasonography or fetal scan till date. The patient gave birth to a male child weighing 2.5 kg by vaginal delivery. The child had large omphalocele containing intestines, liver and spleen. He breathed poorly, had a poor cry, and was cyanotic immediately after birth but responded well to oxygen therapy. No other gross congenital anomalies were found. Seven hours after birth, the child received a surgery to excise the entire amniotic sac, remove the spleen and approximately 30 percent of the liver, and replace the abdominal organs in the abdominal cavity.

(1) What is the difference between physical herniation and omphalocele?

(2) How does omphalocele cause breathing difficulty?

(3) What is the pathogenesis of omphalocele?

（周雯）

第25章 | 泌尿生殖系统的发生

学习目标

（1）能够描述前肾和中肾的发生过程。

（2）掌握后肾的发生过程。

（3）了解前肾管和中肾管的关系和走向。

（4）能够说明生殖腺的发生过程和生殖管道的演变。

（5）掌握生殖腺和生殖管道的分化机理。

（6）能够识别多囊肾、异位肾、马蹄肾、双输尿管、脐尿瘘、隐睾、先天性腹股沟疝、双子宫等先天畸形。

课前问题

（1）肾的组织结构是怎样的？

（2）试着描述一下卵巢和睾丸的组织结构？

（3）泌尿系统和生殖系统各自发生的胚胎原基是什么？

实验材料

大体标本，胚胎模型，仿真视频。

实验观察与思考

1. 泌尿系统的发生

➤ 肾和输尿管的发生

（1）前肾的发生。第4周初，人胚生肾节内形成数条横行的前肾小管。前肾小管外侧端向尾部延伸，连接于一条纵向的前肾管，前肾管尾端开口于泄殖腔。前肾小管和前肾管形成前肾。第4周末，前肾小管退化，而前肾管大部分保留（图25-1A，B）。

（2）中肾的发生。第4周末，前肾小管退化，中肾开始发生。人胚生肾索内形成80对横行的小管，称中肾小管。这些小管逐渐延长形成"S"形小管，内侧端膨大并凹陷形成肾小囊，包绕毛细血管球，形成肾小体；外侧端与向尾端延伸的前肾管相通，此时前肾管改为中肾管，中肾小管和中肾管共同构成中肾（图25-1C，图25-2）。在后肾出现之前，中肾有短暂功能，在第2个月末，大部分中肾退化，仅中肾管和尾端少数中肾小管保留。

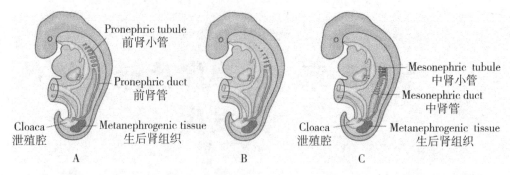

A：前肾的发生（Formation of the pronephros）；B：前肾的退化（Degeneration of the pronephros）；
C：中肾的发生（Formation of the mesonephros）。

图 25 - 1　前肾和中肾的发生
Fig. 25 - 1　Development of the pronephros and mesonephros

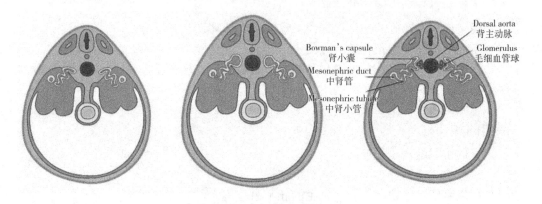

图 25 - 2　中肾小管的发生
Fig. 25 - 2　Development of the mesonephric tubules

思考题

（1）前肾小管在哪里？前肾管如何形成的？前肾小管和前肾管的关系，以及随后的演变过程是怎样的？

（2）中肾小管的位置及其后续演变过程？中肾管来源于哪里？

（3）后肾和输尿管的发生。后肾发生于人胚第5周，有两个起源：输尿管芽和生后肾组织。

输尿管芽是中肾管近泄殖腔处向背外侧发出的一盲管，可长入中肾嵴尾端，诱导中胚层细胞形成生后肾组织。输尿管芽伸长并反复分支，其主干发育为输尿管，末端各级分支先后形成肾盂、肾大盏、肾小盏和各级集合管（图25 - 3）。

生后肾组织在输尿管芽末端形成细胞团，呈帽状包围输尿管芽盲端，随后逐渐弯曲伸长，形成"S"形肾小管，其一端与集合管的盲端相连通，另一端膨大凹陷形成肾小囊，毛细血管长入囊内形成血管球，肾小囊与血管球共同形成肾小体。S形肾小管中段继续迂曲增长，发育形成近端小管、细段和远端小管，肾小管与肾小体共同组成肾单位（图25 - 4）。

后肾发生在中肾嵴尾端，原始位置较低，在盆腔。后因胎儿的生长、输尿管伸展及胚体直立，移至腰部。同时，后肾在上升的同时也沿纵轴旋转，肾门从腹侧转为内侧（图 25 – 5）。

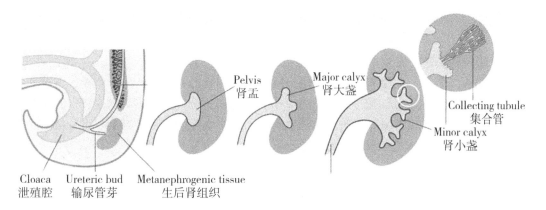

图 25 – 3　后肾的发生

Fig. 25 – 3　Development of metanephros

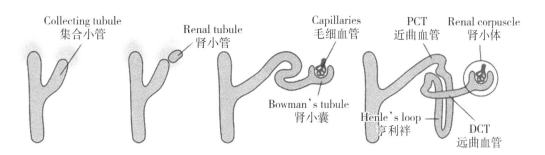

图 25 – 4　肾单位的发生

Fig. 25 – 4　Development of nephron

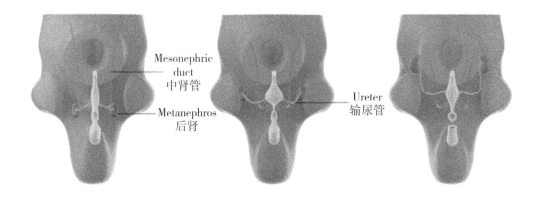

图 25 – 5　后肾位置的变化

Fig. 25 – 5　Changes in position of metanephros during its development

思考题

（1）后肾的发生位置以及其发生的原基是什么？

（2）输尿管芽来源于哪里？它是如何演变的？

（3）输尿管芽和生后肾组织形成后肾的什么结构？

> **膀胱和尿道的发生**

人胚第4～7周，泄殖腔被尿直肠隔分隔为背侧的直肠和腹侧的尿生殖窦，膀胱和尿道主要由尿生殖窦分化而成。尿生殖窦分上、中、下三段。上段宽大发育为膀胱，其顶端与脐尿管相连；中段狭窄，在女性发育为尿道大部分，在男性发育为尿道前列腺部和膜部；下段扁平，在女性发育为尿道下段和阴道前庭，在男性发育为尿道海绵体部（图25-6）。

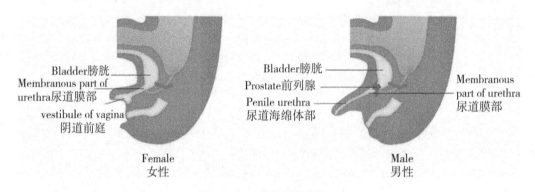

图25-6 尿生殖窦的发生

Fig. 25-6 Development of urogenital sinus

思考题

（1）泄殖腔被尿直肠隔分为哪几个部分？

（2）尿生殖窦分为哪几段？每段在男性和女性分别演变成什么结构？

2. 泌尿系统发育异常

> **多囊肾**

后肾发生过程中，由于集合小管盲端和远端小管未接通，或者是集合小管发育异常，尿液积聚在肾小管内，使肾内出现大小不等的囊泡。囊泡可挤压周围正常肾组织，从而引起肾功能障碍（图25-7）。

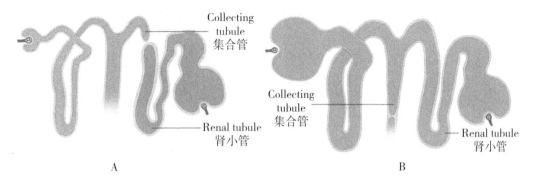

A：集合管和肾小管远端不相通（Disconnection between the collecting tubule and the distal end of renal tubule）；B：集合管结构异常（Abnormalities of collecting tubule）。

图 25 -7　多囊肾
Fig. 25 -7　Polycystic kidney

> **肾位置的异常**

肾上升过程受阻，仍保留在盆腔，为异位肾。有时由于肾上升时被肠系膜下动脉根部所阻，两肾下端融合呈马蹄形，为马蹄肾。

> **双输尿管**

由输尿管芽过早分支或同侧形成两个输尿管芽所致。

> **脐尿管相关畸形**

由于脐尿管未闭锁，出生后尿液可从脐部溢出，称为脐尿管瘘。若仅脐尿管中段未闭锁且扩张，则称为脐尿囊肿。

> **膀胱外翻**

由于表面外胚层与尿生殖窦之间没有间充质长入，下腹正中部与膀胱前壁的结缔组织及肌组织缺如，致使表皮和膀胱前壁破裂，膀胱黏膜外翻暴露于外，并常伴有尿道上裂。

3. 生殖系统的发生

> **生殖腺的发生**

生殖腺（睾丸和卵巢）发生有 3 个起源：内侧生殖腺嵴表面的体腔上皮、上皮下的间充质和原始生殖细胞。

（1）未分化性腺。人胚第 5 周，生殖腺嵴表面上皮增生，向下方的间充质长入，形成指状的上皮性细胞索，为初级性索。原始生殖细胞经后肠背侧系膜，向生殖腺嵴迁移。人胚第 6 周，原始生殖细胞迁入生殖腺嵴的初级性索内，此时尚不能辨认性别，故称未分化性腺（图 25 -8）。

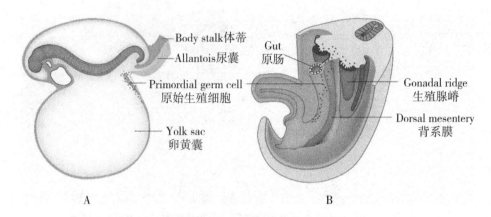

图 25 -8 原始生殖细胞的发生（A）和迁移（B）

Fig. 25 -8 Development（A）and Migration（B）of the primordial germ cells

（2）睾丸的发生。人胚第 7 周，如果胚胎的性染色体为 XY 时，未分化性腺向睾丸方向分化。初级性索与表面上皮分离，向深部继续增生，发育为睾丸索，睾丸索为实性，在门部逐渐形成网状的细胞索（后面演化成睾丸网）。在青春期睾丸索会管化，演变成生精小管、直精小管。人胚第 8 周，表面上皮下方的间充质分化为一层较厚的致密结缔组织白膜，分隔表面上皮和睾丸索。原始生殖细胞发育分化为精原细胞，表面上皮发育分化为支持细胞。睾丸索之间的间充质将演变成睾丸间质和间质细胞（图 25 -9）。

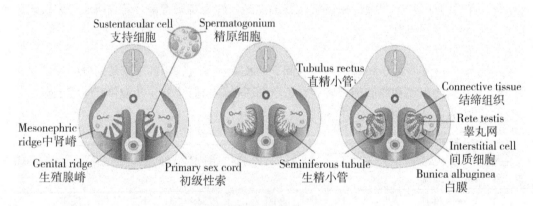

图 25 -9 睾丸的发生

Fig. 25 -9 Development of the testis

（3）卵巢的发生。如果胚胎的性染色体为 XX 时，未分化性腺向卵巢方向分化。人胚第 10 周，初级性索退化，生殖腺嵴表面上皮再度增殖形成次级性索或皮质索。皮质索继续增殖并与表面上皮脱离，形成卵巢皮质，表面上皮下方的间充质形成薄层的白膜。人胚第 16 周，皮质索断裂形成许多细胞团，发育成为原始卵泡，卵泡间的间充质分化为卵巢间质。每个原始卵泡中央有一个由原始生殖细胞分化而成的卵原细胞，周围有多个由皮质索分化而成的卵泡细胞（图 25 -10）。

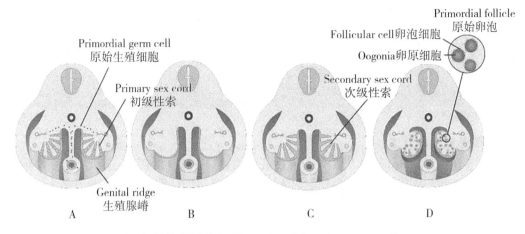

A：初级性索的形成（Formation of the primary sex cord）；

B：初级性索的消失（Disappearance of the primary sex cord）；

C：次级性索的形成（Formation of the secondary sex cord）；

D：原始卵泡的形成（Appearance of the primordial follicle）。

图 25 - 10　睾丸的发生

Fig. 25 - 10　Development of the ovary

（4）睾丸和卵巢的下降。生殖腺最初位于腹后壁，尾端到阴唇阴囊隆起之间，有一条长索状引带。随着胚体逐渐长大，引带相对缩短，导致生殖腺下降。人胚第 3 个月时，卵巢停留在骨盆缘下方，睾丸则继续下降，于胎儿第 7 ～ 8 个月时抵达阴囊（图 25 - 11）。

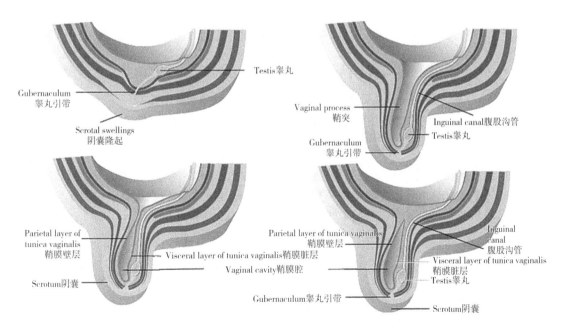

图 25 - 11　睾丸的下降

Fig. 25 - 11　Descent of the testis

思考题

（1）未分化腺如何演变而来？原始生殖细胞来源于哪里？

（2）什么因素决定未分化腺的性别分化？

（3）卵巢和睾丸的发生过程分别是什么？

➤ **生殖管道的发生**

（1）未分化期。人胚第6周，无论男性还是女性，胚胎内有中肾管和中肾旁管两套生殖管道。中肾旁管由尿生殖嵴头端外侧的体腔上皮凹陷后闭合而成。其头端呈漏斗形，开口于腹腔；上段位于中肾管的外侧，两管相互平行；中段跨过中肾管的腹面，弯向中肾管的内侧；下段两侧的中肾旁管在中线处合并形成一管状结构，其末端为盲端，凸入尿生殖窦的背侧壁，在窦腔内形成一结节状隆起，为窦结节（图25－12）。中肾管开口在窦结节的两侧。

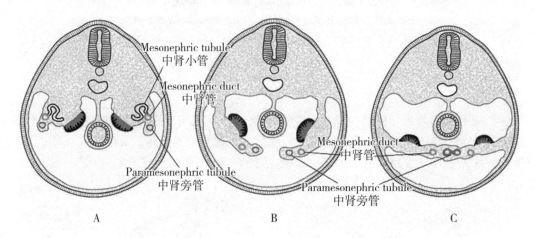

A：上部（Upper part）；B：中部（Middle part）；C：下部（Lower part）。

图25－12　生殖管道不同部位的中肾管和中肾旁管位置关系

Fig. 25－12　Varied locations of the mesonephric duct and the paramesonephric tubule in the different parts of the rudimentary genital duct

（2）男性生殖管道的演变。如果生殖腺分化为睾丸，则中肾管发育，中肾旁管退化。中肾管头段演变为附睾管，中段演变为输精管，尾段演变为射精管和精囊。中肾小管大部分退化，仅靠近睾丸的部分中肾小管发育为输出小管（图25－13）。

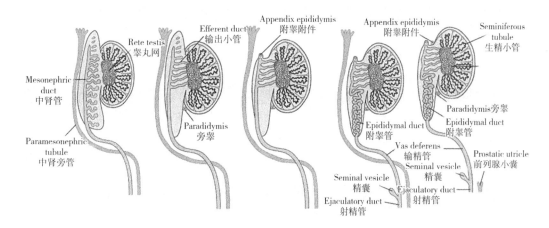

图 25 – 13　男性生殖管道的演变

Fig. 25 – 13　Development of the genital ducts in male

（3）女性生殖管道的演变。如果生殖腺分化为卵巢，则中肾旁管发育称女性主要的生殖管道，大部分中肾管退化，残留部分形成卵巢冠或 Gartner's 囊泡。中肾旁管上段和中段演变为输卵管，下段融合发育为子宫和阴道穹窿部（图 25 – 14）。窦阴道球增生形成阴道板，第 5 个月时，阴道板出现管腔，形成阴道的中段和下段，下段末端对应的尿生殖窦膜形成处女膜（图 25 – 15）。

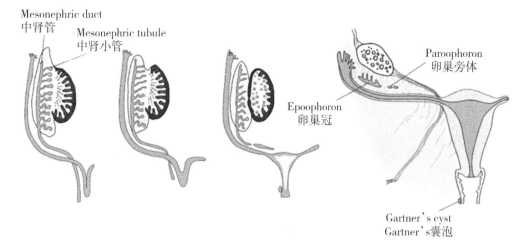

图 25 – 14　女性生殖管道的演变

Fig. 25 – 14　Development of the genital ducts in female

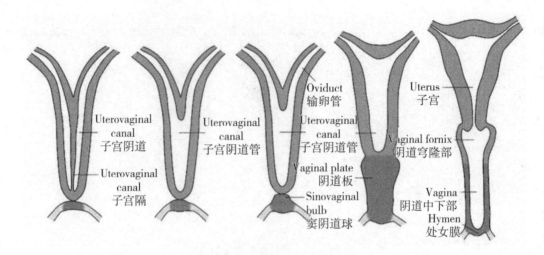

图 25 – 15　子宫和阴道的形成

Fig. 25 – 15　Formation of the uterus and vagina

➢ **外生殖器的发生**

（1）未分化期。未分化期的外生殖器由生殖结节、一对尿生殖褶和一对阴唇阴囊隆起组成。尿生殖褶之间的凹陷为尿生殖沟，沟底为尿生殖膜（图 25 – 16）。在人胚第 6 周末，不能分辨外生殖器的性别差异。

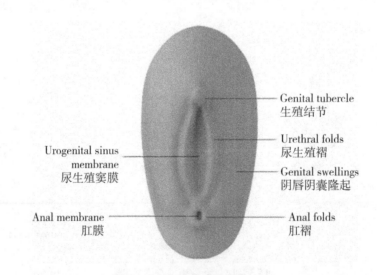

图 25 – 16　未分化期外生殖器

Fig. 25 – 16　Development of the external genitalia at indifferent stage

（2）男性外生殖器的演变。如果生殖腺分化为睾丸，生殖结节伸长和增粗，形成阴茎。左、右尿生殖褶在腹侧中线愈合，形成尿道海绵体部。左、右阴唇阴囊隆起在中线愈合，形成阴囊（图 25 – 17A）。

（3）女性外生殖器的演变。如果生殖腺分化为卵巢，生殖结节略增大，形成阴蒂。左、右尿生殖褶不愈合，发育形成小阴唇。左、右阴唇阴囊隆起大部分不愈合，发育形成大阴唇，其头端合并形成阴阜，尾端合并形成阴唇后连合。尿生殖沟扩展，形成阴道前庭

（图 25 – 17B）。

思考题

（1）未分化期的两套管道是什么？它们是怎么发生的？

（2）两性分化时，中肾管和中肾旁管分别是如何演变的？

（3）什么因素决定生殖管道和外生殖器的两性分化？

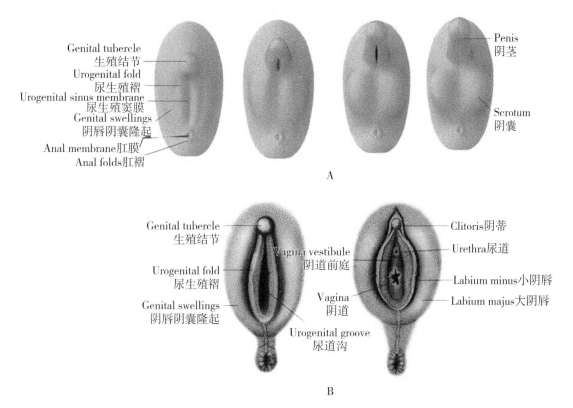

A：男性（Male）；B：女性（Female）。

图 25 – 17 外生殖器的演变

Fig. 25 – 17 Development of the external genitalia in male and female

4. 生殖系统的异常发育

➢ **隐睾**

出生后，睾丸未完全降入阴囊，多停在腹腔内或腹股沟管等处，称为隐睾。

➢ **先天性腹股沟疝**

若腹膜腔与鞘膜腔之间的通道没有闭合或闭合不全，当腹压增大时，部分小肠可突入鞘膜腔内，形成先天性腹股沟疝。

➢ **双子宫和双角子宫**

左右中肾旁管的下段未合并，形成双子宫，常伴有双阴道。若仅上部的中肾旁管未合并，子宫上端呈分叉状，形成双角子宫。

课后作业

填写表 25 –1 中男女性生殖系统的发生的区别。

表 25 –1　男女性生殖系统的发生的区别

胚胎时期		男性生殖系统	女性生殖系统
基因			
分化的因素			
可识别时间			
生殖细胞			
中肾管			
中肾旁管			
尿生殖窦	上段		
	中段		
	下段		

案例讨论题

一位 48 岁男性，因下肢水肿一周而入院。该患者无高血压、糖尿病、肝炎、结核和药物过敏病史。入院后发现 24 小时尿蛋白高达 7540 mg，血白蛋白低至 25 g/L，诊断为肾病综合征。腹部超声提示马蹄肾。患者兄弟也曾患肾病综合征，发现时即已晚期，并无接受肾活检。该患者在超声引导下，进行肾活检术，术后诊断为 PLA2R 阳性 Ⅱ 期膜性肾病。经过泼尼松、环磷酰胺 6 个月治疗后，尿蛋白水平明显降低。

（1）什么是马蹄肾？胚胎期马蹄肾是如何形成的？

（2）相比于正常解剖位置的肾，为什么马蹄肾容易造成泌尿系统紊乱，哪些方面表现异常？

（3）相比于正常解剖位置的肾，为什么对马蹄肾患者施行肾活检有难度？

（张巍）

Chapter 25   DEVELOPMENT OF THE UROGENITAL SYSTEM

Both the urinary system and the genital system develop from the **intermediate mesoderm**, which is forming a pair of longitudinal bulges, along the posterior wall of the abdominal cavity at the fourth week of embryo, called **urogenital ridge** (尿生殖嵴).

The cephalic portion of these bulge are segmented **nephrotomes** (生肾节), which form the **pronephros** (前肾) and gradually degenerates during the development of urinary system. But the medial and caudal portions of these bulges are not segmented, which are subsequently divided into outer **nephrogenic ridge** (生肾嵴) and inner **gonadal ridge** (生殖腺嵴). The gonadal ridge is the rudiment of genital system, and the nephrogenic ridge forms **mesonephros** (中肾). The **ureteric bud** (输尿管芽) and the **metanephrogenic tissue** (**metanephrogenic blastema**, 生后肾原基) are the rudiment of **matanephros** (后肾), which forms the permernant kidney.

Learning Objectives

(1) Be able to describe the process of the development of pronephros and mesonephros.

(2) Be able to grasp the process of the development of metanephros.

(3) Be able to understand the relation and changes of both the pronephric duct and mesonephric duct.

(4) Be able to illustrate the development or the progress of the gonads and the genital ducts.

(5) Be able to grasp the mechanisms of the differentiation for the gonads and the genital ducts.

(6) Be able to identify the reasons of various urinary anomalies, such as the polycystic kidney, ectopic kidney, horseshoe kidney, double ureter, cryptorchidism, congenital inguinal hernia, double uterus etc.

Pre-class Questions

(1) Can you describe the structure of kidney?

(2) Can you describe the structures of ovary and testis?

(3) What's the rudiment of the urogenital system?

Materials

Gross specimens, embryo models, simulation videos.

Observation and Reflection

1. Development of the Urinary System

➢ Development of Kidney and Ureter

（1）**Pronephros**. The pronephros appear in human embryos early in the fourth week of development, several pairs of tubules locate in the cephalic portion of the intermediate mesoderm. These small **pronephric tubules**（前肾小管）, forming in a cephalocaudal sequence, empty laterally on each side into a common duct called the **pronephric duct**（前肾管）. The pronephric ducts run caudally and open into the cloaca. Soon the rudimentary pronephros degenerate, but most of the pronephric tubules retain（Fig. 25 – 1A, 1B）.

（2）**Mesonephros**. At the fourth week of development, the first excretory tubules of the mesonephros appear, which are called mesonephric tubules. They lengthen rapidly, forming S-shaped tubules. A mesonephric tubule develops a cuplike outgrowth into which a tuft of capillaries is pushed. The cup shaped outgrowth from the tubule is termed the **Bowman's capsule**（肾小囊）, and the tuft of capillaries is the **glomerulus**（血管球）. Both structures constitute a **renal corpuscle**（肾小体）. Laterally the tubule enters the longitudinal collecting duct known as the **mesonephric ducts**（中肾管）（Fig. 25 – 1C）. They function until the permanent kidneys develop. By the end of the second month the majority have disappeared, except that the ducts and a part of tubules of the mesonephros participate in the genital development in male（Fig. 25 – 2）.

Reflection

（1）Where are the pronephric tubules? How is the pronephric duct formed? What's anatomical relation between the pronephric tubules and the pronephric duct? And how will both structures change afterwards?

（2）Where are the mesonephric tubules and how do they develop? Where does the mesonephric duct come from?

（3）**Metanephros and Ureter**. The metanephros develops from two sources: **ureteric bud** and **metanephrogenic tissue**, which appear in the fifth week.

Ureteric bud is an outgrowth of the mesonephric duct. It penetrates the metanephric tissue and branched repeatedly. The main stem of the bud forms the ureter, while the distal branches subsequently develop into the renal pelvis, the major and the minor calyces, and millions of collecting tubules of permanent kidney（Fig. 25 – 3）.

Metanephrogenic tissue belongs to the intermediate mesoderm. Under the inductive influence by the terminal branches of the ureteric bud, the cells of the metanephrogenic mesenchyme form small vesicles, which in turn give rise to small S-shaped tubules and differentiate into glomeruli. These tubules, together with their glomeruli, form nephrons. The proximal end of each nephron forms Bowman's capsule. The distal end forms an open connection with one of the collecting tubules, establishing a passageway from Bowman's capsule to the collecting unit（Fig. 25 – 4）.

Due to diminution of body curvature and growth of the body in the lumbar and sacral regions, the metanephric kidney "ascends" from its original location to its mature location (in the retroperitoneum just caudal to the diaphragm) (Fig. 25 – 5).

Reflection

(1) Where are metanephros and what do they develop into?

(2) Where is the ureteric bud derived from? And how does it change?

(3) What structures of metanephros will the ureteric bud and metanephrogenic tissue form?

➢ Development of the Bladder and Urethra

During the fourth to seventh weeks of development, the **urorectal septum** (尿直肠隔) divides the **cloaca** (泄殖腔) into two parts: the **rectum** (直肠) and a ventral **urogenital sinus** (尿生殖窦). The bladder and urethra mainly develop from the urogenital sinus. The urogenital sinus can be divided into three portions. The upper and largest part forms most of the urinary bladder. The middle part is narrow, which becomes the prostatic and membranous parts of the urethra in males, and the entire urethra in females. The lower part is flat, which forms the **vestibule of vagina** (阴道前庭) in females and the **penile urethra** (尿道海绵体部) in males (Fig. 25 – 6).

Reflection

(1) What's the components of the division of the cloaca by urorectal septum?

(2) What're the components of urogenital sinus? And how does its every portion change in male and in female, respectively?

---

2. Anomalies of Urinary System

➢ Polycystic Kidney (多囊肾)

During the development of metanephros, if the collecting tubules are unable to form an open connection with the distal convoluted tubule or they develop abnormally, the renal tubules are filled with fluid. And the kidney becomes cystic because there is no outlet for the fetal urine. This defect is called polycystic kidney (Fig. 25 – 7).

➢ Ectopic Kidney and Horseshoe Kidney

If the kidney does not ascent to the normal level, it still remains in the pelvis, known as **ectopic kidney** (异位肾). Sometimes, the kidneys are pushed so close together during their passage through the arterial fork that the lower poles fuse, forming a **horseshoe kidney** (马蹄肾). The horseshoe kidney is usually at the level of the lower lumbar vertebrae, since its ascent is prevented by the root of the inferior mesenteric artery.

➢ Double Ureter (双输尿管)

The double ureter results from early splitting of the ureteric bud. Splitting may be partial or complete.

> ➤ Urachal Anomalies（脐尿管相关畸形）

If patent of urachus has been persisted, urine may drain from the umbilicus after birth, which is called **urachal fistula**（脐尿管瘘）. If only the middle part of urachus remains patent and dilated, it is called **urachal cyst**（脐尿囊肿）.

> ➤ Exstrophy of Bladder（膀胱外翻）

This is a ventral body wall defect in which the bladder mucosa is exposed. **Epispadias**（尿道上裂）is a constant feature. Exstrophy of bladder may be caused by a lack of mesodermal migration into the region between the umbilicus and urogenital sinus, followed by rupture of the thin layer of ectoderm.

3. Development of the Genital System

> ➤ Development of Gonads

The gonads (testes and ovaries) are derived from three sources: the epithelium covering the inner gonadal ridge, the underlying mesenchyme, the primordial germ cells.

(1) **Indifferent gonads**. During the fifth week, the epithelium on the surface of gonadal ridge proliferates and grow into the underlying mesenchyme, to form finger-like epithelial cords, known as the **primitive sex cords**（初级性索）. The **primordial germ cells**（原始生殖细胞）originate in the wall of the yolk sac and migrate along the dorsal mesentery of the gut to the gonadal ridges (Fig. 25 –8). During the sixth week of development, the germ cells enter the underlying mesenchyme and migrated into the gonadal cords. Before the seventh week of development, the gonads of the two sexes are identical in appearance and are called indifferent gonads.

(2) **Development of testes**. During the seventh week, if the sex chromosome of human embryo is XY, the indifferent gonads may differentiate into the testes. The primitive sex cords are separated from the surface epithelium and continue to proliferate, then they penetrate deep into the medulla to form numerous **testis cords**. Towards the hilum of the gland the cords break up into a network of tiny cell strands that later give rise to tubules of the **rete testis**. Testis cords remain solid until puberty, when they acquire a lumen, forming the **seminiferous tubules**, Later, the seminiferous tubules are canalized and join the **tubulus rectus**. A dense layer of fibrous connective tissue, the **tunica albuginea**, separated the testis cords from the **surface epithelium**. The primitive germ cells may develop into the **spermatogonium**, and the surface epithelium forms the **Sertoli cells.** The original mesenchyme between the testis cords will develop into the interstitial of testis and **Leydig cells** (Fig. 25 –9).

(3) **Development of ovaries**. In female embryos with an XX sex chromosome and no Y chromosome, primitive sex cords dissociate into irregular cell clusters. These clusters, containing groups of primitive germ cells, occupy the medullary part of the ovary. Later they disappear and are replaced by a vascular stroma that forms the **ovarian medulla**. The surface epithelium of the female gonad, unlike that of the male, continues to proliferate. In the seventh week it gives rise to **secondary sex cords**（次级性索）, which penetrate the underlying mesenchyme but remain close to the surface. In the fourth month these cords split into isolated cell clusters, with each surrounding one or more primitive germ cells. Germ cells subsequently develop into **oogonia**, and the surround-

ing epithelial cells, descendants of the surface epithelium, form **follicular cells** (Fig. 25 – 10).

(4) **Descent of the testes and ovaries**. Prior to descent, the gonads are attached to the posterior abdominal wall by a mesentery. The mesentery extends from the caudal end of the gonads towards the scrotal or labial swelling, which becomes fibrous and is then known as the **gubernaculum** (引带). With the enlarged embryo and the relatively shorten gubernaculum, the gonads descend. At the third month of human embryo, ovary retains at the lower surface of pelvis. But testes continue to descend and arrive at the scrotal sac until the seventh to eighth months of embryo (Fig. 25 – 11).

Reflection

(1) What are the indifferent gonads derived from? Where does the primordial germ cell originate?

(2) What factors determine the sex differentiation of the indifferent gonads?

(3) How do the testes and ovaries develop?

> Development of Genital Ducts

(1) **Indifferent Stage**. Initially both male and female embryos have two pairs of genital ducts: **mesonephric ducts** and **paramesonephric ducts** (**Müllerian ducts**, 中肾旁管). The paramesonephric duct forms as the epithelium on the anterolateral surface of the urogenital ridges invaginate. The cranial part of the paramesonephric duct opens into the abdominal cavity with a funnel-like structure. The caudal part crosses the mesonephric duct ventrally to grow caudomedially. In the midline the paramesonephric duct comes in close contact with the opposite one (Fig. 25 – 12). The caudal tip of the combined ducts projects into the posterior wall of the urogenital sinus, inducing the formation of the **sinus tubercle** (窦结节). The mesonephric ducts open into the urogenital sinus on either side of the sinus tubercle.

(2) **Genital Ducts in Male**. If the gonads differentiate into the testes, the mesonephric ducts develop, but the paramesonephric ducts regress. The cranial portion of the mesonephric duct progresses into the epididymal duct. The middle portion forms the vas deferens, while the caudal portion forms the vas deferens and seminal vesicle. Most of the mesonephric tubules regress, and only the cranial mesonephric tubules develop into the efferent ducts of epididymis (Fig. 25 – 13).

(3) **Genital Ducts in Female**. If the gonads differentiate into the ovaries, the paramesonephric ducts develop into the main genital ducts of the female, while the mesonephric ducts almost disappear, except for a small cranial portion found in the **epoophoron** (卵巢冠) and occasionally a small caudal portion that may be found in the wall of the uterus or vagina, called **Gartner's cyst** (Fig. 25 – 14).

The cranial and middle portions of the paramesonephric duct develop into the uterine tube. The caudal parts fuse to form the uterovaginal primordium, which gives rise to the uterus and upper vagina. Shortly after the solid tips of the paramesonephric ducts reach to the urogenital sinus, two solid evaginations, the **sinovaginal bulbs** (窦阴道球), grow out from the sinus tubercle and form a

solid vaginal plate（阴道板）. By the fifth month, the vaginal outgrowth is canalized. The wing-like expansions of the vagina around the end of the uterus, the **vaginal fornix**（阴道穹窿）, are of paramesonephric origin. Thus, the vagina has a dual origin, with the upper portion derived from the uterine canal and the lower portion derived from the urogenital sinus. The lumen of the vagina remains separated from that of the urogenital sinus by a thin tissue plate, the **hymen**（处女膜）（Fig. 25 – 15）.

➤ Development of External Genitalia

（1）**Indifferent Stage**. During the indifferent stage, the external genitalia originates from the mesenchyme around the cloaca. It includes the **genital tubercle**（生殖结节）, a pair of **urogenital folds**（尿生殖褶）, and another pair of **genital swellings**（生殖隆起）, which later form the scrotal swellings in the male and the labia majora in the female（Fig. 25 – 16）. The groove between the urethral folds is the **urogenital groove**（尿生殖沟）. And its bottom is the **urogenital membrane**（尿生殖膜）. At the end of the sixth week, it is impossible to distinguish between the two sexes.

（2）**External Genitalia in the Male**. If the gonads differentiate into the testes, the genital tubercle elongates to form the **penis**and the genital swellings become enlarged to form the scrotum. The urethral groove extends along the caudal aspect of the elongated phallus and form the **urethra penis**. At the end of the third month the two urethral folds fuse ventrally, forming the penile portion of the urethra（Fig. 25 – 17A）.

（3）**External Genitalia in the Female**. If the gonads differentiate into the ovaries, the genital tubercle enlarges slightly to form the **clitoris**. The urethral folds do not fuse, but develop into **labia minora**. Two genital swellings enlarge slightly and form the **labia majora**. The urogenital groove is open and forms the **vestibule**（Fig. 25 – 17B）.

Reflection

（1）What are the two pairs of genital ducts? And how do they develop?

（2）What're the differences in the evolution of the mesonephric ducts and paramesonephric ducts in different sexes?

（3）What factors determine the sex differentiation of the genital ducts and the external genitalia?

---

4. Anormalies of the Genital System

➤ Cryptorchidism（隐睾）

During the first three months postnatally, if one or two testes fail to descend, this anomaly is called cryptorchidism. The testes may stay in the inguinal canal, the abdominal cavity, or somewhere along the usual path of descent of testes.

➤ Congenital inguinal Hernia（先天性腹股沟疝）

If the connection between the abdominal cavity and the processes vaginalis in the scrotal sac fails to close normally, intestinal loops may descend into the scrotum, causing a congenital inguinal hernia.

> ➤ Double uterus and bicornuate uterus（双子宫和双角子宫）

If the caudal parts of both paramesonephric ducts do not fuse, double uterus form, usually with double vagina. If only the above half of their caudal parts do not fuse, bicornuate uterus form.

Post-class Task

Fill in the Tab. 25 – 1 about the developmental differences of the genital system between a male and a female.

Tab. 25 – 1　The developmental differences of the genital system
between a male and a female

Embryonic period		male	female
Gene			
Factors for the differentiation			
Identifiable time			
Germ cell			
Mesonephric duct			
Paramesonephric duct			
Urogenital sinus	Upper		
	Middle		
	Caudal		

Case-based Learning

A 48-year-old male patient was admitted at our hospital because of edema of both the lower limbs for 1 week. He had no history of hypertension, diabetes, hepatitis, tuberculosis, and drug allergy. The patient was diagnosed with nephrotic syndrome due to abnormal 24 h urine protein (7540 mg) and blood albumin (25 g/L) levels. Abdominal ultrasonography revealed horseshoe kidney (HSK). The patient's brother had a history of end-stage renal disease due to nephrotic syndrome. But his brother didn't accept renal biopsy. The patient was diagnosed with PLA2R-positive stage II membranous nephropathy through renal biopsy under abdominal ultrasonography guidance. He was administered with adequate prednisone and cyclophosphamide, and after 6 months of treatment, urinary protein excretion levels significantly decreased.

(1) What is HSK? And how is HSK formed during the embryonic stage?

（2）Compared with the normally anatomic kidney, which urinary disorders are prone to be caused in the patients with HSK?

（3）Do you think whether if the renal biopsy in the HSK patients easily, when compared with the patients containing normally anatomic kidney?

（张巍）

第26章 神经系统的发生

学习目标
（1）能够识别神经管形成过程中的主要结构。
（2）能够描述神经上皮细胞的分化，神经元和神经胶质细胞系的分化。
（3）能够描述脊髓的发生过程，以及相关出生缺陷的胚胎学基础。
（4）能够识别脑曲。
（5）能够说明5个脑泡的发生和衍生物，以及相关出生缺陷的胚胎学基础。

课前问题
（1）神经管在胚胎发育的什么时间及如何形成？
（2）脊髓是如何发生的？
（3）你能描述大脑的解剖结构吗？大脑是如何发生的？

实验材料
大体标本，胚胎模型，仿真视频。

实验观察与思考

1. 神经管的发生

1）神经板

第3周，在脊索的诱导下，神经板出现在胚胎的外胚层中线（图26-1A）。

2）神经沟和神经褶

第18天，神经板的中间内陷形成神经沟，神经褶在两侧形成（图26-1B）。

3）神经管

第21天，神经褶开始愈合，神经管开始形成（图26-1C）。

4）神经孔的闭合

第25天，前神经孔闭合（第18至20体节期）（图26-1D），而后神经孔在第27天闭合（第25体节阶段）（图26-1F）。神经管是中枢神经系统的原基。

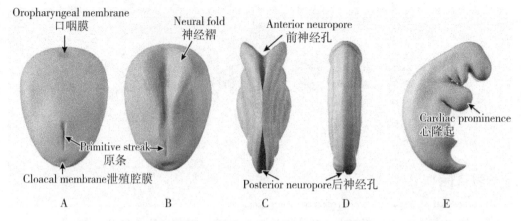

A：第 14 天（At day 14）；B：第 18 天（At day 18）；C：第 21 天（At day 21）；
D：第 25 天（At day 25）；E：第 27 天（at day 27）。

图 26 -1　神经管的发生

Fig. 26 -1　Development of neural tube

2. 脊髓的发生

神经管的管壁由假复层柱状神经上皮组成。一旦神经管闭合，神经上皮细胞就开始分裂和分化。子细胞向外迁移，形成套层，套层发育成脊髓灰质。来自套层细胞的神经纤维形成边缘层，边缘层发育成脊髓白质。原来的神经上皮细胞成为室管膜层，形成衬贴中央管的室管膜细胞（图 26 -2）。

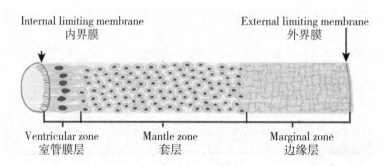

图 26 -2　神经上皮的分化

Fig. 26 -2　Differentiation of neuroepithelium

由于成神经细胞的增殖和分化，神经管套层的腹侧增厚形成基板，背侧增厚形成翼板。基板和翼板分别发育成脊髓的腹角和背角。一条纵向的沟，即界沟，将翼板与基底板分开。神经管的中线部分很薄，称为顶板和底板。神经管的管腔构成脊髓的中央管（图 26 -3）。

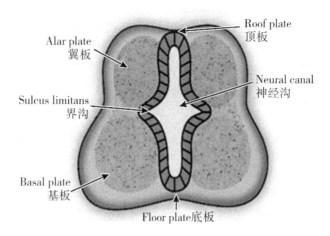

图 26 - 3　脊髓的发生

Fig. 26 - 3　Development of spinal cord

思考题

(1) 请描述脊髓的解剖结构。

(2) 脊髓在胚胎时期是如何发育的?

(3) 请描述脊髓的解剖结构。

(4) 脊髓在胚胎时期是如何发育的?

---

3. 脑的发生

1) 脑泡的发生

第 4 周,神经管的头端形成 3 个初级脑泡 (图 26 - 4A):前脑、中脑、菱脑。

第 5 周,前脑衍生出端脑和间脑,中脑不变,菱脑衍生出后脑和末脑,5 个次级脑泡形成 (图 26 - 4B)。

思考题

(1) 请描述大脑的解剖结构。

(2) 脑泡是如何发育形成大脑的各个组成部分的?

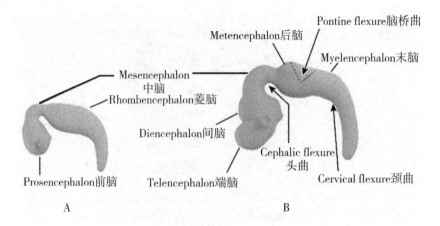

A：第4周（At week 4）；B：第5周（At week 5）。

图 26 - 4　脑泡和脑曲

Fig. 26 - 4　Brain vesicles and brain flexures

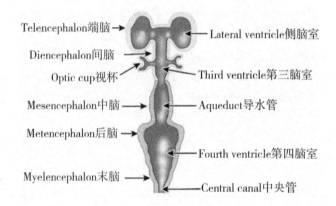

图 26 - 5　脑室系统的发生

Fig. 26 - 5　Development of ventricular system

2）脑曲的发生

在第5周，大脑迅速生长并向腹腔弯曲，形成3个脑曲（图26 - 4B）：①头曲，在中脑的腹侧；②颈曲，在后脑与脊髓交界处的腹侧，相当于枕骨大孔的水平；③脑桥曲，位于后脑和末脑交界处的背侧。

3）菱脑的发生和演变

➢ 末脑

末脑演变为延髓。

末脑的尾端（闩以下）：神经管的管腔形成延髓的中央管。与脊髓不同的是，末脑的背侧边缘层含有来自翼板的成神经细胞，形成灰质区，包括内侧的薄束核和外侧的楔束核。延髓的腹侧部分包含一对锥体，由皮质脊髓束组成。

末脑的头端（闩以上）：宽而平，像一本打开的书（图26 - 6）。神经管管腔成为第四脑室的下半部分。翼板位于基板的侧面，因此感觉核一般位于运动核的侧面。

延髓基板的成神经细胞发育成运动神经元，并在每侧形成3个细胞柱。从内到外，这些细胞柱是：①一般躯体运动核，即舌下神经核（CN Ⅻ）；②特殊内脏运动核，即舌咽神经（CN Ⅸ）、迷走神经（CN Ⅹ）和副神经（CN Ⅺ）的疑核；③一般内脏运动核，包括舌咽神经的下泌涎核（CN Ⅸ）和迷走神经的背核（CN Ⅹ）。

胚胎第 7 周，特殊内脏运动核的神经元向腹外侧迁移，到达网状结构内。

延髓翼板中的成神经细胞在每侧形成 4 列细胞柱。从内到外，这些细胞柱包括：①一般内脏感觉核，即孤束核下部，接受舌咽神经（CN Ⅸ）和迷走神经（CN Ⅹ）传入的内脏冲动；②特殊内脏感觉核，即孤束核上部，接受来自面神经（CN Ⅶ）和舌咽神经（CN Ⅸ）的味觉冲动；③一般躯体感觉核，即三叉神经脊束核，接受三叉神经（CN Ⅴ）、面神经（CN Ⅶ）和舌咽神经（CN Ⅸ）以及迷走神经（CN Ⅹ）传入的头部一般感觉。④特殊躯体感觉核，即前庭神经（CN Ⅷ）的前庭核和耳蜗核，接受听觉和平衡觉。

一些来自翼板的成神经细胞向腹侧迁移，形成橄榄核。

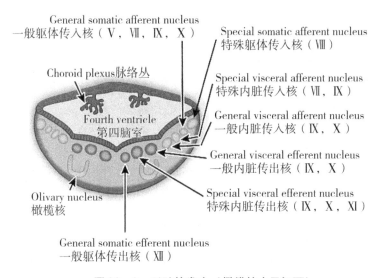

图 26 - 6　延髓的发生（橄榄核水平切面）

Fig. 26 - 6　Development of myelencephalon（transverse section at the level of olivary nucleus）

> **后脑**

后脑演变成脑桥和小脑，后脑的神经管腔形成了第四脑室的上半部分。

脑桥：宽而平（图 26 - 7）。基板上的成神经细胞发育成运动核，从内侧到外侧每侧三列：①一般躯体运动核，即展神经核（CN Ⅵ）；②特殊内脏运动核，即三叉神经运动核（CN Ⅴ）和面神经核（CN Ⅶ）；③一般内脏运动核，即面神经（CN Ⅶ）的上泌涎核。

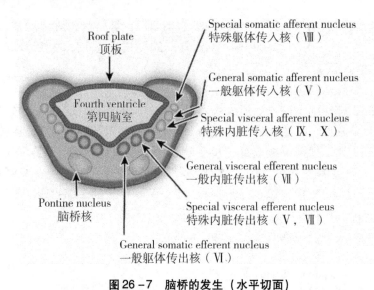

图 26 – 7　脑桥的发生（水平切面）

Fig. 26 – 7　Development of pons（transverse section）

从内侧到外侧，来自翼板的成神经细胞发育为感觉核，包括：①特殊内脏感觉核，即舌咽神经（CN Ⅸ）和迷走神经（CN Ⅹ）孤束核，接受味觉冲动；②一般躯体感觉核，即三叉神经（CN Ⅴ）脑桥核；③特殊躯体感觉核，即前庭蜗神经（CN Ⅷ）的耳蜗核和前庭核。来自翼板的细胞还形成脑桥核。

小脑：后脑翼板背侧部分增厚形成小脑（图 26 – 8、图 26 – 9）：①翼板的背侧部分形成菱唇；②菱唇在中线融合，形成小脑板，由室管膜层、套层和边缘层组成。小脑板的外侧部分形成小脑半球；④蚓部出现在中线区域；⑤蚓部和半球的下方出现绒球和小结。

第 3 个月，一些成神经细胞迁移到小脑表面，形成外颗粒层。外颗粒层的细胞向内迁移，形成内颗粒层。室管膜层的成神经细胞迁移分化成浦肯野细胞、星形细胞、篮状细胞、高尔基细胞和中央核。

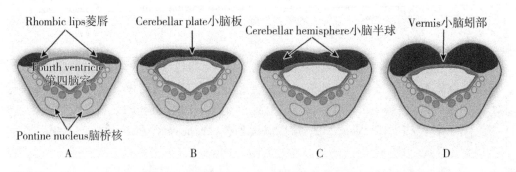

A：第 5 周（At week 5）；B：第 7 周（At week 7）；C：第 9 周（At week 9）；D：第 12 周（At week 12）。

图 26 – 8　小脑的发生（水平切面）

Fig. 26 – 8　Development of cerebellum（transverse section）

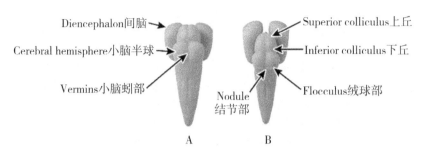

A：第 12 周（At week 12）；B：第 13 周（At week 13）。

图 26 - 9　小脑的发生（背面观）

Fig. 26 - 9　Development of cerebellum（dorsal view）

4）中脑的发生和演变

从内侧到外侧，基板每侧含有两组运动核（图 26 - 10）：①一般躯体运动核，即动眼神经核（CN Ⅲ）和耳蜗神经核（CN Ⅳ），支配眼肌；②一般内脏运动核，即动眼神经的 Edinger-Westphal（埃丁格 - 韦斯特法尔）核（CN Ⅲ），支配瞳孔括约肌。

基板的成神经细胞形成中脑的被盖。基板相邻的边缘层形成大脑脚。

翼板的成神经细胞迁移到相邻的边缘层，形成上、下丘。翼板的成神经细胞还形成三叉神经中脑核（CN Ⅴ），含有一般躯体传入神经元。

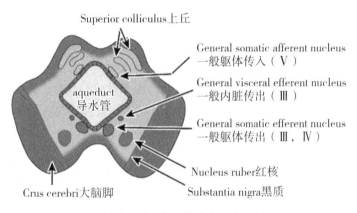

图 26 - 10　中脑的发生（水平切面）

Fig. 26 - 10　Development of midbrain（transverse section）

5）前脑的发生

➢ **间脑**

间脑形成视杯和视柄、上丘脑、丘脑、下丘脑、乳头体、垂体和松果体（图 26 - 11）。

间脑的神经管管腔形成第三脑室。第三脑室的侧壁形成丘脑、下丘脑和上丘脑。丘脑在中线处融合，形成丘脑间黏合。

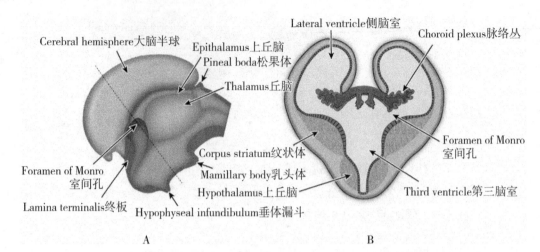

A：第7周前脑的右半侧（The right half of prosencephalon at week 7）；

B：图 A 中虚线对应的水平切面（Transverse section at the level of the broken line in "A"）。

图 26 - 11　间脑的发生

Fig. 26 - 11　Development of diencephalon

> **端脑**

端脑两侧膨大形成端脑泡，端脑的中间部分为终板（图 26 - 11A）。

连合：前神经孔由终板封闭。终板演变形成端脑的连合部，包括胼胝体、前连合、穹窿连合。

大脑半球：端脑泡是大脑半球的原基。当大脑半球向背侧和尾侧扩展并在中线相遇时，它们构成 "C" 形，并依次覆盖间脑、中脑和后脑。

皮质：端脑泡的顶部形成大脑皮质，而端脑泡的底部形成纹状体。大脑皮质分为三个区域（图 26 - 12）：①旧皮质，位于腹侧，形成嗅球和结节；②原皮质，位于背侧，形成齿状回和海马；③新皮质，是大脑中最大和进化中最新的部分。

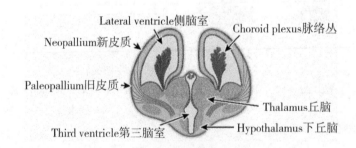

图 26 - 12　大脑皮质的发生（水平切面）

Fig. 26 - 12　Development of cerebral cortex（transverse section）

> **新皮质的组织发生**

第 5 周，大脑半球的壁有 2 层：室管膜层和边缘层（图 26 - 13A）。成神经细胞从室管膜层迁移到两层之间，形成中间层。第 6 周末，室管膜下层在室管膜层和中间层之间形成。第 7 周时，在中间层和边缘层之间形成皮质板。皮质板中的神经元首先分布在深层，后形成的神经元向上迁移到浅层（"由内向外"分层）。第 10 周，室管膜层分化为室管膜细胞，停止产生成神经细胞，室管膜下层继续形成神经元。第 12 周，中间层和皮质板之间形成板下层。中间层形成白质。在出生后的几个月，室管膜下层消失。板下层和皮质板形成灰质。边缘层形成大脑皮质的分子层（图 26 - 13B）。

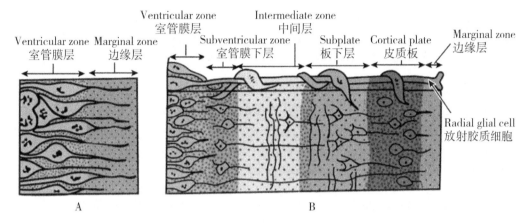

A：第 5 周（At week 5）；B：第 12 周（At week 12）。

图 26 - 13　新皮质的组织结构发生

Fig. 26 - 13　Histogenesis of neocortex

4. 神经系统的异常发育

1）神经管缺陷

神经管缺陷，包括脊柱裂和无脑畸形，是神经管未正常闭合造成的。脊柱裂影响神经弓，可能影响也可能不影响脊髓结构。无脑畸形的特点是颅骨畸形和大脑不发育（图 26 - 14）。

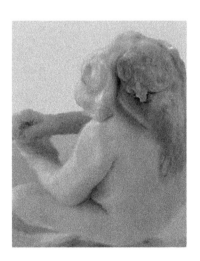

图 26 - 14　脊柱裂和无脑儿

Fig. 26 - 14　Spina bifida and anencephaly

2）小脑畸形

小脑畸形的特点是颅顶和颅盖比正常人小，而脸部大小正常。

3）脑积水

脑积水是由于脑脊液循环或吸收受阻，脑脊液在脑室系统内异常积聚导致。

课后作业

绘制次级脑泡的示意图。

案例讨论题

一位 35 岁的女性怀孕 30 周。经超声检查，她腹中胎儿被诊断为胎儿无脑畸形。她有羊水过多的病史，没有补充叶酸。既往无妊娠高血压、糖尿病、心脏病和肾脏疾病。病人接受了引产手术终止妊娠。胎儿显示无头皮和颅盖，缺陷延伸至颈椎，眼睛突出，鼻宽，耳折叠，颈部和躯干短，肩部宽，无其他相关的缺陷。

（1）无脑畸形的胚胎学基础是什么？

（2）无脑畸形的解剖学特征是什么？

（3）导致无脑畸形的原因有哪些？

（4）女性备孕期间补充叶酸的益处是什么？

（周雯）

Chapter 26 DEVELOPMENT OF NERVOUS SYSTEM

The nervous system develops from the **neural plate** （神经板）. The neural plate invaginates to form **neural groove** （神经沟） which is then converted into the **neural tube**. Neural tube develops into central nervous system （CNS）. The **neural crest** （神经嵴） cells migrate away from the neural folds to form ganglion and neuroglia of peripheral nervous system （PNS）, and chromaffin cells of the adrenal medulla.

The anterior part of the neural tube is expanded to form three primary brain vesicles:

prosencephalon （forebrain, 前脑）, **mesencephalon** （midbrain, 中脑）, **rhombencephalon** （hindbrain, 菱脑）. During the 4th week, brain flexures develop. In the 5th week, five secondary vesicles form: **telencephalon** （端脑）, **diencephalon** （间脑）, **mesencephalon**, **metencephalon** （后脑）, **myelencephalon** （末脑）.

The posterior end of the neural tube forms spinal cord. Neuroepithelium of neural tube forms **ventricular zone** （室管膜层）, **mantle layer** （套层）, and **marginal zone** （边缘层）.

The **neural canal** （神经管腔） is modified to form the ventricular cavities of the brain, and the central canal of the medulla oblongata and spinal cord.

Learning Objectives

（1） Be able to identify the major structures during the formation of neural tube.

（2） Be able to describe the differentiation of neuroepithelium, the differentiation of neuronal and glial cell lineages.

（3） Be able to illustrate and describe the development of spinal cord, and the embryological basis of related birth defects.

（4） Be able to identify the brain flexures.

（5） Be able to illustrate the development and derivatives of 5 brain vesicles, and the embryological basis of related birth defects.

Pre-class Questions

（1） When and how does neural tube form?

（2） How does spinal cord develop?

（3） Can you describe the anatomical structure of definitive brain? How does the brain develop?

Materials

Gross specimens, embryo models, and simulation videos.

Observation and Reflection

1. Development of Neural Tube

1) Neural plate

At the beginning of the 3rd week, the **neural plate** is induced by the developing notochord, appearing as a thickening of the embryonic ectoderm at the midline (Fig. 26 – 1A).

2) Neural groove and neural folds

At day 18, as the neural plate invaginates, the **neural groove** develops in the median region and the **neural folds** form on each side (Fig. 26 – 1B).

3) Neural tube

At day 21, neural folds begin to fuse and the **neural tube** starts to form (Fig. 26 – 1C).

4) Closure of neuropores

At day 25, the **cranial neuropore** closes (18- to 20-somite stage) (Fig. 26 – 1D), whereas the posterior neuropore closes at day 27 (25-somite stage) (Fig. 26 – 1F). Neural tube is the primordium of the CNS.

2. Development of Spinal Cord

The wall of the neural tube is composed of pseudostratified columnar **neuroepithelium** (神经上皮).

Once the neural tube closes, neuroepithelial cells divide and differentiate.

The daughter cells migrate outside to form **mantle zone** which develops into gray matter of the spinal cord.

Nerve fibers emerging from the cells of the mantle layer form **marginal zone** which would develop into white matter of the spinal cord.

The original neuroepithelium becomes the **ventricular zone** (ependymal layer) which will form the ependyma lining the central canal (Fig. 26 – 2).

As a result of proliferation and differentiation of neuroblasts, the mantle zone of neural tube shows ventral thickenings called the **basal plates** (基板) and dorsal thickenings called the **alar plates** (翼板). Basal plates and alar plates give rise to ventral horns and dorsal horns of spinal cord respectively. A longitudinal groove, the **sulcus limitans** (界沟), separates the alar plate from the basal plate. The midline portions of the neural tube are thin, called the **roof plate** (顶板) and **floor plate** (底板). The **neural canal** (神经沟) forms the central canal of spinal cord (Fig. 26 – 3).

Reflection

(1) Can you describe the anatomic structure of definitive spinal cord?

(2) How does the spinal cord develop embryologically?

---

3.   Development of the Brain

1）Development of brain vesicles

In the 4th week, identify 3 **primary brain vesicles**（Fig. 26 – 4A）in the cranial portion of the neural tube：①forebrain（**prosencephalon**），②midbrain（**mesencephalon**），③hindbrain（**rhombencephalon**）.

In the 5th week, identify 5 **secondary brain vesicles**（Fig. 26 – 4B, 5）：①**telencephalon** and **diencephalon** derived from the prosencephalon；②the **mesencephalon** remaining undivided；③the **metencephalon** and **myelencephalon** derived from rhombencephalon.

Reflection

（1）Can you describe the anatomic components of definitive brain?

（2）How does the brain vesicles develop into each components of brain?

2）Development of brain flexures

During the 5th week, the brain grows rapidly and bends ventrally, and 3 brain flexures form（Fig. 26 – 4B）：①**cephalic flexure**（头曲），at the ventral side of midbrain；②**cervical flexure**（颈曲），at the ventral side of the junction between the hindbrain and the spinal cord, and roughly at the level of foramen magnum；③**pontine flexure**（脑桥区），at the dorsal side of the junction between the metencephalon and myelencephalon.

3）Development of hindbrain

➢ Myelencephalon

The myelencephalon becomes the **medulla oblongata**（延髓）.

The myelencephalon caudal to the obex：The neural canal forms the central canal of the myelencephalon. Unlike that of the spinal cord, the dorsal region of marginal zone in the myelencephalon contains neuroblasts from the alar plates and form gray matter areas—the **gracile nuclei**（薄束核）medially and the **cuneate nuclei**（楔束核）laterally. The ventral part of the medulla contains a pair of **pyramids**（锥体）that consist of corticospinal fibers.

The myelencephalon rostral to the obex：It is as wide and flat as an opened book（Fig. 26 – 6）. The neural canal of this part becomes inferior part of fourth ventricle. The alar plates lie lateral to the basal plates, so that the sensory nuclei generally are lateral to the motor nuclei.

Neuroblasts in the basal plates of the medulla develop into motor neurons and organize into 3 cell columns on each side. From medial to lateral, the columns are：①**general somatic efferent nuclei**（一般躯体运动核），i. e., the nucleus of hypoglossal nerve（CN XII）；②**special visceral efferent nuclei**（特殊内脏运动核），i. e., nucleus ambiguus of glossopharyngeal nerves（CN IX），vagus nerve（CN X），and accessory nerve（CN XI）；③**general visceral efferent nuclei**（一般内脏运动核），i. e., inferior salivatory nucleus of glossopharyngeal nerves（CN IX），and dorsal nucleus of the vagus nerve（CN X）.

At 7 weeks of embryo, the neurons of special visceral efferent nuclei migrate ventrally and laterally into **reticular formation** （网状结构）.

Neuroblasts in the alar plates of the medulla form 4 columns on each side. From medial to lateral, the columns are: ①**general visceral afferent nuclei** （一般内脏感觉核）, i. e. , solitary nucleus receiving impulses from the viscera through glossopharyngeal nerves （CN Ⅸ） and vagus nerve （CN Ⅹ）; ②**special visceral afferent nuclei** （特殊内脏感觉核）, i. e. , solitary nucleus receiving taste impulses from facial nerve （CN Ⅶ） and glossopharyngeal nerves （CN Ⅸ）; ③**general somatic afferent nuclei** （一般躯体感觉核）, i. e. , spinal trigeminal nucleus receiving impulses from the surface of the head through trigeminal nerve （CN Ⅴ）, facial nerve （CN Ⅶ） and glossopharyngeal nerves （CN Ⅸ） and vagus nerve （CN Ⅹ）; ④**special somatic afferent nuclei** （特殊躯体感觉核）, i. e. , vestibular nucleus and cochlear nucleus of vestibulocochlear nerve （CN Ⅷ） receiving impulses from the ear.

Some neuroblasts from the alar plates migrate ventrally and form **olivary nuclei** （橄榄核）.

➢ Metencephalon

The metencephalon forms the pons and cerebellum, and the cavity of the metencephalon forms the superior part of the fourth ventricle.

Pons （脑桥）: The pons is wide and flat like rostral part of the myelencephalon （Fig. 26 - 7）. Neuroblasts in each basal plate develop into motor nuclei and organize into three columns on each side from medial to lateral: ①**general somatic efferent nuclei**, i. e. , abducens nucleus of abducent nerve （CN Ⅵ）; ②**special visceral efferent nuclei**, i. e. , motor nucleus of trigeminal nerve （CN Ⅴ） and nucleus of facial nerve （CN Ⅶ）; ③**general visceral efferent nuclei**, i. e. , superior salivatory nucleus of facial nerve （CN Ⅶ）.

From medial to lateral, neuroblasts from the alar plates develop into sensory nuclei: ①**special visceral afferent nuclei**, i. e. , solitary nuclei receiving impulses from the viscera through glossopharyngeal nerves （CN Ⅸ） and vagus nerve （CN Ⅹ）; ②**general somatic afferent nuclei**, i. e. , pontine nuclei of the trigeminal nerve （CN Ⅴ）; ③**special somatic afferent nuclei**, i. e. , cochlear nucleus and vestibular nuclei of vestibulocochlear nerve （CN Ⅷ）.

Cells from the alar plates also give rise to the **pontine nuclei** （脑桥核）.

Cerebellum （小脑）: Thickenings of dorsal parts of the alar plates develop into cerebellum in the following steps （Fig. 26 - 8, Fig. 26 - 9）: ① dorsal parts of the alar plates form **rhombic lips** （菱唇）; ② rhombic lips fuse in the midline and form **cerebellar plate** （小脑板） which consists of ventricular, mantle, and marginal layers; ③ the lateral parts of cerebellar plate form cerebellar hemispheres; ④ vermis appears in the midline area; ⑤ the flocculus and nodule appear inferior to the vermis and the hemispheres.

In the 3rd month, some neuroblasts migrate to the surface of the cerebellum to form the **external granular layer** （外颗粒层）. Cells of the external granular layer migrate inward and give rise to granule cell layer, while neuroblasts from ventricular zone give rise to Purkinje cells, stellate, basket and Golgi interneurons, and the central nuclei.

4) Development of midbrain

Mesencephalon forms the midbrain （Fig. 26 - 10）.

From medial to lateral, basal plate contains two groups of motor nuclei on each side: ① general somatic efferent nuclei, i. e. , nucleus of oculomotor nerve（CN Ⅲ）and nucleus of trochlear nerve（CN Ⅳ）which innervate eye musculature；②general visceral efferent nuclei, i. e. , nucleus of Edinger-Westphal of oculomotor nerve（CN Ⅲ）which innervate sphincter pupillary muscle.

Neuroblasts from the basal plates form neurons in the **tegmentum** of midbrain.

The marginal zone of each basal plate develops into the **crus cerebri**（大脑脚）.

Neuroblasts of alar plates migrating into the marginal zone and form **superior colliculus**（上丘）and **inferior colliculus**（下丘）. Neuroblasts of alar plates also form mesencephalic nucleus of trigeminal nerve（CN V）, containing general somatic afferent neurons.

5）Development of forebrain

➤ Diencephalon

Diencephalon forms the optic cup and stalk, epithalamus, thalamus, hypothalamus, mammillary bodies, pituitary, and pineal body（Fig. 26－11）.

The neural canal of diencephalon forms 3rd ventricle. Lateral walls of the 3rd ventricle become the thalamus, hypothalamus, and epithalamus. The thalami meet and fuse in the midline, forming **interthalamic adhesion**（丘脑间黏合）.

➤ Telencephalon

The telencephalon forms two lateral out pockets-the **cerebral vesicles**, and a median portion-the **lamina terminalis**（终板）（Fig. 26－11A）.

Commissures（连合）: The anterior neuropore is closed by the lamina terminalis. The lamina terminalis develops into the commissures of the telencephalon including corpus callosum, anterior commissure, and commissure of fornix.

Cerebral hemispheres（大脑半球）: The cerebral vesicles are the primordia of the cerebral hemispheres. As the cerebral hemispheres expand dorsally and caudally and meet in the midline, they become C-shaped and cover successively the diencephalon, midbrain, and hindbrain.

Pallium（皮质）: The arched roofs of the cerebral vesicles form the cerebral covering, i. e. , the pallium. The floor, i. e. , the subpallium, forms the corpus striatum. The pallium forms the cerebral cortex and it has three regions（Fig. 26－12）: ①the **paleopallium**（旧皮质）, ventrally located, forming olfactory bulb and tubercle；②the **archipallium**（原皮质）, dorsally located, forming dentate gyrus and hippocampus；③ the **neopallium**（新皮质）, forming neocortex.

➤ Histogenesis of neocortex

At the 5th week, the wall of the cerebral hemisphere has two layers: the ventricular zone and the marginal zone（Fig. 26－13A）. Neuroblasts migrate from ventricular zone to form the intermediate zone in the between. At the end of 6th week, **subventricular zone**（室管膜下层）forms between ventricular zone and intermediate zone. At 7 weeks, the **cortical plate**（皮质板）forms between intermediate zone and marginal zone. The neurons in the cortical plate first occupy the deeper layers, and those formed later migrate upward into the more superficial layers（"inside-out" layering）. At 10 weeks, the ventricular zone differentiates into ependyma and stops producing neuroblasts, and subventricular zone continues the formation of neurons. At 12 weeks, the **subplate**（板下层）forms between intermediate zone and cortical plate（Fig. 26－13B）.

The intermediate zone forms the white matter. During the first months after birth, the subventricular zone disappears. The subplate and cortical plate form the grey matter. The marginal zone forms the molecular layer of neocortex.

4. Anormalies of the Nervous System

1) Neural tube defects (NTD, 神经管畸形)

Neural tube defect, including spina bifida (脊柱裂) and anencephaly (无脑畸形), results from abnormal closure of the neural folds. Spina bifida affects the neural arches, and may or may not affect underlying neural tissue. Anencephaly is characterized by malformed cranial bones and rudimentary brain (Fig. 26 – 14).

2) Microcephalus (小脑畸形)

Microcephalus is characterized by cranial vault and calvaria smaller than normal, while the face is normal size.

3) Hydrocephalus (脑积水)

Hydrocephalus is characterized by an abnormal accumulation of CSF within the ventricular system due to obstruction of CSF circulation or absorption.

Post-class Task

Draw a diagram of secondary brain vesicles.

Case-based Learning

A 35-year-old female with 30 weeks of gestation was diagnosed with a fetus having anencephaly by ultrasonography. She had a history of polyhydraminios (羊水过多) and did not take folic acid supplementation. She had no history of pregnancy induced hypertension, diabetes mellitus, cardiac and renal disease. She was given medical termination of pregnancy. The fetus revealed absence of scalp and cranial vault and the defect extended up to the cervical vertebrae. The eyes were protruding. The nose was broad and ears were folded. The neck with trunk was short and shoulders were broad. No other associated defects were observed.

(1) What is the embryological basis of anencephaly?

(2) What are the anatomic features of anencephaly?

(3) What are the causes of anencephaly?

(4) What are the benefits of folic acid supplement for a woman who prepares for pregnancy?

(周雯)

第 27 章 | 眼和耳的发生

学习目标

（1）能够描述眼的发生过程和相关畸形。
（2）能够描述耳的发生过程和相关畸形。

课前问题

（1）视网膜、视神经、晶状体和角膜发生过程。
（2）内耳、中耳和外耳发生过程。

实验材料

大体标本，胚胎模型，仿真视频。

实验观察与思考

1. 眼的发生

胚胎发育第 4 周时，神经管前端闭合形成前脑，前脑两侧向外膨出一对囊泡状结构，称视泡。视泡腔与脑室相连，视泡远侧端增大，并与表面外胚层相连，视泡向内凹陷形成双层杯状结构，称为视杯。视泡近端变细，称为视柄。靠近视泡的表面外胚层在视泡的诱导下细胞增生，形成晶状体板，随后晶状体板向视杯内凹陷，并与表面外胚层分离，形成晶状体泡。眼睛各组织结构由视杯、视柄、晶状体泡和周围的间充质分化而来（图 27 - 1）。

1）视网膜的发生

视网膜由视杯内、外两层细胞分化而来。视杯外层细胞分化为视网膜色素上皮层。视杯内层细胞增厚，分化为神经上皮，从胚胎第 6 周开始，视网膜内层细胞分化为节细胞、视锥细胞、无长突细胞、水平细胞、视杆细胞和双极细胞。视杯内、外两层之间的视泡腔逐渐缩小最终消失，分化为视网膜视部。视杯内层上皮靠近杯口边缘部不再增厚，直接与视杯外层分化而来的色素上皮相连，同时沿着晶状体泡与角膜之间的间充质延伸，形成视网膜盲部，即睫状体部与虹膜部。睫状体部内层上皮分化为非色素上皮。虹膜部内层上皮分化为色素上皮，虹膜的外层上皮还分化瞳孔括约肌和瞳孔开大肌（图 27 - 1）。

2）玻璃体的发生

从胚胎第 5 周开始，视杯及视柄下方内陷，形成一条纵沟，称脉络膜裂。脉络膜裂内含有间充质、玻璃体动脉和静脉，其中玻璃体动脉为晶状体和玻璃体在胚胎发育时提供营养。玻璃体动脉还发出分支支配视网膜。脉络膜裂在胚胎第 7 周闭合，玻璃体动和静脉远端退化，形成一残迹结构，称玻璃体管。玻璃体动脉和静脉近端分别分化为视网膜中央动脉和静脉。

3）视神经的发生

视柄分内、外两层，与视杯相连。伴随着视网膜发育，节细胞不断增多，其突触向视柄聚集，导致视柄内层不断增厚，并与外层融合。视柄内、外层细胞分化为星状细胞和少突胶质细胞，并与节细胞突触聚集在一起，因此，视柄演变为视神经（图27-1）。

4）晶状体的发生

晶状体由晶状体泡分化而来，早期晶状体泡为单层细胞，后期演变为双层细胞，晶状体泡的前层细胞为立方形，后层细胞为高柱状细胞，并延伸至前层，形成初级晶状体纤维，泡腔慢慢变小最后消失，晶状体演变为实体结构。晶状体赤道上的上皮细胞增生并延长形成次级晶状体纤维，早期形成的初级晶状体纤维以及其细胞核退化形成晶状体核。新的晶状体纤维逐渐延伸到晶状体核的周边，因此，晶状体核和晶状体不断增大。这个过程终身存在，但是随着年龄增加速度放缓（图27-2）。

5）角膜、虹膜和眼房的发生

在晶状体泡的诱导下，与晶状体泡相连的表面外胚层细胞分化为角膜上皮，角膜上皮后面的间充质分化为角膜其余四层结构。在晶状体前面视杯口周围的间充质分为虹膜基质，虹膜基质中央薄边缘厚，封闭视杯口，称瞳孔膜。视杯两层上皮的前缘组织分化为虹膜上皮层，与虹膜基质共同发育为虹膜。位于晶状体泡与角膜上皮之间间充质内的腔隙，即前房。虹膜和睫状体形成后，虹膜、睫状体和晶状体之间的腔隙为后房。由于出生前瞳孔膜被吸收，因此，前房和后房通过瞳孔相连（图27-2）。

6）血管膜和巩膜的发生

胚胎第6～7周，视杯周围的间充质分化为内层和外层。内层含有较多的血管和色素细胞，分化成眼球壁的血管膜。血管膜的大部邻近视网膜外面，称为脉络膜；靠近视杯口边缘部的间充质分化为虹膜基质和睫状体的主体。视杯周围间充质的外层分化为巩膜。脉络膜与视神经周围的软脑膜相延续，巩膜与视神经周围的硬脑膜相连接（图27-2）。

7）眼睑和泪腺的发生

胚胎第7周，与眼球前面角膜上皮相连的表面外胚层上、下部分形成两个皱褶，分别分化为上眼睑和下眼睑。反折至眼睑内表面的表面外胚层分化为复层柱状的结膜上皮，与角膜上皮相连。位于眼睑外的表面外胚层分化为表皮。皱褶内的间充质分化为眼睑的其他组织。胚胎第10周时，上眼睑与下眼睑的边缘融合，到胚胎第7或第8个月时眼裂又重新张开。上眼睑外侧部表面外胚层的上皮内陷到间充质内，分化为泪腺的腺泡和导管。出生后第6周泪腺才开始分泌泪液（图27-2）。

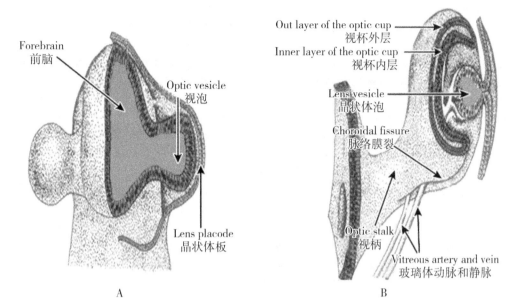

A：第 4 周（In the 4th week）；B：第 5 周（In the 5th week）。

图 27 - 1　视杯和晶状体的发生

Fig. 27 - 1　Development of the optic cup and lens

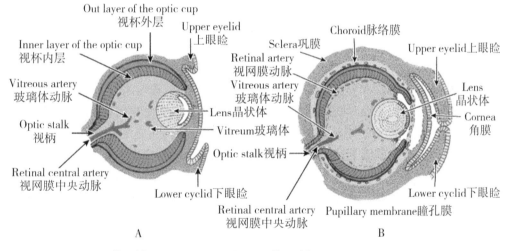

A：第 7 周（In the 7th week）；B：第 15 周（In the 15th week）。

图 27 - 2　眼球和眼睑的发生

Fig. 27 - 2　Development of the eyeball and eyelid

思考题

（1）视网膜发生过程？

（2）角膜、虹膜和眼房的发生过程？

（3）血管膜的发生过程？

---

2. 眼的畸形

1）先天性无虹膜

为常染色体显性遗传，多为双侧性。目前形成的确切机制还不清楚，可能是由视杯前缘生长和分化障碍，虹膜不能发育所致。由于无虹膜，瞳孔特别大。

2）瞳孔膜残留

由于瞳孔膜未能全部退化消失，在瞳孔处可见薄膜或蛛网状细丝覆盖在晶状体前面，轻度残留不影响视力和瞳孔活动。

3）先天性白内障

指晶状体的透明度发生异常。多为遗传性，也可能是由于母体在妊娠早期感染风疹病毒、母体甲状腺机能低下、营养不良和维生素缺乏等因素造成。

4）先天性青光眼

属常染色体隐性遗传性疾病，目前发病机制不明确，可能是由于巩膜静脉窦或小梁网发育障碍导致。患儿房水排出受阻，导致眼内压增高，眼球胀大，角膜突出，造成眼球增大，又称牛眼。

思考题

眼睛畸形有哪些类型？各种畸形形成原因？

---

3. 耳的发生

1）内耳的发生

胚胎第4周初，菱脑诱导其两侧的表面外胚层增生，形成听板，听板然后内陷形成听窝，最终听窝封闭，与表面外胚层分离，形成囊状的听泡。听泡早期呈梨形，后期向背腹方向增生延伸分别形成背侧的前庭囊和腹侧的耳蜗囊，背端内侧出现一小囊管，成为内淋巴管。前庭囊形成三个半规管上皮和椭圆囊上皮；耳蜗囊形成球囊上皮和耳蜗管上皮。听泡和周围的间充质分化为内耳膜迷路。胚胎第3个月，膜迷路周围的间充质形成软骨囊，包绕膜迷路。胚胎第5个月，软骨囊骨化形成骨迷路。因此，骨迷路套着膜迷路，两者之间的腔隙为外淋巴间隙（图27-3）。

2）中耳的发生

胚胎第9周时，第1咽囊向背外侧方向延伸，远侧端为盲端，增大形成管鼓隐窝，近侧段形成咽鼓管。管鼓隐窝上方的间充质分化为3个听小骨原基。胚胎第6个月，3个听小骨原基骨化成为3块听小骨。同时，管鼓隐窝增大形成原始鼓室，听小骨周围的间充质被吸收而形成腔隙，并与原始鼓室共同形成鼓室，听小骨位于鼓室内。位于管鼓隐窝顶部的内胚层与第1鳃沟底部的外胚层分别形成鼓膜内上皮和外上皮，两者之间的间充质形成鼓膜内的结缔组织（图27-3）。

3）外耳的发生

外耳道由第1鳃沟演变而成（图27-3）。胚胎第2个月末，第一鳃沟向深部内陷，形成外耳道外侧段。管道的底部外胚层细胞增生形成上皮细胞板，称为外耳道栓。胚胎第7个

月，外耳道栓内部细胞退化被吸收，形成管腔，成为外耳道内侧段。胚胎第 6 周，位于第一
鳃沟周围的间充质增生形成 6 个结节状隆起，称为耳丘。耳丘围绕外耳道口排列，形成
耳郭。

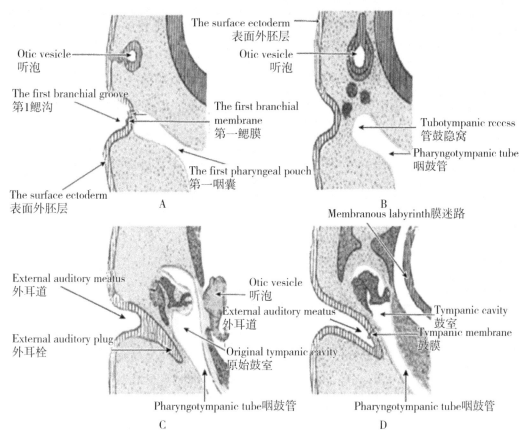

A：第 4 周（In the 4th week）；B：第 5 周（In the 5th week）；
C：第 6 月（In the 6th month）；D：成体耳（The definitive ear）。

图 27 - 3　耳的发生
Fig. 27 - 3　Development of the ear

> **思考题**
> 内耳是如何发生的？

4. 耳的畸形

1) 先天性耳聋

较为常见，分遗传性和非遗传性两类。遗传性耳聋属常染色体隐性遗传，主要是由不同
程度的内耳发育不全、耳蜗神经发育不良、听小骨发育缺陷与外耳道闭锁等因素导致。非遗
传性耳聋与药物中毒、感染、新生儿溶血性黄疸等因素相关。这些原因都可能损伤胎儿的内
耳、耳蜗神经节、耳蜗神经和听觉中枢。先天性耳聋患儿由于听不到语言，不能进行语言学

习与锻炼，所以伴有哑。

2）副耳郭

由于耳丘发生过多所致，常见位于耳屏前方。

3）耳漏

位于耳屏前方，可能是由于第 1 鳃沟的背部闭合不全，或第 1、第 2 鳃弓发生的耳丘融合不良导致，形成皮肤性盲管向下延伸，与鼓室相通，可挤压出白色乳酪状液体，常常导致感染。

思考题
耳的畸形有哪些类型及其发生原因？

课后作业

描述视网膜的发生过程。

病例教学

患者，女性，一周岁半岁，出生后对外界声音刺激无反应，偶尔发出嘶哑声。查体：对外界声音刺激无应答，不能说话。听觉诱发电位确认诊断为先天性耳聋。

（1）先天性耳聋的发病因素有哪些？

（2）为什么先天性耳聋伴有哑？

（陈雄林）

Chapter 27   DEVELOPMENT OF EYES AND EARS

The eyes and ears develop at the beginning of the 4th week. The eyes develop from two germ layers-ectoderm and mesoderm, while the ears are derived from three germ layers-ectoderm, mesoderm, and endoderm.

Learning Objectives

(1) Be able to describe the process of the eye development and related malformations.

(2) Be able to describe the process of the ear development and related malformations.

Pre-class Questions

(1) The development of retina, optic nerve, lens and cornea.

(2) Development process of inner ear, middle ear and outer ear.

Materials

Gross specimens, models, simulation videos.

Observation and Reflection

1. Eye development (眼的发生)

At the 4th week of embryonic development, a pair of vesicular structures called **optic vesicles** (视泡) protrude from both sides of the forebrain. The cavities of the optic vesicles are continuous with that of the forebrain (前脑), and the distal end of the optic vesicle is enlarged and connected with the surface ectoderm. The optic vesicle become concave inward to form a double-layer cup structure called the **optic cup** (视杯). The proximal ends of the optic vesicles become thinner, which are called **optic stalks** (视柄). The optic vesicles induce the surface ectoderm to proliferate and form **lens placodes** (晶状板), and then the lens placodes sink into the optic cup and separate from the surface ectoderm to form **lens vesicle** (晶状体泡). The eyes develop from the optic cup, optic stalk, the lens vesicle and the surrounding mesenchyme (Fig. 27 – 1).

1) Development of the retina

The retina (视网膜) develops from the cells of the optic cup (Fig. 27 – 1).

(1) The outer layer of the optic cup differentiates into pigment layer of retina (视网膜色素细胞层). The inner layer of the optic cup proliferates to form neuroepithelium.

（2）From the 6th week, the inner layer of the retina begins to differentiate into ganglion cells （节细胞）, cone cells （视锥细胞）, amacrine cells （无长突细胞）, horizontal cells （水平细胞）, rod cells （视杆细胞） and bipolar cells （双极细胞）.

（3）The optic vesicle cavity between the inner and outer layers of the optic cup gradually shrinks, and eventually disappears.

（4）The inner epithelium of the optic cup no longer proliferates near the edge of the optic cup mouth. At the same time, it extends along the mesenchyme between the lens vesicle and the cornea, forming the blind part of the retina including the epithelium of ciliary body and that of the iris.

2）Development of the hyaloid vessels

In the 5th week, the optic cup and optic stalk invaginate to form a longitudinal groove, which is called **choroid fissure** （脉络膜型）. The choroid fissure consists of mesenchyme, hyaloid artery （玻璃体动脉） and hyaloid vein （玻璃体静脉）. The hyaloid artery sends branches to nourish the lens, vitreous body, and retina. The choroid fissure is closed in the 7th week. The distal end of the hyaloid artery and hyaloid vein degenerate to form **vitreous canal** （玻璃体管）. The proximal end of the hyaloid artery and hyaloid vein differentiate into the retinal central artery and vein respectively.

3）Development of the optic nerve

The optic stalk is divided into inner and outer layers, which are connected with the optic cup. With the development of retina, ganglion cells increase continuously in number, and their axons converge into the optic stalk to form the optic nerve fibers. T inner and outer layer of the optic stalk fuse together. The inner and outer cells of the optic stalk differentiate into astrocytes （星型胶质细胞） and oligodendrocyte （少突质细胞）. Therefore, the optic stalk develops into optic nerve （视神经）（Fig. 27 - 1）.

4）Development of the lens

（1）**Lens vesicle**：The lens （晶状体） develops from the lens vesicle. The anterior cells of the lens vesicle are cubic, and the posterior cells are tall columnar.

（2）**Primary lens fibers** （初级晶状体纤维）：The posterior cells extend to the anterior layer and lose their nuclei to form primary lens fibers. The cavity of the lens vesicle gradually becomes smaller and finally disappears, and the lens develops into a solid structure.

（3）**secondary lens fibers** （次级晶状体纤维）：The epithelial cells on the equator of the lens proliferate and extend to form secondary lens fibers, and primary lens fibers and their nuclei degenerate to form lens nuclei. The secondary lens fibers gradually extend to the periphery of the lens nucleus, so that the lens nucleus continue to grow （Fig. 27 - 2）.

5）Development of the cornea, iris, ciliary body and eye chambers

（1）**Cornea** （角膜）：By the induction of lens vesicles, the surface ectoderm connected with lens vesicles differentiates into corneal epithelium, and the mesenchyme behind corneal epithelium differentiates into the other four layers of cornea.

（2）**Iris** （虹膜）：The mesenchyme around the mouth of optic cup differentiates into iris matrix. The mesenchyme sealing the mouth of the optic cup is called the **pupillary membrane** （瞳孔

膜）. The pupillary membrane is absorbed before birth.

（3）**Ciliary body**（睫状体）: The mesenchyme around the mouth of optic cup also differentiates into matrix and ciliary muscle.

（4）**Eye chambers**: The anterior chamber is located in the space between the lens vesicle and the corneal epithelium. After the formation of iris and ciliary body, the cavity between iris, ciliary body and lens is posterior chamber. After the pupillary membrane regresses, the anterior chamber and posterior chamber are connected through the pupil（瞳孔）（Fig. 27 – 2）.

6）Development of the choroid and sclera

At 6 ～ 7 weeks, the mesenchyme around the optic cup differentiates into inner and outer layers（Fig. 27 – 2）.

（1）**Choroid**（脉络膜）: The inner layer contains more blood vessels and pigment cells, which differentiate into the choroid of the eyeball wall. The choroid is connected with the cerebral pia mater around the optic nerve.

（2）**Sclera**（巩膜）: The outer layer of the mesenchyme around the optic cup differentiates into sclera. The sclera is connected with the cerebral dura mater around the optic nerve.

7）Development of the eyelids and lacrimal glands

（1）**Eyelids**（眼睑）: During the 6th week, the upper and lower parts of the surface ectoderm in front of the eyeball form two folds, which differentiated into the upper and lower eyelid. At the 10th week, the edges of the upper and lower eyelids fuse, and the eye fissure reopens at the 7th or 8th month of the embryo.

（2）**Lacrimal glands**（泪腺）: The epithelium of the surface ectoderm on the lateral surface of the upper eyelids invaginates into the mesenchyme and differentiates into acini and ducts of the lacrimal glands. At the 6th week after birth, the lacrimal glands began to secrete tears（Fig. 27 – 2）.

Reflection

（1）Please describe the development process of retina?

（2）Please describe the development of cornea, iris and eye chamber?

（3）Please describe the development process of vascular membrane?

---

2. Eye deformity（眼的畸形）

1）Congenital aniridia（先天性无虹膜）

Congenital aniridia is an autosomal dominant genetic anomaly that usually affects both eyes. In most cases aniridia originates from a mutation in the PAX6 gene, Because of aniridia, the pupils are very large.

2）Persistent pupillary membrane（瞳孔膜存留）

Because the pupillary membrane has not completely degenerated, the membrane can be seen in front of the lens. Mild residue does not affect vision and pupil activity.

3）Congenital cataract（先天性白内障）

Congenital cataract refers to a clouding of lens that presents at birth. This may be caused by maternal infection with rubella virus in early pregnancy, maternal hypothyroidism, malnutrition, vitamin deficiency and other factors.

4）Congenital glaucoma（先天性青光眼）

Most cases of congenital glaucoma are sporadic in origin, while some are autosomal recessive inherited. The patient's aqueous humor is blocked, which leads to increased intraocular pressure, eyeball swelling, corneal protrusion, and eyeball enlargement（bovine eye）.

Reflection

（1）How many types do eye malformations have?

（2）What are the causes of various eye malformations?

---

3. Ear development（耳的发生）

1）Development of the internal ear

（1）**Otic vesicles**（听泡）：Early in the 4th week, the rhombencephalon induces the proliferation of the surface ectoderm on both sides of the embryo to form **otic placodes**（听板）. The otic placodes then sink inward to form **otic pits**（听窝）. Finally, the otic pits close and separate from the surface ectoderm to form vesicular otic vesicles.

（2）**membranous labyrinth**（膜迷路）：The otic vesicle proliferates and extends to the dorsal-ventral direction and form the dorsal utricular component and the ventral saccular component respectively. A small cystic duct appears at the medial side of the dorsal end and becomes the endolymphatic vessel. The utricular component and the surrounding mesenchyme form three semicircular canals and the utricle. The saccular component and the mesenchyme form the saccule and cochlear duct. The otic vesicles and the surrounding mesenchyme differentiate into the membrane labyrinth.

（3）**osseous labyrinth**（骨迷路）：At the third month of the embryo, the mesenchyme around the membranous labyrinth forms cartilaginous otic capsule. At the fifth month of the embryo, the cartilaginous otic capsule ossifies to form osseous labyrinth. Therefore, the osseous labyrinth is sheathed with the membranous labyrinth, and the space between them is the perilymphatic space（外淋巴间隙）（Fig. 27 – 3）.

2）Development of the middle ear（中耳）

（1）**Tubotympanic recess**（咽鼓管鼓室隐窝）：In the 5th week, the first pharyngeal pouch extends to the dorsolateral direction. Its distal end develops into the tubotympanic recess and the proximal segment forms the **pharyngotympanic tube**（咽鼓管）.

（2）**Auditory ossicles**（听小骨）**and muscles**：The neural crest cells from the 1st and 2nd pharyngeal arches differentiate into anlage of three auditory ossicles. At the 6th month of embryo, anlage of three auditory ossicles is ossified into 3 auditory ossicles. The mesoderm from the 1st and

2nd arch forms the middle ear muscles.

（3）**Tympanic cavity**（鼓室）：The tubotympanic recess is enlarged to surround the auditory ossicles and form the original tympanic cavity. The mesenchyme around the ossicles is absorbed to produce the tympanic cavity.

（4）**Tympanic membrane**（鼓膜）：The endoderm at the top of the tubotympanic recess and the ectoderm at the bottom of the first branchial groove（鳃沟）form the inner and outer epithelium of the tympanic membrane respectively, and the mesenchyme between them forms the connective tissue in the tympanic membrane（Fig. 27 – 3）.

3）Development of the external ear

The external auditory meatus（外耳道）develops from the first branchial groove（第 1 腮沟）（Fig. 27 – 3）.

（1）Lateral segment of the external auditory meatus：At the end of the 2nd month of the development, the first branchial groove was invaginated to form the lateral segment of the external auditory meatus.

（2）Medial segment of the external auditory meatus：Epidermal cells at the bottom of the meatus proliferate to form epithelial plates（上皮板）, which are called external auditory meatal plug（耳栓）. In the 7th month, the cells inside the external auditory meatal plug degenerate and form a lumen which becomes the medial segment of the external auditory meatus.

（3）The auricle（耳郭）：At the 6th week of the embryo, the mesenchyme around the first branchial groove proliferates to form 6 nodular protuberances called **auricular hillocks**（耳丘）. The auricular hillocks fuse to form the auricle.

Reflection

How does the inner ear develop?

---

4. Ear deformity（耳的畸形）

1）Congenital deafness（先天性耳聋）

Congenital deafness is relatively common, which can be divided into hereditary and non-hereditary. Hereditary deafness is an autosomal recessive inheritance, which is mainly caused by various factors such as internal ear hypoplasia, cochlear nerve dysplasia, auditory ossicles development defect and external auditory meatus atresia. Non-hereditary deafness is related to drug poisoning, infection, neonatal hemolytic jaundice and other factors. These reasons may damage the inner ear, cochlear ganglion, cochlear nerve and auditory center of the fetus. Children with congenital deafness can not hear or learn to speak language, so they usually have speech delay.

2）The accessory auricle（副耳郭）

The accessory auricle is usually located in front of the tragus due to excessive development of the auricular hillocks.

3）Preauricular sinuses（耳漏）

The preauricular sinuses are located in front of the tragus（耳屏）, which may be caused by the incomplete closure of the dorsal part of the 1st branchial groove, or the poor integration of the auricular hillocks. The preauricular sinuses form a blind tube that extends downward and connects with the tympanic cavity, and can extrude white and cheese-like liquid, which often leads to infection.

Reflection

What kinds of the ear malformations are there? And what are the causes of the ear malformations?

Post-class Task

Describe the development of retina.

Case-based Learning

The patient, a female, was one and a half years old. After birth, she did not respond to external sound stimuli and occasionally made hoarse sounds. Physical examinations showed she had no response to external sound stimulation and was unable to speak. Auditory evoked potentials confirmed the diagnosis of congenital deafness.

(1) What are the pathogenic factors of congenital deafness?

(2) Why is congenital deafness accompanied by speech delay?

（陈雄林）

参考文献 │（References）

白咸勇，谌宏鸣. 组织学与胚胎学案例版［M］. 2 版. 北京：科学出版社，2010.

成令忠. 现代组织学［M］. 上海：上海科学技术文献出版社，2003.

符皎荣，郑小桃，钟南田，等. 组织学与胚胎学实验指导［Z］. 海南医学院组织学与胚胎学教研室，2005.

李继承，曾园山. 组织学与胚胎学［M］. 9 版. 北京：人民卫生出版社，2018.

石玉秀. 组织学与胚胎学彩色图谱［M］. 4 版. 北京：高等教育出版社，2022.

唐军民，李继承. Textbook of histology and embryology［M］. 北京：北京大学医学出版社，2011.

谢小薰，孔力. 组织学与胚胎学［M］. 2 版. 北京：高等教育出版社，2019.

曾园山，常青，杨雪松. A laboratory manual of histology and embryology［M］. 北京：人民卫生出版社，2012.

BAUMANN J L, PATEL C. Enteric duplication cyst containing squamous and respiratory epithelium：an interesting case of a typically pediatric entity presenting in an adult patient［J］. Case Rep Gastrointest Med，2014：790326.

BROWN J W. Prenatal development of the human nucleus ambiguus during the embryonic and early fetal periods［J］. Am J Anat.，1990，189（3）：267 – 283.

BUCHANAN R W, CAIN W L. A case of a complete omphalocele［J］. Ann Surg.，1956，143（4）：552 – 556.

CLEARY M, RUIZ D, EBERMAN L, et al. Dehydration, cramping, and exertional rhabdomyolysis：a case report with suggestions for recovery［J］. J Sport Rehabil，2007，16（3）：244 – 259.

DAVIS D L, MORRISON J J. Hip arthroplasty pseudotumors：pathogenesis, imaging, and clinical decision making［M］. J Clin Imaging Sci，2016，29（6）：17.

GLEESON P. Spontaneous gingival haemorrhage：case report［J］. Aust Dent J. 2002，47（2）：174 – 175.

GUNDUZ M, UNAL O. Dysmorphic facial features and other clinical characteristics in two patients with PEX1 gene mutations［J］. Case Rep Pediatr.，2016：5175709. DOI：10. 1155/2016/5175709.

HOLLAND G R, MOXHAM B J. Oral anatomy, histology and embryology［M］. 5th ed. Elsevier，2017.

LANDSEND E C S, LAGALI N, UTHEIM T P. Congenital aniridia：a comprehensive review of clinical features and therapeutic approaches［J］. Surv Ophthalmol.，2021，66（6）：1031 – 1050.

LI T T, QIU F, WANG Z Q, et al. Rare case of Helicobacter pylori-related gastric ulcer: malignancy or pseudomorphism? [J]. World J Gastroenterol, 2013, 19 (12): 2000-2004.

LI Y, DING Y. Embryonic development of the human lens [J]. Pediatric Lens Diseases, 2016: 1-9.

LIAO L, LI L, ZHAO R C. Stem cell research in China [J]. Philos. Trans. R. Soc. Lond. B Biol. Sci., 2007, 362 (1482): 1107-1112.

LIN J W, LIN M S, LIN C M, et al. Idiopathic syringomyelia: case report and review of the literature [J]. Acta Neurochir Suppl, 2006 (99): 117-120.

MESCHER A L. Junqueira's basic histology: text and atlas [M]. 15th ed. McGraw-Hill Education, 2013.

MESCHER A L, 李和, 陈活彝. Textbook of histology and embryology [M]. 2版. 北京: 科学出版社, 2021.

NAME L, NAME F, TRAINING O, et al. Langman's medical embryology [M]. 12th ed. Lippincott Williams & Wilkins, 2014.

SADLER T W. Langman's Medical Embryology [M]. 8th ed. Lippincott Williams & Wilkins, 2000.

SADLER T W. Langman's medical embryology [M]. 14th ed. Wolters Kluwer Health, 2018.

SANGEETA S K, VIJAYKUMAR S K. Anencephalic fetus with craniospinal rachischisis: case report [J]. IJASHNB, 2022, 8 (3): 2581-5210.

SHI S S, YANG X Z, ZHANG X Y, et al. Horseshoe kidney with PLA2R-positive membranous nephropathy [M]. BMC Nephrol (case reports), 2021, 22 (1): 277.

SHOJA M M, TUBBS R S, LOUKAS M, et al. Marie-François Xavier Bichat (1771-1802) and his contributions to the foundations of pathological anatomy and modern medicine [J]. Ann Anat, 2008, 190 (5): 413-420.

SILVERMAN M G, BLAHA M J, KRUMHOLZ H M, et al. Impact of coronary artery calcium on coronary heart disease events in individuals at the extremes of traditional risk factor burden: the multi-ethnic study of atherosclerosis [J]. Eur Heart J, 2014, 35 (33): 2232-2241.

TEPPER M L, GYLLY P R. Viral hepatitis: know your D, E, F, and G [J]. Can Med Assoc J, 1997 (156): 1735-1738.

TONG D Z, WU S Q, YE Y E, et al. Yuleixibao he Deyizhi. Nuclear transplantation of fish [J]. Kexuetongbao (Chinese Science Bulletin), 1963 (7): 60-61.

VIVES C J L, ALBARÈDE S, FLANDRIN G, et al. Haematology Working Group of the European External Committee for External Quality Assurance Programmes in Laboratory Medicine. Guidelines for blood smear preparation and staining procedure for setting up an external quality assessment scheme for blood smear interpretation. Part I: control material [J]. Clin Chem Lab Med, 2004, 42 (8): 922-926.

致　谢

本教材由海南医科大学教材出版基金资助出版。我们向所有为本书的编写和出版做出贡献的人员致以衷心的感谢。他们的奉献精神和专业知识为本书的编写和出版奠定了坚实的基础。

我们向海南医科大学教务处的谢协驹教授、李其富教授和牛莉娜教授表示最诚挚的感谢。他们的支持和悉心指导塑造了本书的内容和结构。

特别感谢参加本书编写的所有老师。在整个编写过程中，他们的细致编写、专业见解和坚定支持在确保本书的全面性和准确性方面发挥了重要作用。

我们也感谢山东数字人科技股份有限公司提供的组织学与胚胎学图片，以及为实验室材料准备做出贡献的实验技术人员。

最后，我们感谢参与并提供宝贵反馈意见的学生。他们的参与和热情对本书的编写至关重要。

这本书是所有参与者合作努力的证明，我们真诚地感谢他们对创作本书的贡献。

由于我们的专业水平和写作能力有限，本教材难免存在不足或错误之处，欢迎使用本教材的老师和学生提供宝贵意见，以便及时更正。

谢谢！

Acknowledgments

This textbook is sponsored by the Textbook Publication Fund of Hainan Medical University. We extend our heartfelt gratitude to all those who have contributed to the development and realization of this book. Their dedication and expertise have been invaluable in creating a resource that enriches the learning experience of students in the field of life sciences.

We would like to express our deepest appreciation to Professor Xieju Xie, Professor Qifu Li, and Professor Lina Niu from Academic Affairs Department of Hainan Medical University, whose guidance and mentorship have shaped the content and structure of this manual.

Special thanks go to all members of the writing team for their meticulous editing, invaluable insights, and unwavering support throughout the development process. Their wealth of knowledge and commitment to education have been instrumental in ensuring its comprehensiveness and accuracy.

We are also grateful to Shandong Digihuman Technology Coorperation for providing Histology and Embryology Images, as well as to the technical staff and assistants who have contributed to the preparation of laboratory materials.

Finally, we acknowledge the students who have participated in pilot testing and provided valuable feedback for refining the content and usability of this manual. Their engagement and enthusiasm have been instrumental in shaping its final form.

This book stands as a testament to the collaborative efforts of all those involved, and we sincerely appreciate their contributions to its creation.

Thank you!